osocial

apy

# The Practice of Psychosocial Occupational Therapy

## 3rd Edition

Linda Finlay

T

First published in 1987 as *Occupational Therapy Practice in Psychiatry* by:
Chapman and Hall
Second edition published in 1997 by:
Stanley Thornes (Publishers) Ltd

This edition published in 2004 by:
Nelson Thornes Ltd
Delta Place
27 Bath Road
CHELTENHAM
GL53 7TH
United Kingdom

04  05  06  07  08 / 10  9  8  7  6  5  4  3  2  1

A catalogue record for this book is available from the British Library

ISBN 0 7487 7257 X

Page make-up by Acorn Bookwork Ltd, Salisbury

Printed and bound in Spain by Graphycems

# CONTENTS

# PREFACE

Mental health care in the United Kingdom has changed dramatically over the last decade. Driven particularly by the National Health Service Framework for Mental Health (Department of Health, 1999), we are experiencing shifts in practice towards health promotion, social inclusion and partnerships with users, their carers and agencies within the community. The introduction of clinical governance has fuelled calls for evidence-based practice, coinciding with demands for a needs-led, rather than profession-led, service.

In the main, these changes have been in tune with our professional person-centred philosophy. As occupational therapists we have readily embraced new community orientated opportunities for care management, user advocacy and crisis outreach. Paradoxically, while our professional boundaries have been under challenge, our confidence in our collaborative role and occupation-focused contribution has grown. As we strive to become evidence-based practitioners, we are increasingly aware of research and more comfortable embracing occupational models, theory and standardised protocols.

In this restructured third edition, I have tried to reflect these trends. All the chapters have been substantially rewritten. I have also added two new chapters to reflect users' experience of mental health problems and the collaborative, person-centred nature of the therapeutic relationship.

Another change has been my self-conscious use of language. To fit our person-centred practice and holistic concerns, I strive to refer to service users as individual people, rather than as patients or clients. Where it fits the context being discussed, however, I might talk about 'patients in hospital' or 'auditing service users' views'. To reflect the shift away from more traditional remedial activities in hospitals towards the occupational therapist being a facilitator and adviser in the community, I prefer to use the term 'intervention' rather than 'treatment'. I have also taken care in my choice of pseudonyms for the individuals in the various case studies, where I deliberately emphasise cultural diversity. At the same time, I have not always specified people's social class, ethnicity, age or gender. I only mention these factors where they seem to be particularly pertinent to the interventions being discussed. In these ways I seek to reflect broader cultural patterns and contemporary discourses.

I have tried to retain something of the style and approach of both previous editions. I continue to emphasise the practical application of occupational therapy through numerous case studies, practical illustrations and examples of research. I also continue to acknowledge areas of our practice that remain open to debate (such as our choice of theoretical approach and specifying our new roles in the community). At the end of each chapter, a 'conclusion and reflections' section sets out my personal view with the aim of stimulating further thought, discussion and debate. In each chapter the text slides between three different 'voices': my *occupational therapist's* voice, my *academic-researcher* voice and my more *personal sharing* voice.

**Part One** explores the theory underpinning our practice. Chapter 1 examines the occupational therapy role focusing primarily on mental health practice. (While I recognise that psychosocial dimensions are also relevant to physical practice and in the field of physical learning disabilities as principles can be applied across boundaries, I fall short of doing justice to the full spectrum of our practice.) Chapter 2 shifts the focus from professional perspectives to user perspectives and explores individuals' experiences of mental health problems. Chapter 3 spotlights our special use of occupation, while Chapters 4 and 5 explore, respectively, occupational therapy models and different psychological approaches. **Part Two** examines the occupational therapy process, starting with a chapter on therapeutic relationships and moving through stages of assessment, planning, intervention and evaluation.

It remains for me to acknowledge my debts. First, I am indebted to all the therapists and service users who shared their stories with me. These stories helped ensure that the content of the book remained properly grounded in contemporary practice and lived experience. Secondly, I would like to thank Beth McKay for sharing her wisdom and contributing the case study of 'Pat' to Chapter 2. Thirdly, special gratitude goes to two people who continue to help me in my work and to push me to write better – Sue Ram for her invaluable editing advice and Mel Wilder for being my foundation. Finally, my thanks must be extended to Helen Broadfield, Commissioning Editor at Nelson Thornes, and her team, who have ably steered this project to its completion. Needless to say, in the last analysis I alone remain responsible for errors of content.

A quotation from a service user:

*My occupational therapist, Janet, believes that we are what we do – that 'doing' life makes us what we are. It can be cooking dinner, visiting friends or building a house – it is the doing that is important. Doing life makes us people and doing a new life makes us new people. If we get sick, disabled or old, sometimes we cannot do our old life any more and we have to find a new life. That comes from doing. 'You start again,' she said to me, 'decide what possibilities you have, then try them to see if they work for you.'*

*After my breakdown, Janet made me look at myself – my beliefs, capabilities, habits, traditions, expectations, interests and ambitions, and then rebuild them anew. I had to reconstruct my self-belief and self-respect. I didn't really believe her at first. I guess I was still in shock – traumatised by my lost abilities, my lost personality, my powerlessness in the face of my breakdown. Now I see that way of thinking as looking backwards. I learned to become a new person. I always liked to build stuff so Janet helped me restart to build things again. The first step was to make some toys for the kids in the hospital to play with. It gave me a purpose again and problems to solve. And the kids liked playing with my toys. It was a start.*

*I was in a terrible place when Janet found me. All I could see was the devastation of what was once me. The ruin of everything I thought I was. Janet helped me stand and plot a route to another life, another me. She convinced me I should do things. Now I, too, believe that if you can start with the 'doing' then the 'being' will follow.*

# PART ONE

# THEORY FOR OCCUPATIONAL THERAPY PRACTICE

# 1 OCCUPATIONAL THERAPY: ROLE CHALLENGES AND OPPORTUNITIES

*Defining occupational therapy is a perilous pursuit.*

Duncan

Over the course of our profession's evolution there have been many debates about the nature of occupational therapy: what we do and what we should become. Mary Reilly (1962) captured the imagination well when she suggested, almost half a century ago, that 'occupational therapy can be one of the great ideas of 20th century medicine'. Now, in the 21st century, it seems that our ideals (valuing occupation for health and quality of life) are becoming even more pertinent. Yet concern has been expressed about our ambiguous role and how, as a profession, we have a tendency to be misunderstood, undervalued and negatively stereotyped. Some would say that confusion about our role identity has led to occupational therapy being a 'profession in crisis'. We are faced with the challenge of working within a rapidly changing health and social care context that has generated a huge variety of practice. What special contribution do we make? What opportunities can be embraced?

This chapter addresses these questions. First, I review the core aims, values and processes of occupational therapy. The second section extends this discussion to consider the place of occupational therapy within the interprofessional team. It offers ideas about our unique contribution, our shared values and how our division of labour can be negotiated. The third section focuses specifically on psychosocial occupational therapy and briefly analyses our role in different contexts. The chapter ends with an examination of some of the threats and opportunities confronting us as a profession.

## 1.1 DESCRIBING OCCUPATIONAL THERAPY

### Core values

Following their national survey of mental health occupational therapy managers' views, Craik *et al.* (1999) argue that the most 'critical issue' for the future is to identify our core skills and roles. The exact nature of these has been hotly debated in our literature over the last two decades, with the following six aims and values emerging as rough consensus:

- Occupational therapists believe in '**occupation for health**' (Wilcock, 1999). We are concerned with individuals' quality of life in terms of how they engage in satisfactory and meaningful occupations. We have a deep appreciation of the occupational nature of humans, of the relationship between health and occupation, and of how occupations can be used to influence health. While our profession has evolved considerably over the last century, the enduring theme that has provided continuity for our identity has been our celebration of occupation.

- Occupational therapists focus on **occupational performance**. We are centrally concerned with how individuals function in their work, leisure, domestic life and personal self care. For us, a healthy person is one able to perform his or her daily occupations to a satisfying (for that person) and effective level. A person's occupational performance may well be disrupted or impaired when he or she becomes ill or disabled in some way. We work with these individuals who experience some difficulty in their daily life functioning. As Molineux notes (2002), we have a unique ability to assess occupational performance and to use occupations to improve or maintain that performance.

---

*Research example 1.1*

**The value of occupations and occupational therapy**

Lyons and colleagues (2003) studied the experiences of 23 people in an Australian hospice. Occupations were found to promote doing, being and becoming – demonstrating the value of activity. **Doing** was evident in the accounts of losing and maintaining valued occupations (such as hobbies and driving) and striving to maintain physical/mental functioning. **Being** emerged through occupational engagement focused on social relationships and self-exploration, which enhanced feelings of self-worth. Occupation promoted **becoming** by providing fresh learning opportunities and encouraging a sense of contributing to others' welfare.

Fieldhouse (2003) explored the subjective meanings of nine clients with serious mental health problems who attended a horticultural allotment group in Britain. The study concludes there are particular qualities of the person-plant relationship which promote individuals' well being and interactions with the environment. He demonstrates how the embeddedness of allotments within communities offers a mechanism to increase social inclusion and promote health.

---

- Occupational therapists believe in the **importance of participation** and of **being active** in life situations. The *National Services Framework for Mental Health* (Department of Health, 1999) requires services to promote health and social inclusion by enabling participation in the community. In occupational therapy terms we focus here on 'occupational participation' (Kielhofner, 2002c). This involves helping individuals to actively engage in personally significant activities and culturally meaningful social roles. We aim to enable individuals who feel excluded, isolated, empty or worthless to feel part of their social world. We help by trying to ensure that the person's environment and social networks are as supportive as possible towards maintaining participation.

- Occupational therapists value the **therapeutic potential of purposeful and meaningful activities** to promote health and well being. We believe that people are innately active beings. Through being active we learn about ourselves, develop our capabilities and maintain our physical/mental health. Reilly (1962) captured this idea well in her famous statement, 'Man, through the use of his hands as energised by mind and will, can influence the state of his own health'. Thus, occupational therapy is premised on the idea that purposeful activity can be therapeutic and can be used to improve individuals' functioning when used in a way that is meaningful to the person. One of our core skills is being able to apply activity in the treatment process. This process values the inherent properties of activities, the experience of 'doing' and the end product. We employ two main types of therapeutic activity: activities of daily living (such as cooking) and therapy activities (such as group work). Treatment often involves grading and adapting these activities and their inherent properties.
- Occupational therapists view service users holistically as **unique individuals** who have particular life experiences, interests, needs, skills, problems and motivations arising out of their particular social and cultural background. We aim to view and treat individuals as complex, whole beings rather than seeing their problems in isolation. We try to attend to emotional, cognitive, physical and social dimensions, in the context of the person's wider lifestyle. In practice this means we need to negotiate therapeutic interventions in individualised ways: one person's treatment cannot be transferred wholesale to another. It also means that we resist stereotyping our patients and clients (for instance, we try to avoid categorising a person by diagnosis).
- Occupational therapists aim to take a **person-centred approach** to practice. The collaborative relationship between service user and therapist is stressed and service users are invited to participate fully in negotiating their therapy. Therapy is guided by service users who, ideally, are enabled to identify their own priorities and needs and to set their own agenda (mirroring their increasing role in guiding wider health service development). They are placed at the centre of decision making. We aim to offer individuals choice, and we seek to ensure that they engage in activities that are meaningful to them. The notion of 'empowerment' is a key value: therapists seek to enable and empower service users by embracing egalitarian ideals and democratic relationships.

## The occupational therapy process

Occupational therapists put these values into action through a therapeutic process that involves intertwining the therapeutic relationship with a special clinical reasoning and problem solving process.

The **therapeutic relationship** between therapist and client is probably the most significant dimension of any therapy. Of course the nature and level of the relationship developed varies according to the kind of intervention involved. In general, occupational therapists try to communicate genuine interest and empathy for the service users' experience. The impact of this can be powerful.

Through our very *presence* we can help an individual feel safe, comfortable, worthy, valued, nurtured, perhaps even inspired. Then, as we collaborate with service users, we motivate them to engage in therapy. Mattingly (1998) describes something of this when she says: 'Therapists work to create significant experiences for their patients because if therapy is to be effective, therapists must find a way to make the therapeutic process matter to the patient, to make it meaningful' (1998, p. 82).

In tandem with the therapeutic relationship we develop with each service user, occupational therapists engage in a complex and multilayered **clinical reasoning** process. Here, we think about the individual's needs/problems and the therapeutic interventions that might be positively applied. Mattingly and Fleming (1994) suggest that therapists engage in a range of reasoning strategies, including procedural, interactive and conditional reasoning. *Procedural* reasoning is the type of thinking we use when thinking scientifically about an individual's problems and how to solve them. *Interactive* reasoning is the thinking that emerges through the relationship with the individual. *Conditional* reasoning is the way therapists seem to build images of the individual's past, present and, importantly, future life as we seek to understand and treat the 'whole' person.

As part of the clinical reasoning process the occupational therapist, in negotiation with the service user, engages in what can be regarded as a **problem-solving cycle**. The first stage of this cycle is *assessment*, where we aim to identify, in partnership with the individual concerned, their occupational needs and functioning, given their particular environment and social context. We then *plan* our therapeutic intervention by considering numerous options of what could be done to enhance a person's occupational performance. As part of our clinical reasoning and in collaboration with the individual, we consider their skills, needs and way of life and select the most promising problem solving strategy that can be realistically applied at the *implementation* stage. We then *evaluate* the intervention, being alert to the need for further problem solving if necessary (Figure 1.1). This process is a complex one where each stage blends into the next – for instance, from the first moment we enter into assessing individuals we simultaneously engage them therapeutically. The process can be viewed as a spiral where each stage is revisited progressively and simultaneously.

Case example 1.1 shows the occupational therapy process in practice. In this example we see how Mr Weiss is helped towards better physical and mental health through a combination of being involved in structured activity and having a change in his social environment. The occupational therapy role with Mr Weiss is primarily one of assessment, with the aim of referring him on to another appropriate agency to increase his community participation. At the same time, the therapist has to engage Mr Weiss in the intervention and motivate him to take up new occupations. As you read the case study, you might find it useful to consider the extent to which the six occupational values discussed in section 1.1 are applied.

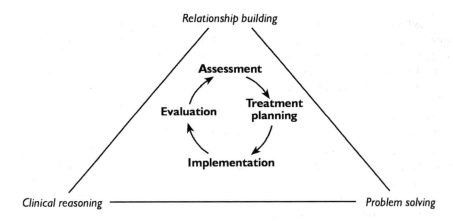

**Figure 1.1** The occupational therapy process

---

### Case example 1.1   The impact of activity and changing environments

Mr Weiss, an 80-year-old widower, has deteriorated both physically and mentally over the last two years since the death of his wife. Living alone, he has become increasingly dependent on his daughter, who lives nearby. Concerned about her father's health, safety and isolation, the daughter seeks help.

The community mental health team decides that the occupational therapist is best placed to manage Mr Weiss's care. The occupational therapist visits Mr Weiss at home for an initial assessment. As they talk together, Mr Weiss becomes tearful when he speaks of his wife. He admits that he is finding it difficult to take care of himself and that he 'can't be bothered' to do anything. He agrees to cook a light lunch of soup and toast so that the therapist can observe how he copes. He says he misses his wife's cooking – he has never really learned to do more than open a tin.

The therapist observes that Mr Weiss is unshaven, sloppily dressed, physically slow and seems slightly confused and absent-minded, confirming his daughter's report that he seems to be neglecting himself. She suggests that his lack of motivation to do anything comes from his depression, where he is still grieving for his wife, and that this is aggravated by being both inactive and socially isolated. The therapist suggests that Mr Weiss might benefit from attending a day unit three times a week where he could meet others and be involved in different activities. 'You'll even be given a hot meal,' she says, to give him further encouragement. Initially, Mr Weiss is reluctant to go to the day unit, although he is tempted by the idea of having a hot lunch cooked for him. The therapist acknowledges that it is difficult to try something new. She suggests that he try it for just two weeks. She asks what would make it easier for him to attend. When he replies, 'Knowing people', she offers to go with him the first day.

Once at the day unit, Mr Weiss is encouraged to take part in different practical and social activities. Somewhat to his surprise, he finds that he enjoys his time there. He particularly appreciates the warm, friendly environment and the company of others.

After a month, the therapist pays Mr Weiss a follow-up visit. She is pleased to see that he seems quite transformed. In addition to looking dapper in a new blazer, he admits to being more alert now that he has more purpose to and in his day. Today, he is going to the unit and he is looking forward to meeting his friends.

**Summary**: We can define occupational therapy as a person-centred, collaborative, problem-solving process which involves the therapeutic use of purposeful activity to enable individuals to participate in social life and to perform their daily occupations to a satisfying and effective level.

## 1.2   OCCUPATIONAL THERAPY WITHIN THE TEAM

Government policies in the UK over the last few years have called for new approaches to health and social care (see, for example, the *National Service Framework for Mental Health*, Department of Health, 1999). Particular emphasis has been placed on providing 'seamless care' across health and social care boundaries and on interprofessional collaboration. The Care Programme Approach (CPA) has become the foundation for mental health services. It commits the multidisciplinary team to a 'needs-led', community-orientated service. Here, team members (ideally) collaborate with service users *and* their carers to plan and regularly review care (Theory into practice 1.1).

*Theory into practice 1.1* _____

**A needs-led approach**

A 'needs-led', as opposed to 'profession-led' or 'service-led', approach requires first that individual problems or needs are identified in collaboration with the person themselves. Then, possible solutions are explored and agreed. Four examples of such an approach are shown in the following questions asked by the team:

- Adam is troubled by his voices, which tell him he is 'bad'. What will make them go away? Can he be helped to live with them? Would medication or cognitive-therapy help? Does he have a preference?'
- After being discharged from a lengthy admission to hospital, Paris feels lonely, isolated and bored without friends and productive occupations. He is at risk of relapsing. What will enable greater social inclusion? Would he be interested to join a group or take up a new leisure hobby?'

- Maya wants help to stop cutting herself. Would she prefer individual therapy or to work with other young women who are self-harming?
- Clare cares for her mother who is physically frail and in the early stages of dementia. The mother lives with Clare, having refused to consider going into a nursing home. What practical and emotional support does Clare need to help her cope?

To a growing extent, then, with the explosion of community services, occupational therapy is being practised and developed in the context of the 'team'. The 'team' here consists of various professionals plus the user and his/her family or carers. It is a fluid category that depends on the context, circumstances and needs of the person concerned. New variants of interprofessional teamwork have evolved. Increasingly, team members are being required to work out, sometimes from scratch, how they are going to blend, co-operate and communicate with each other while exercising their distinctive contributions. The challenge is to accommodate unique roles and tasks while sharing and developing new skills. At the same time, we are all required to remain fluid in our roles to adapt to changing demands and requirements of both service users and providers.

Along with other team members, our contributions as occupational therapists have become much less fixed and clear-cut. In general terms, we tend to find ourselves either in teams that operate generic or shared *care management* systems or in teams that have discrete, separate, specialist *professional* input. In both cases, we still need to actively negotiate our specific contribution.

## Care management and teamwork

Since the beginning of the 1990s (with the National Health Service and Community Care Act 1990) mental health care has moved increasingly into the community. Community teams have mushroomed and various models of care have evolved, including **care management** (sometimes called 'case management') and key worker ('care co-ordinator') systems designed to deliver total care for service users. The requirement for integrated health and social care services has reinforced this trend. There now exist Care Trusts/Primary Care Trusts (called Local Care Groups in Wales) that commission and provide, via pooled budgets, specifically tailored care packages (NHS and Social Care Act 2001). Interprofessional collaboration is centrally on the agenda.

These policies have continued to impact on the way teamwork is organised. Many teams now operate a *Care Programme Approach*, where one team member co-ordinates and follows through the service user's care. The key worker has responsibility for maintaining contact and monitoring the implementation of a team's agreed care plan. Specialist practitioners are then brought in as necessary. This trend has meant that occupational therapists may find themselves working as care managers employing **generic mental health worker skills**, such as mental state examinations, needs assessments, medication education, client advocacy, counselling, anxiety management training and so forth. At other times, we might be specifically brought in as **specialist consultant** occupational therapists to deliver discipline-specific services, for instance carrying out an in-depth functional and occupational performance assessment.

This trend has sparked much debate and has taxed the profession profoundly in the last decade (as evidenced by the many letters on the subject in the *British Journal of Occupational Therapy* – see, for instance, the issues of January–March 2002). Some within the profession argue that generic therapists have lost sight of their unique contribution and that this is a loss to both the team and service users. In response, generic therapists have argued that attending to the needs of service users is more important than focusing on professional concerns. Valuing their mental health worker role, they may seek extra training and move away from occupational therapy.

In practice, most therapists, particularly those working in the community, are now obliged to do some generic work. The question that continues to be debated is: what is the ideal balance between generic and specialist roles? The challenge is to supply discipline-specific services within a generic care management service. Questions, too, are raised about our professional education and how, without extra training, certain 'generic' tasks may be beyond our professional competence (Craik *et al.*, 1998a). Increasingly, new models of education delivery (e.g. work-based and distance learning) and professional skills development (e.g. generic skills courses) are evolving.

## Demarcating team roles

An alternative way of working within a team, often found in more traditional hospital settings, involves combining professional contributions. Here, the team as a whole aims to offer holistic interventions or treatment packages. Different team members focus on different needs of the individual service user, using specific professional knowledge and skills as relevant. A common pattern involves nurses taking on the acute care and behavioural management of a newly admitted patient, while the occupational therapist focuses on long-term issues related to occupational function and discharge. In the specific case of a patient having a violent outburst, a doctor might review what sedating medication would be suitable, a nurse might explore how best to contain and manage the behaviour, while an occupational therapist might seek to identify what activity seemed to precipitate the outburst or what might have a calming effect.

Of course, reality it is not quite as simple and clear cut as this. Role territory still needs to be demarcated and professional boundaries established. While we can comfortably say that our central concern, which offers us our unique role, is occupation, what this actually means in practice requires some negotiation. Nurses and other professionals may well attend to activities of daily living or use activities in treatment (ward activity groups, for instance). However, such interventions do not constitute these professionals' primary focus. Occupational therapists privilege occupation and *purposeful* activity – others do not. Alternatively, we sometimes encroach on other professionals' territory: we might work on managing a person's mental state (really the domain of doctors and nurses, using a medical model) or we use therapy techniques such as systematic desensitisation (normally the province of the psychologist). While these types of intervention could be part of our therapeutic tool bag, they do not constitute the core of our contribution.

The fact that roles often need to be negotiated within a team means that an element of competition or conflict between members may surface (Finlay, 2000). One professional group may feel that they are not being valued as highly as another or that their roles are being usurped. As a result, professionals can also become territorial and defensive about their role. In addition, as Hyde (2002) has recognised, behaviours of team members can reflect the psychological difficulties service users face. Staff conflict may have a defensive function and arise out of unconscious dynamics.

There are no easy solutions to these problems of team-working. Staff dynamics and internal politics can be powerful destructive factors. However, I suggest that we are in a stronger position if we remember, and act upon, four things:

- The service should be 'needs-led' and less focused on professional perspectives
- Occupational therapists' special contribution is the focus on 'occupation for health'
- When other team members focus on or use 'activity' we should not feel threatened; perhaps we are being handed a compliment
- We need to keep focused on the central question: *does the service user think they are getting a 'good deal' from the way the team is functioning?*

It is worth remembering the opportunities afforded by a team approach in whatever manifestation. Surely it is better to be able to draw upon multiple perspectives, knowledge and skills of different team members rather than be restricted to the abilities of one isolated practitioner? The team is also a core source of support and learning. The challenge is how best to operate as a team to ensure an effective and properly needs-led service.

## 1.3 PSYCHOSOCIAL OCCUPATIONAL THERAPY

While occupational therapists are relatively unified in their focus on 'occupation for health', how this is operationalised in the field varies. In some settings we exercise our discipline-specific skills more fully, while in others we draw on generic skills.

Research reviewing current mental health practice (for instance, Lloyd *et al.*, 2002 with reference to Australian practice) suggests that there are two distinct groups of occupational therapists. One group – mostly working in special units or **hospital** environments – is engaged in what could be described as traditional rehabilitation activities. These therapists carry out functional assessments, are focused on activities of daily living and involve patients/clients in group work and other activity treatments. The second (increasingly common) group tends to be found in a range of **community** settings (from day units to people's homes). Here, therapists embrace more generic roles and engage in a broader range of interventions as necessary for service user care management. The *practice context*, then, largely determines the occupational therapist role.

This section will briefly describe the roles seen typically in a range of psycho-social contexts and practice fields. We start with community mental health – our largest field of practice.

## Community mental health

A great variety of community mental health services (both home- and unit-based) are offered in the UK. New services based around primary care, crisis inter-vention and assertive outreach work now exist, supplementing the care that takes place in various day units. Services have become more intense and rapid as they aim to reach out to individuals and to establish more supportive community environments. Mental health is a priority for the government and new investment has been earmarked to provide for more primary care teams and new mental health liaison and 'gateway' workers (as laid out in *Mental Health: Fast-Forwarding Primary Care in Mental Health*, Department of Health, 2003).

A number of studies have examined the occupational therapy role within community mental health (e.g. Harries and Gilhooly, 2003; Craik *et al.*, 1998b). These studies reveal diversity of practice in terms of the way therapists balance their **generic** and **specialist** roles. For example, Harries's (2002) study of 40 therapists practising in the UK revealed that the percentage of time devoted to generic work ranged between 5% and 100%! Half the occupational therapists in the survey felt that their generic role was too prominent in relation to their specialist role while the other half felt that their role balance was about right (Research example 1.2).

---

### *Research example 1.2*

**Generic versus specialist interventions for people with severe mental health problems**

Cook (2003) investigated the type and frequency of occupational therapy and care management interventions delivered to people with severe mental health problems who were being treated in a primary care service. The occupational therapy interventions of 25 people with enduring psychotic conditions were recorded over a 12-month period. Findings revealed that 60% of the 1877 interventions categorised were specialist interventions (54% occupational therapy; 6% psychological) and 40% were generic care management interventions.

In her discussion, Cook suggests that clients with severe and enduring mental health problems might be better served by increasing the proportion of specialist occupational therapy interventions. The costs of having insuffi-cient functionally focused interventions when a single occupational therapist is working in a team, she says, are too high.

---

A diversity of practice is also evident in the **wide range of interventions** that seem to be employed. In Craik *et al.*'s (1998b) study of 137 therapists practising in the UK, the most frequently employed interventions were leisure pursuits, counselling, anxiety management, activities of daily living and creative activities. Meeson's (1998) study of 12 therapists in England found that supportive counselling, anxiety management and problem-solving were most popular. What such statistics disguise are the considerable variations of practice between individuals. For instance, Meeson points out how one participant used counselling 92% of the time, while another offered counselling 22% of the time plus many other types of intervention.

To get a feel for this diversity, consider how the following three therapists describe their community mental health role:

**Care management** – *I'm a* generic *key worker in our community mental health team and much of our work is in primary care. Referrals are randomly assigned to members in the team. Mostly, the people who get referred tend to have depression or anxiety and usually they've had little previous contact with mental health services. On receiving a referral, I'll visit the client in their home for a general mental health and needs assessment. From there I might offer weekly or fortnightly counselling. I work eclectically, doing both* client-centred counselling *and* cognitive–behavioural *work. I might see a person over the course of several months, giving support and helping them to develop confidence. Others I'll just see for a few sessions, taking a problem-solving approach and teaching key* coping strategies, *perhaps doing some anxiety management or 'solution-focused brief therapy'.*

**Sessional therapy** – *I carry out a range of treatment sessions in different community locations, seeing people on a one-to-one and group basis. I run a range of* activity groups *at the day hospital. I also act as a* consultant adviser to *a social services day centre. I hold a weekly women's evening support group at a local community centre. Working with a community psychiatric nurse, I run a weekly anxiety management group and a* psychotherapy *group in a local day unit that runs on therapeutic community lines. I enjoy working with different sorts and levels of user and being part of several different units and multidisciplinary teams. I really feel part of the community.*

**Rehabilitation** – *I'm in a Rehabilitation and Community Living Unit, which also runs a Community Outreach programme. As a team we work with people who have long-term mental health problems: they are either in and out of hospital regularly or have drifted into homelessness. We focus on their personal, domestic and social needs, and when we feel we can do something we look at their work too. My role mostly involves practical* groupwork, *while the nurses concentrate on individual care. In a typical week I'll probably run a domestic cooking group, a social skills training group, an assertiveness group and a gardening allotment group. I also do a lot of domestic rehabilitation, teaching* independence *and* life skills *such as cooking, shopping, budgeting and DIY.*

## Acute psychiatry

Occupational therapy in acute psychiatry may begin in in-patient settings but it is usually oriented to community living. Here, these therapists have a key **discharge planning** function and this serves as a bridge to community-based care. As part of the team, they are also involved in **educating** users about mental health and coping with illness. Eaton (2002), for instance, describes running a psychoeducational group designed to provide information (e.g. on managing stress and using community resources) and to facilitate supportive interactions.

People who are admitted to hospital are usually severely ill or disturbed: they may be a danger to themselves or to others. Their ability to cope with everyday life is severely impaired – if only temporarily – by extreme feelings (such as anxiety) or by disturbed cognitive–perceptual processes (e.g. delusions). Patients are often discharged home or transferred within a month. Prompt therapeutic intervention, then, is essential.

When a patient is acutely ill, occupational therapists are limited in what they can do. The actual medical/psychiatric condition and symptomatology (e.g. delusions and hallucinations) are usually best treated by medication. Our role is usually limited to offering activities that help to '**contain**' the person's behaviour (e.g. using relaxing, concrete activities to help the person focus on the here and now) and that encourage them to express themselves (e.g. through the use of creative therapies). We also have an **assessment function** to observe the person while he or she is engaged in activity. Often, such assessment can assist with differential diagnosis and when assessing risk.

As soon as (or sometimes before) patients 'feel better' – or are reasonably stabilised on medication – they are discharged. Assessing the optimum time for discharge (given the pressures for beds) is a crucial decision for the team, which must ensure that patients are adequately prepared to cope safely in their expected environment. The team role then shifts to longer-term support and assertive outreach with crisis intervention towards enabling social inclusion and recovery. Occupational therapists, by offering ongoing **outpatient support** to bridge the gap between hospital and community, play a key role here.

Patients with enduring mental health problems typically suffer functional problems associated with their psychotic, affective or organic disorder along with problems of institutionalisation (passivity, dependence, apathy). Usually, all areas of their occupational performance (work, domestic, leisure and self-care) are impaired. These problems are exacerbated by the hostile social environments in which such individuals are forced to live, including unemployment, poverty, isolation, exclusion and lack of social support. There is often a history of repeated crises and hospital admissions (the 'revolving door' syndrome).

The main occupational therapy aims with individuals with severe and enduring mental health problems are to maintain independence and functional skills and to develop productive occupations. Interventions focus on enhancing personal, domestic, work or social aspects, aiming to be realistic about what can be achieved. The emphasis throughout is on enabling social inclusion, recovery,

**rehabilitation** and, where necessary, resettlement. Most people will be discharged home (be it to an existing home or a new location), ideally with extra support such as going to a day centre to give them a daily structure and work role. Others might be referred on to specialist rehabilitation units. Occupational therapists, alongside other team members, are also likely to work with the patients' and clients' family or carers, offering support and advice.

## Learning disabilities

The needs of people with learning disabilities vary according to their level of disability and functioning. It is appropriate to distinguish between those individuals who are profoundly and multiply handicapped, who may need life long institutional care, and those with special needs who can live relatively independent, if sheltered, lives in the community, given some support.

The occupational therapist's role with individuals who are profoundly and/or multiply handicapped is varied. We might use **sensorimotor activities** to stimulate and develop skills. Here, activities involving light, movement, noise and touch are used to stimulate sensory awareness. In addition, the occupational therapist may be involved in supplying adaptive equipment for any physical disabilities and to increase functional ability (e.g. to assist an individual to sit or eat independently). Alongside other team members, the occupational therapist may also be involved in implementing a range of programmes to manage 'problem' behaviour in the short term and to advise on long-term care and placement. Paediatric occupational therapists may be called in to assess sensorimotor function, encourage play and develop skills.

Where individuals are more independent, the occupational therapist acts as teacher, facilitator and advocate. The aim is develop the individual's skills – cognitive, social and practical; to enable them to make choices and to be independent; and to protect the individual's interests.

Therapists will often be involved in the long-term **habilitation** (rather than rehabilitation) – for example, enabling the service user to live independently or in a sheltered housing scheme. In these circumstances the person's wider **occupational performance** will need attention – both to develop skills and to facilitate opportunities for work, leisure and social participation. Whatever the focus, the occupational therapist is likely to work both with carers (e.g. helping carers to avoid being over-protective) and with the local community (where hostile social reactions may need to be dealt with).

## Combining psychosocial and physical interventions

All occupational therapy involves some psychosocial intervention. Developing relationships with service users and engaging them in treatment always entails a psychosocial process: how we focus on individuals' experience of meaningfulness in their occupations requires an appreciation of psychosocial aspects; in seeking to empathise with an individual and enter their life-world we embark on a psychosocial exploration. Increasingly, with the requirements for 'seamless' care across health and social care boundaries, our practice in the community spans both physical and mental health. In physical hospitals, too, posts in *liaison psychiatry* are on the increase.

The crossover between mental health and physical disability is particularly evident when occupational therapists become involved in treating older persons and individuals who have sustained organic damage such as is seen with dementia, head injuries and neurological conditions. Here we have a particular role in assessing behavioural, social, cognitive and perceptual functioning. Care programmes need to be developed in conjunction with family members and/or carers. Often, the focus will be on risk assessment, for example assessing the risk of falls and safety in the home generally. Service users with a wide range of other neurological conditions (from epilepsy to multiple sclerosis) also benefit from interventions focused on **occupational performance** geared to helping them cope emotionally and practically with the impact of chronic, progressive conditions.

Palliative care also offers particular opportunities and challenges for occupational therapists, with new standards for specialist palliative care recommending the provision of psychological services (Department of Health, 2000). Along with other team members we can help remove the stigma of mental health problems. We can encourage individuals to express difficult emotions such as hopelessness, grief and fear (e.g. through **creative and projective** activities). We may also be involved in symptom reduction, such as using relaxation for pain management. Our unique contribution in this field, however, is in encouraging positive, **meaningful occupations**, helping individuals to enjoy what they can do now – in the present (see Research example 1.1).

In the mental health field therapists often offer a combination of psychosocial and physical interventions (Everett *et al.*, 2003). Evidence is accumulating which links physical activity and exercise to improvements in psychological well being and quality of life (Mutrie and Faulkner, 2003). Therapists may well encourage service users to engage in exercise – perhaps joining a group at the local leisure centre – as part of encouraging social inclusion.

## 1.4 THREATS, CHALLENGES AND OPPORTUNITIES

The previous sections have presented the occupational therapy role as being relatively clear cut. The reality of practice is, of course, considerably more messy and sometimes problematic. In this section we explore some of the threats, challenges and opportunities currently confronting our profession in terms of our role in a fast-changing context.

### Role confusion?

The confusion, insecurity and anxiety that has dogged our sense of professional role and identity has been much commented on. Duncan (1999) sees this confusion as reminiscent of an 'adolescent identity crisis', especially in view of the fact that we are a relatively young profession. As Creek and Ormston point out: 'Through three decades of professional publication, the same writing has appeared on different walls: warnings that we need to clarify our role and become more proficient in expressing our unique practices, and to establish a firmer scientific theoretical base' (Creek and Ormston, 1996, p. 7).

Taylor and Rubin's (1999) interviews with 19 community mental health occupational therapists exposed considerable role confusion. Their responses revealed a lack of uniformly used words/concepts when defining their work and often their definitions just applied to their own specific role rather than describing the role of occupational therapists in general. Fortune (2000) argues that occupational therapists stand in danger of being simply 'filling gaps', depending on others to define our role rather than anchoring our practice within a unifying professional paradigm – a theme reminiscent of the argument presented by Barris and Kielhofner in 1986, when they identified the absence of unifying theory as the problem.

As far back as 1977, Kielhofner and Burke suggested that our profession was 'in crisis'. Commenting on the diversity and fragmentation of practice, they argued that occupational therapy lacked a common core; without a central organising philosophical base, it was in danger of being ambiguous and incoherent. They saw these confusions as the result of shifting *paradigms*: occupational therapy had passed through two paradigms and was now engaged in a third.

The first paradigm, which emerged at the start of the 20th century, involved principles of moral treatment, where occupation was seen as central to human life. The second paradigm, lasting into the 1970s, had pronounced reductionist and mechanistic features as occupational therapy became subverted by the medical model and the application of technology. The profession fragmented into different specialties. By the end of the 1970s, this was being rejected and Kielhofner and Burke (1977) foresaw a shift to a new paradigm – one that was more holistic and that placed a greater emphasis on occupation as distinct from the functioning of body parts. They argued that by returning to a more holistic philosophy and by embracing new theory related to human occupations, therapists could clarify their role and once again unite as a profession.

Over the past 20 years, others, too, have sought to persuade us to re-engage with our history and values. They argue that a **focus on occupations** offers therapists a distinct and clear identity and that we should seize the opportunity (e.g. Molineux 2002). Golledge (1998a, b) concurs, arguing that occupational therapists need to clarify their unique contribution if the profession is to survive. She exhorts therapists to reflect on their current somewhat disparate professional practice and unite under the banner of 'occupation'.

With the explosion of literature and developing evidence base around the value of occupations, some would argue that our professional crisis has now largely passed. If anything, they would say, healthcare practice in general has begun to catch up with occupational therapy's person-centred values. That the new International Classification of Functioning, Disability and Health (ICF) acknowledges the dynamic interaction between functioning and disability and between individual and contextual factors only strengthens our position.

## Threats or ideal opportunity?

Blom-Cooper's independent commission report, entitled *An Emerging Profession* (1989), characterised occupational therapy as a 'submerged profession'. Hagedorn echoes this idea, arguing that: 'Our professional visibility is being camouflaged by our continuing difficulty in expressing the processes and purposes of occupational therapy. There is still a gap between our professional perceptions of the scope and potential of our interventions, and the distorted image that others perceive' (Hagedorn, 1995, p. 324).

Occupational therapy literature is full of practitioners protesting against the **negative images** of the profession and misconceptions about its practice and purpose. Sometimes therapists can be seen to struggle against traditional images of basket-making and entertainment – of providing diversion instead of active treatment. Such images endure in the minds of the public, service users and other professionals. For instance, Harries and Caan (1994) found that patients viewed occupational therapy as merely something to keep them busy or even to give the ward staff a break. Significantly, 82% of the psychiatric patients surveyed in their study believed that entertainment was part of the occupational therapy role – a view with which all of the therapists surveyed disagreed.

At other times, therapists contend with generic work and **blurred team roles**; it is often difficult to identify positive, profession-specific contributions (Harries, 2002). Kaur *et al.* (1996) surveyed 89 multidisciplinary team members in mental health and solicited their views about occupational therapy. They found that each discipline saw an overlap between its own work and that of occupational therapists. The study also revealed that, while others could recognise key occupational therapy functions, they were not confident that they really understood the occupational therapy role and – more significantly in terms of practice – did not apply their knowledge in their referrals.

More recently, the literature has focused on the fast-changing nature of health and social care services and impact on professional roles. In particular, practice is becoming increasingly fragmented and determined by local agencies with their own particular agendas. Some workforce confederations, for instance, are moving away from funding profession-specific training programmes towards programmes designed to train generic health and social care workers. While other allied health professional groups have also come under some degree of threat, occupational therapy seems particularly vulnerable. If our role is too opaque we stand in danger of fading away entirely. Doyal and Cameron sound a warning knell: 'From our observations the group that appears to be most at risk from future developments are occupational therapists [who are] farthest away from the medical power base. Many occupational therapists are now managed by physiotherapists. This has further weakened their capacity to market their services and determine their own practice' (Doyal and Cameron, 2001, p. 379).

With comments like this, the message is clear. We need to make a more concerted effort to develop a more robust **evidence base** and to **positively market** our role and value. Specifically, we need to focus on what we do well and withdraw from peripheral services where we don't really make a difference. We also need to communicate our contribution more clearly, both to our managers and to other professionals. To do this we should draw on our growing research base to demonstrate the efficacy of our services. The use of standardised assessments, clear outcome measures and focused, effective interventions validated by research are all required if we are to survive in the modern professional world.

On the positive side, there remains a chronic national shortfall of occupational therapists. Our profession – given our person-centred values and breadth of skills – is particularly well placed to adapt to changing health-care contexts and demands. The loss of traditional hospital roles offers us exciting possibilities to attend more to new community roles, including health promotion, advocacy, care management and crisis outreach. The development of needs-led provision requires us to be flexible and responsive and allows us to positively exploit the malleability of our role (Harrison, 2003). New opportunities are also opening up for therapists to become consultants in clinical, education or research fields. Craik and McKay (2003) describe the post of 'Consultant Therapist' as offering expert practice (characterised by deep tacit knowledge and vision); professional leadership; training; and service development. These practitioners are likely to have Master's degrees and to be involved in research.

## 1.5 CONCLUSION AND REFLECTIONS

This chapter has offered some ideas about our distinctive professional identity and contribution. While the role of psychosocial occupational therapy varies according to the different teams and health care contexts in which we work, the concept of 'occupation for health' gives us a unique and unifying focus. Our central aims are to enable individuals to engage in meaningful occupations and to cope better with daily life.

Team collaboration is the key to working in health and social care. Our task is to find a way of co-operating with others while being clear about our distinctive contribution. The challenge is how to accommodate traditional professional roles and habits while collaborating with other team members in a new and changing world. We need to find a sustainable balance between generic and specialist roles – a balance that works for us, the team and our service users. We need to develop a strong generic skills base while being confident about our specific contribution related to community living and occupations. At the same time, we need to recognise that change is ongoing. We need to continually evolve our services according to the different trends and challenges that arise.

In my view, the changes and reforms to health and social care should be viewed as an exciting opportunity, not a threat. We are being given an ideal opportunity to explore new ways of interprofessional working that aim to provide integrative, needs-led care. It is time to move away from our acute hospital work towards offering more community-oriented services, expanding into new areas such as consultancy, health promotion and service-user advocacy.

It is time to celebrate the way that occupational therapy ideals are being embraced across different health care professions and contexts.

It is, also, more than time to end any angst about our role. Such professional navel-gazing can only take energy away from our more important work with service users. I agree with Hagedorn (1995) when she implores occupational therapists to cease the endless introspection. Indeed, she argues, we should take some responsibility for perpetuating negative images. I would add that we need to be clear about, and proud of, our 'occupation for health' values and roots. Focusing on the needs of our service users, we need to move on, to concentrate on the business of providing a high quality service – one that is underpinned by a solid theory and research base. It is time, finally, to replace *defensive* practice with *defensible* practice.

# 2  MENTAL ILLNESS: LISTENING TO USERS' EXPERIENCE

*Linda Finlay and Elizabeth McKay*

*Pain sure brings out the best in people, doesn't it?*

Bob Dylan

The previous chapter on the 'occupational therapy role' focused on the professional's perspective. This chapter, in contrast, emphasises service users' perspectives. If we are to provide a truly 'needs-led' service, our first concern as therapists should be to try to understand service users' experiences and priorities. We need to learn to listen to their life stories.

We take this point seriously and this chapter is the result. We move away from occupational therapy towards exploring individuals' journeys through mental illness. While the individuals in this chapter make some references to therapy, their focus is on struggles to cope and to recover mental health.

---

**Case example 2.1   A personal account: extract from Ojomo's diary**

I vaguely remember being taken into hospital kicking and screaming. I thought everyone was out to get me. They tell me I wasn't making any sense. But I was just trying to tell them what was going on. You see, I just knew I had to keep touching wooden things. They grounded me cos anything metal was a conduit for evil. I had been given the gift to see this and my mission was to help others to see it too. But people didn't want to listen. Also, I had to be careful who I told cos 'they' might have been listening. So I'd test people and watch if they touched metal. If they did, I'd know they were 'on the other side'.

Ojomo is a house painter. He lives with his wife, two children and a dog. Mostly, he stays well.

---

A considerable literature is available on the lived experience of disability in general (e.g. Charmaz, 2000; Kleinman, 1988) and of mental illness in particular (e.g. Walton, 1999; Godschalx, 1989; Solomon, 2001). Numerous qualitative studies on chronic illness – whether it be physical or mental – have demonstrated the potentially devastating impact it can have on individuals' lives where illness threatens to 'unmake the world' (Good, 1992, p. 42). Charmaz (2000) focused on the 'loss of self' and self-esteem that occurs with chronic illness, which makes the reconstruction of a valued self a daunting project.

This chapter explores the experience of mental illness. We offer three narratives from individuals who have lived with mental health problems. Through these narratives we take an 'insider' view, describing the individual's perspective. We have focused on their experiences without particular reference to treatment or the potential role of occupational therapy. All too often, the research and literature on mental health and illness is written from the outside. As David Karp (1996) notes in his excellent book on depression, *Speaking of Sadness*, 'The essential problem with nearly all studies of depression is that we hear the voices of a battalion of mental health experts ... and never the voices of depressed people themselves' (Karp 1996, p. 11). Drawing on the experiences of over 20 people (including himself), Karp offers a rich, in-depth exploration of the anguish of depression.

The three narratives in this chapter tell us how becoming ill is just one part of the story. The individuals involved are also *people*, with lives, loves, strengths and projects beyond their illness. Yet when they become ill their whole lives, and those of their families, are affected and it is a struggle to find a way back to health. We catch glimpses of both their struggle and the way they have survived and come through.

At one level, these are 'ordinary', everyday stories. In part, this is why these particular narratives were chosen. Stories like these have been told time and time again by many people who have suffered from mental health problems. At another level, the stories are unique and they are profoundly powerful. They tell of pain, torment, confusion, fear, loss. They tell of the devastation, however temporary, of people's lives.

The three narratives were selected and constructed in different ways: We chose the first narrative – Linda's story – because it offered a graphic account of acute 'madness', revealing something of what it is like to be caught up in hallucinations and delusions. It is a short extract taken from Linda Hart's powerful autobiography (Hart, 1994). The second narrative – Pat's story – came out of Elizabeth McKay's PhD research (McKay, 2002) on narratives of women with enduring mental health problems. The quotes were taken from two research interviews she undertook with Pat and an attempt was made to mould these into a coherent, if co-constructed, story. Kenny's story similarly came out of a research interview, this time carried out by Linda Finlay. Over the course of several years Linda has had a small but ongoing role in supporting Kenny. He was keen to share his experiences in the hope of helping others. (In order to preserve their anonymity, Pat and Kenny's names are pseudonyms. As we are using Linda Hart's own published piece we have retained her name.)

Frank (1998) pleads for health-care professionals to listen empathetically to each individual's story: 'The greatest clinical gift to the ill is to appreciate them as the "good stories" they are. In these stories there is nothing to fix, only a great deal to listen to' (Frank, 1998, p. 210). We are urged to *honour* individuals' experience – to truly listen. Listening has to be the first step in helping a person work through their difficulties.

## 2.1 LINDA HART'S STORY: 'THE ROLLER COASTER OF MY ILLNESS'

---

**Case example 2.2    Extract from Phone at Nine Just to Say You're Alive
by Linda Hart**

*That Wednesday evening when my GP left, I took 100mgs chlorpromazine, had a bath and went to bed.*

*I found it difficult to get to sleep but finally dropped off at around midnight. I awoke at 3am. Wide awake. It was still dark so I went down to the kitchen to make some tea.*

*As I sat at the kitchen table, drinking tea, I kept my eyes on the floor. There were spiders, cockroaches and vermin. I would suddenly catch sight of a tail, a black body, a leg, out of the corner of my eye. My stomach was filled with maggots; I was rotting. I could hear my father's voice telling me to drink bleach or use a Stanley knife to cut open my belly to let the maggots out.*

*I sat at the table with my feet on the chair opposite. I could smell the maggots and my decomposing flesh; I could see the infested floor and I could hear my father's voice.*

*It was a long time till dawn.*

Hart, 1994, p. 26

---

Linda first became ill in 1985. She remembers those first few months:

> *I had had what felt like a shadow behind me for a few months. On odd occasions I had heard the voice of my dead father. One March morning I was driving to work when he told me to drive faster and faster, that my car could fly. As the day progressed, his voice became more insistent. He told me my skin was coming off and that I could disappear. He said I should return to London, my home until 1981, and jump under a tube train. He wanted me to join him in death.*
>
> Hart, 1994, p. 27

Linda was admitted to Ward 20 of the General Hospital that evening. It was the start of many admissions. She remembers her husband (Gordon) and two sons, Jack and William, aged 16 and 15 respectively, coming with her to the hospital. She remembers how becoming ill shattered her and her family's illusions that she was 'Wonder Woman'.

She tells of how the years went by, with periods of good health 'interrupted by the ravages' (p. 28) of her illness. It was not easy to cope: 'For several years I tried to cope with an illness which had been diagnosed as schizophrenia. Drugs used to treat me often had disastrous side effects and alongside the psychotic element I also developed a deep and lasting period of depression' (p. 28).

In her autobiography (Case example 2.2), she talks of how her life became, fundamentally, a series of losses:

> *Gordon, who bore the brunt as a carer, met Ann and left me to set up home with her. The house we spent so much time and money on became obsolete and I needed to leave it to live elsewhere. This coincided with Jack and William leaving home to set up independent lives, one in London and one in Luton. I had to give up my job in 1986 so it seemed that I had lost my husband, my children, my home and my job.*
>
> Hart, 1994, p. 28.

Linda also acknowledges the positive aspects:

> *On the plus side I remained good friends to this day with Gordon and also have a good relationship with his wife, Ann. The lads are settled in their careers. One is happily married and the other has wedding bells beginning to register in his mind for the future. We sold the big house and I was able to buy a cottage in the same village. In 1990 I obtained a part time job working for Social Services in the field of mental health.*
>
> Hart, 1994, p. 28

She values her supportive friends and family: 'I have many friends and family members who have ridden with me on the roller coaster of my illness' (p. 28).


## 2.2   PAT'S STORY: 'IT LEFT ITS MARK ON ME'

### Home life – hard times

Pat was born in 1938. She and her twin sister had an elder brother and a younger sister. They lived in a small town in the north-east of Scotland. She describes life at home as very difficult. Her father suffered from depression. 'He was bothered with his nerves quite a bit. He had treatment every two or three years'. In addition, his mother was considered by the family to be 'a bit loopy'.

Pat recalls her mother 'was never off father's back ... she never stopped nagging him'. Her mother ruled the household. She had strict guidelines that had to be observed. The children were involved in the general upkeep of the house, each with their own tasks. Pat remembers not being able to have friends over or to visit her friends out of school hours. She realised early on that she and her twin sister were treated differently from their eldest brother, who was clearly their mother's favourite child. 'I've an older brother, his childhood was totally different from Jane's and mine'.

Pat reflects on the emotional and physical damage her critical, abusive mother meted out:

> *You two will never be any good, you will never get anywhere. You are hopeless. She never ever gave a word of praise. ... Of course, when you are a twin, this thing 'the terrible twins', I used to think I had done something bad,*

*though I couldn't think what it was. To be called that, it leaves its mark on you. ... She had a half-size walking stick she used to lay into us with. ... I always used to wonder why the school never said anything. But of course, in a small town, they must have wondered about the bruises on us and you had nobody to go to.*

As a child, Pat loved animals. She had her own dog, a present from her father. She took great pride in training her West Highland terrier. She enjoyed holidays she spent with an aunt who had a farm. She loved working with the animals there.

The twins both wished to be nurses. However, at that time, the admission policy of the local nursing school stated that only one family member at any time could join the course. So Jane went off to the nursing college. Pat stayed another year at school. As school came to a close, she organised a job on a local farm, where she would live in. But her mother objected – 'She wouldn't let me do that'. She had had a different plan for Pat, organising a job for her as an assistant in a nursing home in Edinburgh. This post paid minimal wages but it included board and lodging.

At 16, Pat set off for Edinburgh. She missed her twin sister, her home and the hills very much. However, she soon made friends with one of the other staff members. This girl's sister worked in kennels near Glasgow and Pat was intrigued. She enquired about the possibility of a job there and was offered one.

Moving to the outskirts of Glasgow, she really enjoyed her work in the kennels and was happy there for several years. Then, her mother became unwell and Pat returned home to look after her. When her mother had recovered, Pat, now 19, moved on to different jobs working with animals around the country. After a few years she returned home to the north-east. Pat, at 26, decided that she would pursue her earlier idea of nursing and enrolled in 1964 on the pupil nurse-training course.

In 1966, aged 28, Pat got married. She fell pregnant quickly and was unable to finish her nurse training, leaving at the end of her second year. She explains calmly, 'My ex-husband tried to'kill me when I was expecting my first child. He tried to strangle me'. Pat left him and returned home to her parents. In a difficult birth, her son was born in 1967. Someone informed her husband that the baby had arrived. She remembers, 'He got down on his knees and cried and promised. ... My marriage vows meant a lot to me, for better or worse.'

They got back together and the family then moved to Glasgow, where her husband had secured a new job. A second child was born, this time a girl. However, the marital relationship continued to be abusive. 'I had to in the end get away and make a life for the children and myself. ... He had started turning on them as well as me'.

In June 1970, aged 32, she took the children and set up a new home in a council house in Glasgow. She recalls, 'It was really quite bad. You just kind of plodded on from bit to bit. Sometimes it felt like from hour to hour'. At this time, she was pregnant with her third child, another son.

Life for Pat then was very arduous and her main concern was the children's welfare. She explains: 'Well, you've got to pay the rent and at that time you paid full rent. It came in your money. ... All that is in your mind is you've got to pay the rent. You've got to pay the bills, you've got to put food in your children's stomachs and you've got to feed and clothe them and you've got to give them heat and light. ... That was the main thing on your mind. ... You dreamt about it'.

Pat's life revolved around caring for the children. She had little time for herself. She recalls, 'I was never out. I couldn't afford to go out.' On one occasion, a friend convinced her to go out for the evening dancing. Pat organised a babysitter for the children. However, on her return home she found her children misbehaving. 'They were making so much noise they never heard me come in the door the three of them got the fright of their lives.' The following day her elder son announced 'that it wasn't fair that mum had gone out'. Pat explained, 'He thought I had no right to be going out to do something I wanted to do. ... I said to myself, "I'll never go out again until they are grown up." ' Ruefully, she reflects that, in a way, she didn't go out again.

As she continued to look after the family struggling to make ends meet, without realising it her mental health began to suffer. 'Now, I know it was a culmination of my childhood and everything. It caught up with me in my late thirties. The strain of trying to bring up three children on a limited income on my own. It just all caught up with me.'

Although she attended a psychiatric day hospital in Glasgow, Pat felt that she did not receive any help. She remembers that she was asked by her general practitioner to consider giving up her children but she resisted: 'I gave birth to them and even when things are difficult at times, it's my job to bring them up.'

## Giving it up

Pat was admitted voluntarily to a Glasgow psychiatric hospital in 1981. She felt that she could no longer cope with her life and her situation. She was divorced, bringing up her three children in a council flat on a housing estate with no support. She had suicidal thoughts and these were a prime motivator for her to seek admission. She recalls, 'I was crying. I didn't even know what I was crying about. I got frightened to go out. I started getting panic attacks.' She was fearful about the children, especially what would happen to them if she was not there. 'I had nobody to look after the children ... they went into care.'

This was the start of a long admission. Approximately three and a half years of Pat's life was spent in a range of wards in the hospital. Her memories of that time are clear, although she has difficulty recalling exact dates. She recognises that these memory gaps will have been affected by her mental state, as well as by medication she took throughout this period.

Her time in psychiatric care was anything but uneventful and, she believed, not conducive to helping her progress. Her relationships with the staff, and especially her psychiatrist, were strained at the best of times. At the worst times she experienced open conflict with the psychiatrist. She found him unhelpful and she felt threatened by him. 'He just wanted to fill you up with injections and pills until you were just a zombie. He didn't want to know at all. I mean if you've got somebody gazing at their shoes or gazing just over the top of your head, you get the message.' Pat remembers challenging her consultant about her medication during a ward round: 'You are supposed to ask me if I am willing to take a drug that you're trying out for a drug company.' She recalls him 'near spluttering with rage, he couldn't speak'.

Pat also remembers being put under pressure by both nurses and doctors to give up the family home. 'For three months it went on ... "Give up your house. Give up your house."' Pat felt threatened by her psychiatrist particularly: 'The feeling that came from him was this unspoken threat of what he would be able to do.' Eventually she agreed to put her house into her elder son's name.

Pat considered that the nursing staff were generally unhelpful. She remembers their response when she had an item of clothing stolen. 'I had a bra nicked out of my locker. I went to the duty room. They weren't doing anything, they were just sitting, drinking tea. You could stand there for hours waiting, then they would shut the door on you.'

One day, a member of the nursing team held Pat against her will. Pat had made arrangements to go to a review of one of the children and she informed the staff that she would be off the ward. She was told that she could not leave the ward as she was expected to attend a meeting with her consultant. She reminded the ward sister, 'I'm a voluntary patient, I can go out when I want.' At the main entrance of the admission unit the nurse put her back against the door to keep her from going out.

She remembers with sadness and guilt how throughout her time in hospital the children were in care. 'I actually thought the children would have been better off without me because I felt I wasn't being a proper mother because I was in here.' The boys had initially remained together in a children's home but her daughter had been placed in a different children's home. Pat did query this. ' I thought social work policy was to keep children together, not separate them.' Pat maintained contact with the children with regular visits. On one occasion, she recalled that one woman, a member of staff at the home the boys were in, called her an unfit mother and told Pat: 'I don't have to listen to you. You're a nutcase.' However, she became increasingly aware that her younger son in particular seemed ill at ease. 'He was sort of closed off ... he was so closed in on himself.' Pat didn't want to make things difficult for the boys after she had left the home. 'I had to shut my mouth a lot. ... I knew something was going on.' Her younger son was later placed with foster parents – a decision that surprised Pat. 'I never gave my consent to it and I hadn't given them up. ... I don't know how that was worked.'

## Getting it back

Pat's return to better health was slow. She did not have a confirmed diagnosis for several years. Much later, once discharged, she asked for her diagnosis to be clarified. Her consultant stated 'endogenous depression'. Notwithstanding this lack of diagnosis, she was given medication, which caused difficulties, especially the side effects. 'I felt like a zombie. I was massive with the tablets. ... I put on weight and weight and weight. I was nearly 14 stone. I was so slow.'

As Pat's mental health improved she was involved in an active rehabilitation process. She was moved from the admission ward to the rehabilitation unit. She recalls this unit being 'quite good'. She attended occupational therapy. On the whole she found the environment in the occupational therapy department beneficial for several reasons. 'Patients feel that the occupational therapist is their ally. Its not so frightening there as it is on the wards and other departments ... they [patients] would voice things a lot there that they wouldn't voice anywhere else.' That said, Pat felt that for the most part occupational therapy didn't meet her needs. She recalled, 'I used to walk in the occupational therapy (department) and out the other door. See, if I was asked if I'd been to occupational therapy, I wasn't lying when I said yes. I hadn't lied. I'd been in it and straight out again.' However, Pat did have a good relationship with the head occupational therapist: 'I know I told her things I would never voice to him [her psychiatrist] ... but I felt it was safe, it was all right to tell her.'

At the end of her hospital admission, Pat was transferred from the hospital to a group home in the local community. Although the residents in the group home had some professional support, Pat felt that much of the responsibility for the running of the house fell upon her. She found herself caring for one woman in particular: 'I used to take her for walks and that kind of thing. I was very fond of her. ... You had to tell her to change her clothes. ... She couldn't manage it,' Pat believes that her physical health suffered because of her time in the group home. 'A lot of it is to do with the strain of keeping that house going for six years.'

Throughout these years, Pat still maintained contact with her children. Her younger son Mark, now 17, had been housed in an independent living flat fairly near to Pat. He decided that he would move into the group home to be with his mother. Although this was not officially sanctioned, he lived with his mother for about 18 months before being found out during a routine social work visit. Pat, meanwhile, had found alternative accommodation and in March 1991 she and her son moved into their new home. This was to be a new beginning for Pat.

## Starting over

Pat had been in the group home for well over six years when she and her son moved to their new flat in March of 1991. The flat is in a development with an active social programme. Pat set about establishing herself in her new community, taking part in the available activities. So, too, did her son, who currently sits on the committee.

She did not tell people about her time in hospital or in the group home. 'Nobody knows, by the way. My next door neighbour is one of those who thinks people in mental hospitals shouldn't get out.' She banned her Community Psychiatric Nurse, who previously had broken confidentiality, from coming to her house. 'I told her when I moved here, "You're not coming near me at all at any point.'" Pat maintains that the CPN would tell 'everybody who she is and who she was coming to see'. Pat was happy for other staff to visit her at home.

Pat also decided to change her GP. She had to negotiate terms with her proposed GP, who agreed to take Pat on to her list for a month's trial. If there were no problems, they would continue, otherwise Pat would have to find another doctor. However, things worked out well for Pat. She was well pleased with her new GP: 'I'll tell you what she did for me. I'm fed up with the stigma that there is if you have been in a mental hospital or attended one. I asked her to take all references out of my file ... and she did.'

Nowadays, Pat's family is very significant to her. Pat has a good relationship with her daughter, who is married with her own son. Both her grandson and her daughter visit regularly. Pat feels that she is a useful sounding board for her. In the last year, Pat has been supporting her daughter through a family crisis. 'I don't mind if she bends my ear for an hour. She is talking out any worries she has. She realises now that I have always been there.'

However, her relationship with her elder son remains strained, with little contact between them. Pat finds this difficult, especially because she is unable to see her three grandchildren, a boy and identical twin girls. Pat feels that her elder son blames her for how his life has turned out: 'He's still convinced that all of his troubles were me.' But she is also determined that he has to take responsibility for his life. 'I'm not going to feel guilty. ... I'm not going to dig myself into an early grave worrying about it. He is a grown man.'

Over the past few years, Pat has had to come to terms with the devastating knowledge that both boys were sexually abused while in care. She found out about the abuse only when the boys came out of care: 'It nearly took me apart when I discovered it. It was only a chance remark from the oldest one that I discovered it. It nearly took me apart at the seams.' She has asked her younger son why he did not tell her what was going on when she visited. 'He said he was frightened of what would happen once I'd left him.'

Pat reflects, 'I was a voluntary patient. I wouldn't have gone back to the hospital. I would have taken him out of there straight away. He didn't know that and I didn't know.' Pat says of the abuser, 'I can't forgive him for what he did. ... He abused his position in the home, in a place they were meant to be safe.'

As a result of this abuse and its effects, Pat worries about her younger son's future, especially his future relationships. However, Pat really enjoys her relationship with him and finds him a constant support to her, both emotionally and physically. He often accompanies her to hospital appointments, goes shopping with her and is generally active in her life.

In recent years, Pat has suffered from myalgic encephalomyelitis (ME) and she has become an active member of a ME support group with meetings being held in her flat. Until fairly recently she was still attending the mental health drop-in in the city. Here she met up with friends and attended the creative writing group. The women all support each other not only in the centre but informally, especially over the phone.

Pat has started to write poetry. She has been a participant in the creative writing class run at a mental health centre. 'I did sort of write my life story when I lived up the road in the group home. ... I put it away for about two years and then looked at it. I thought it was total dross and tore it up.' Now, Pat writes humorous stories about animals. About her poetry she now laughs: 'Quite often I would be getting in the bath and the whole thing was there by the time I got out of it. There's not been so much poetry coming since I got my walk-in shower.'

## 2.3  KENNY'S STORY: 'CHIPPING AWAY AT THAT CONCRETE BLOCK TO REDISCOVER YOUR CONFIDENCE AGAIN'

### Rock bottom

Five years ago Kenny was at 'rock bottom': 'I was absolutely terrified. I was jumping at me own shadow. I was frightened to be in a room with people. I was frightened of people – which is amazing because most of me adult working life was with people, I'd worked with people.'

He realised something was wrong when he would wake up in the morning and pray there was something wrong with him. 'Anything, just so I didn't have to go to work.' Suddenly one morning, it was all too much. 'That's it', he said, 'I've had enough'. He walked out of his workplace and never went back. He describes his mental state at this time thus:

> I was just shaking the whole time, having panic attacks. I locked myself in the bedroom. It took weeks and weeks before I would go out. I would read, submerge myself in books, escape. I wasn't interested in anything. I just wanted to be in my bed. I suppose in some ways it was my little nest. I was safe in my bedroom and nobody could get to us. The worst part of it was when I was thinking. Then it seemed to get worse. 'What's happening to me? What am I doing?' Then I would get into a panic. I was scaring myself. It was a dreadful experience – one that I wouldn't wish on anyone. To be scared is one of the worst things. It is a method of torture. I had this desperation of what was happening. One minute I was all right and the next I could just go into a rage about the simplest thing. It could be a trivial thing and I'd lose it completely. Again I sought the sanctuary of the bedroom. I knew that there, I couldn't hurt people. The worse thing about it was that I was feeling guilty and that made get more angry.

The doctor put Kenny on medication and encouraged him to see a counsellor. Kenny describes his first counsellor as being very good and sympathetic in that she listened. He began to realise that, for all his depression and anxiety, there was some hope in there keeping him hanging on. 'There was still something at the back of my mind, clinging on by the fingertips, it was still there: "We can go on from this."'

The counsellor then referred him to another counsellor who offered something different. Kenny describes being challenged and confronted by this new counsellor.

*The sessions I had with him were at first quite brutal. Although he was sympathetic he was trying to get me to see what I was doing. 'We have to start looking at what you're doing and start looking for triggers. You've got to face it,' he'd say. And he was encouraging, too. I had no problem, he was being honest and straight. Because you don't like hearing your faults told to you, I thought he was brutal.*

Unfortunately, after six months this counselling had to be curtailed.

*I was with him for six months and then it stopped because of the money allowed – just when I was starting to make some improvements, starting to look at myself and think about things. I took two steps forward and four back because I'd lost the support. I think being able to talk to someone – somebody who only had a professional, not personal, interest. And you knew he wasn't going to be in the pub and bandying it about to all and sundry, you could get everything out and he would listen.*

When this counselling ended, Kenny had two years in 'limbo'. He describes how he was got out a bit more but that he still had problems.

*I was still very fearful. Didn't like to go into crowded places. I wouldn't go to the pub or club, or anywhere on my own. I didn't like to go out anywhere on my own. I wouldn't even go to the shops – I needed someone with me. I was still jumping at my own shadow. I couldn't understand why. I was very much in a shell. Without a doubt. I definitely wasn't myself. It took a long, long time. I suppose you just fumble along.*

## Doing something

Suddenly one morning, something in his head shifted. He suddenly found himself thinking: 'You've got to get out of this! You've got to do something!'. On this same day, his wife came home with the news that a friend of a friend had some repairs that needed doing to a van and would Kenny like to have a go? Kenny describes thinking, 'Well it can't do any harm to have a look. It will give you something to do.' Previously Kenny had been a senior hotel manager but he had always liked working with his hands, so he decided to give it a go. As he said, 'I'm going to try cos I need to do something.' He recognised how destructive it had been to have 'done nothing' for so long. 'I was beginning to feel useless,' he admitted. He gave himself a pep-talk: 'This is not right. I'm 45 year old and I'm not stupid. I can get back into work. You don't have to be working in hotels.' He made the decision that day that he was going to get back into work somehow. That was the beginning of his recovery.

On the first day of his new 'work', he went out to look at the van. Mark, the owner, had said 'Here are the keys and here is the tool room. Don't worry about anything. See what you can do.' To Kenny's surprise at the end of this day he found that he had quite enjoyed himself.

Mark then invited him to do some more odd jobs around the house. He offered Kenny casual but ongoing employment, should he want to take this up.

Kenny decided to accept the challenge: 'It will give me a reason to get out of bed,' he thought. They agreed that Kenny would work at his own pace, without pressure, fixed hours or 'rules'. He could come and go as he pleased, doing only what he felt ready to do. Kenny appreciated this relaxed approach: 'That was just great for me because I was in control. I had the control to do what I wanted.'

One of the worrying aspects for Kenny was that he didn't know what odd jobs he'd have to do day to day. While that was 'frightening', he found Mark an exceptional teacher – one who patiently explained things and encouraged him step by step. As Kenny says, 'I was pleased with myself. I was proud of what I was achieving. He believed I could do it and it was the encouragement which pulled me through.'

Kenny explains how Mark would encourage him by telling him to focus on today: 'Tomorrow will take care of itself. Just get through today. Set realistic targets.' Kenny listened to this advice. He'd think to himself: 'Right, if I get that, that and that done today, that would be good.' So he set himself small targets. But, as he notes, they had to be achievable. 'If you pushed yourself too far, you'd give yourself too much pressure. But it couldn't be too simple either. You had to set yourself achievable targets so that you could measure yourself. You needed to be able to think, 'I'm getting good at this now.' Even today, Kenny still applies this advice.

One of the next turning points for Kenny was when Mark went away and trusted Kenny with a list of jobs to do on his own. 'The first time it happened', Kenny explains, 'I thought "That's not a list it's the Gettysburg address! The man's a fool to leave me with all this to do!"' At the same time, to have someone believe in him was a terrific boost to his confidence. He explains: 'You get to the point when you wonder if anyone is going to take a chance on you. It's one of the barriers.' But Mark did take a chance and Kenny found that he rose to the occasion. He remembers how he found himself tackling different jobs. 'I wasn't too sure what I was doing, but I had enough basic skills and I thought, "I should be able to do this."'

Some jobs, he acknowledges, were 'very, very frightening':

> *They were quite daunting because I hadn't done anything like that before. I was thinking, 'I hope I get this right.' That pressure was there. But I found that I wasn't so frightened to tackle it. I would try, have a go, see how far I would get. Then I'd surprise myself and I'd finish them. I'd think, 'Well you've done well there. You've got it finished. Give yourself a pat on the head!' Although there was no real pressure in what I was doing, it was there for me. I wanted to do it right, to do the best job that I could. So that was pressure. But I learned to say that if that meant jobs took a bit longer then that was okay as the end result would prove I was right.*

Kenny reckons that it was doing things at a *practical* level that made the difference. He describes his state before his slow rehabilitation as having had his confidence stripped away and hidden in a big cement block.

*The only thing to do is to chip at it, until you start seeing your confidence come out. If you can imagine the block and you chip away and get one letter at a time and you build. You see the letter 'C' and you think 'Yes, I can go and get the rest of it.' But you have to watch the pressure and take it one step at a time.*

The practical *doing*, and the *confidence* he gained from it, helped to chip away at the 'confidence block'. As Kenny puts it, 'It gave me the inner strength to go on.'.

## Back in the pond of life

After a couple of years of developing his skills and confidence with Mark, Kenny was ready to stop his medication and get back to work 'properly'. As he describes it, it was time to 'live my life properly. It was time to stop looking into the pond and jump back in.'

Kenny registered at the Employment Office and began his work retraining and resettlement in earnest. First, he was sent to a local sheltered employment scheme, which enabled him to learn some new skills and to cope with working with lots of different people. Then he moved on to a special retraining scheme where he was trained to be a NVQ Assessor.

In his new work as an Assessor, he coped with a number of challenges. However, he found the job unsatisfying and stressful. He recognised that he didn't need to put himself in this position. He decided to move on. He settled on a job at the local factory. He has stayed in this job now for several months and he is content:

*I feel immensely proud of myself that I've managed to get back to where I am today in full-time employment. I'm quite content. It's not the job I trained for. But I've found that it's not a hardship to go to work. I don't wake up and think I don't want to go to work today. I go there. I have no pressure to deal with other than getting there and getting home again. I think one of the loveliest things is that I've regained my sense of humour. I was quite proud of myself. One chap come up to me and said – as you know the place is notorious for people not lasting more than a day – this fella came up to me and said 'We never thought you'd still be here after the first week. We've nicknamed you "the ice man". No matter what anyone asks you to do you never get ruffled. You just go and do it. You don't get flustered.'*

On getting this feedback, Kenny thought to himself:

*That'll do for me. One little chat with him made me realise that I had beaten it! I had sorted it! I just enjoy meself now. Me and the wife still have a lot of worries but we'll sort them in time. I'm aware of how easy it is to slip back if you don't confront things then and there. If you do that they stew and you get worked up. I have found now I can just say something and be done with it.*

He describes enjoying the security and structure of his new job:

*There is no stress, I'm not in charge. I'll do it to the best of me ability and I use my commonsense and me skills. And I get on with it. We have a bit o' fun. I know when I wake up what I'm going to do. I think that's really important. Earning lots of money is not important. Let's settle for something that's steady and that's going to be there. It's in my control to decide how long I want this job. I'm quite happy where I am. I have my self-respect.*

Kenny reflects on where he is now:

*I'm very aware how quickly you can descend into depression and I try very very hard to never go there again. But I don't think I'd get down there so far now, with my past experience. Now I know how to cope. I'm really immensely proud of myself because I've had to kick down a lot of barriers – both personally and professionally. It showed me one thing. I was determined. I wasn't going to be beaten. I wasn't going to lie down. But you can't do it on your own. I couldn't have done it without all the support I got from the family and from Mark and others. We got through it together. I think as a family we're stronger.*

'You've got to put the effort in', Kenny advises.

*You're in a big pit and there's a ladder there. And as long as you don't look down, just look up and keep trying, step by step, you'll get out the pit. You can do whatever you want. I look at it as an achievement. I was down and out but I made the conscious decision to stop the rot. And I did.*

## 2.4   COMPARING AND CONTRASTING EXPERIENCES

### About mental health and illness

Each of the three stories has focused on different aspects of mental health and illness as the individuals move, in various ways, through trauma, withdrawal, loss, emergence and reconstruction. Although the accounts are brief and selective they have given us a glimpse of the individuals' experiences. From Linda we learned something of the horrific living nightmare experienced in an acute stage of a psychotic episode. Here, we witness the power and darkness of her voices and visions. From Pat we hear a story of social hardship and lost years. We are confronted by her experience of abuse – at the hands first of her mother, then of her husband, and then of a brutalising, disempowering health-care system. From Kenny we gain insight into the long struggle to re-claim a life and re-make an identity. We catch a glimpse of the paralysing effect of his intense emotions and can only guess at the impact of this on his sense of self-worth.

The three stories also highlight how mental health problems can manifest in very different ways. Mental health and illness can be viewed on a continuum. At one end of the illness spectrum lie emotional stresses. Kenny's struggle with anxiety can be seen as an extreme version of the kinds of emotional state all of us can identify with. Linda Hart's psychosis, at the other end of the spectrum, illustrates what happens to people when disordered thinking and perception predominate. Linda and Pat have illnesses where biochemical imbalances (requiring medication) seem to play a much bigger part. At the same time, environmental stresses clearly play a role in all their stories.

Although these narratives offer contrasting accounts, they also contain similar elements – elements that would be familiar to most users of mental health services. Three particular shared themes stand out:

- Feeling out of control
- The struggle beyond the illness
- The power of the social context.

## Shared themes

### Feeling out of control

In different ways each individual experienced a sense of feeling 'out of control'. Linda, at the mercy of her voices and visions, was forced to take medication to control these experiences, and this created further symptoms. More than the immediate acute symptoms, however, the loss of Linda's marriage, home and job reinforce her sense that her life is not under her control. Pat's entire life, and that of her children, has similarly felt out of her control and she has struggled to wrest a degree of control in her relationships, whether with her mother, her husband, her children or, indeed, with health-care professionals. Only latterly, it seems, has she been able to assert her needs and identity. Kenny's emotions were out of control. In common with the other two, he had to face his fear, not knowing if, or when, the nightmare was going to end. Even though each has reclaimed their mental health, they live with a constant wariness, if not fear, about what may happen in the future.

A particular theme that comes up in each of the narratives repeatedly is loss – losses that were out of the narrator's control. All three have lost 'time', relationships, valued occupations and, to a greater or lesser extent, their self-respect, self-worth and self-confidence. Their struggle, then, was to reclaim a positive identity and life. Deegan (2001, p. 18) describes it well: 'For those of us who have struggled for years ... recovery is not about going back to who we were. It is a process of becoming new. ... Transforming, rather than restoration, becomes our path.'

### The struggle beyond the illness

In their stories, all three individuals also make the point that mental illness is just one dimension of their struggle. Each person has had to cope with problems beyond, or resulting from, their illness. Linda had to cope with all her losses, which, as she says, were themselves enough to push someone over the edge into depression. Pat had to struggle to simply survive as a single mother, living in poverty with insufficient support in an inner city. Kenny's story told of the long road clawing his way back to full-time employment. We don't hear him say it, but we can well imagine the impact the unemployment had on him personally (given his sense of being a breadwinner and provider) and on his family (creating unaccustomed financial hardship).

## The power of the social context

All the stories reveal the power of the social context – both in the creation of mental health problems and in the healing process. In other words, mental health and illness can be understood to be **socially constructed**. Williams and Collins (2002), for instance, show how many of the problems of schizophrenia arise from associated experiences such as social isolation, stigma and unemployment. They urge professionals to challenge undermining social stereotypes and to guard against having expectations which are too low.

In our society, mental illness is still surrounded by considerable ignorance, fear and stigma. Pat's story shows how people with a history of mental health problems may be denied employment, good housing and other opportunities. At a less tangible level, service users face invidious prejudice such as the way our society routinely judges and labels. The very health-care system purporting to care for Pat turns out, at least in part, to be disempowering and abusive (Research example 2.1).

---

### *Research example 2.1*

### Being labelled

O'Loughlin (1999) carried out a phenomenological investigation of Ana's lived experience of emotional trauma and chronic pain. The following excerpt relates to Ana's experience of being labelled:

> *Ana believed that explicit or implicit labels had been applied to her in relation to her health status since an early age. The underlying meaning implied in such labels had a significant effect on her perception of herself and on the way she believed she was perceived by others. The labels she believed most commonly applied to her were 'sick', 'chronic pain patient' and 'psychiatric' or 'ex-psychiatric patient'.*

Ana recalled experiencing chest pain and difficulty breathing while driving home one day. The pain was unfamiliar and she began to wonder whether it was related to her heart, so she reluctantly drove herself to the Accident and Emergency Department of a large hospital. When she told the receptionist she had chest pain the response was immediate. All the usual procedures for checking out chest pain were commenced. However this came to a rapid halt when her file arrived:

> *My file had finally been collected. And what do I hear? A couple of nurses saying to the sister in charge, 'Have you seen her file?' The next minute I get the sister coming in: 'You can't take up this bed all day.' ... Now I don't know if anybody knows what that feels like but it feels like shit.*

O'Loughlin, 1999, pp. 133–134

---

Pat's story also highlights the significance of relationships: the abuse she suffered at the hands of both her mother and husband contributed to her low self-esteem, stress and distress.

However, the social context may also be a force for good. The individuals in each of the narratives confirm the importance of good support systems in the form of family, friends, community and caring professionals. For each person, empowering, supportive relationships with others provided the route back to mental health. In tandem with these relationships were health-promoting occupations and social roles that enabled participation in community life. Pat, for instance, reclaimed a valued life through the support gained at a mental health drop-in centre and by joining a creative writing group. Kenny gained confidence and self-respect from his sheltered work opportunity. These are the kinds of experience occupational therapists aim to tap into in their interventions. As Deegan (2001, p. 18) notes: 'Because recovery is a unique journey for each individual, there is no cookbook approach. Mental health professionals must explore the special gifts and resources of each individual.'

## Narratives and occupational therapy

Narratives such as those presented in this chapter help us understand our own and others' lives, problems and situations. Life is given meaning and made coherent as we locate ourselves in different stories. The stories offer us a way of integrating the things that happen to us with our past, present and future selves. In some ways, the stories told in this chapter can be seen as 'quest stories' (Frank, 1998). The individuals are engaged in a quest to find a way of living with their illness and they are looking to see what can be learned and how this lesson can be passed on to others. So what are the lessons such stories offer us as occupational therapists?

First and foremost, such narratives offer us a way of **seeing the individual** more deeply. We begin to appreciate not just the impact of a collection of symptoms and problems but something more about the person's life, struggles and relationships. Hearing such stories enables us to treat that individual better. It also provides us with insights into the more effective treatment of other individuals who may have similar experiences. While the person's unique story cannot be generalised, it can serve as a vignette to be returned to when working with others in similar circumstances.

Narratives help us to understand something deeper about a person's **meanings and motives**. It becomes particularly important to identify a person's motivations when we start to engage them in treatment. As Helfrich and Kielhofner (1993) note, occupational therapy can only transform the lives of people if those people feel it has 'meaning and relevance to their own unfolding life story' (p. 324).

Narratives also help us to make sense of our work with clients (Hughes, 2002). Not only do narratives enable both therapist and client to gain insight into current clinical problems, they also help to create stories of different possible *futures*. Mattingly's (1998) work on **narrative reasoning** shows how we use narratives in two distinct ways. Firstly, therapists are seen to retell their clients' stories, either in terms of general pathology 'chart talk' or by relating specific experiences of the person. The telling of such stories, notes Mattingly, is always retrospective. The other use of narrative is in 'story making'. Here, therapists create a possible and desirable future for the person, envisaging how the therapist and the client could work towards that future image. This type of story is always prospective is are shared implicitly as the therapist and the client work together.

Picking up these themes, Kielhofner *et al.* (2002) discuss the need for occupational therapists to focus on clients' **occupational narratives**. They define occupational narratives as the stories, both told and enacted, that integrate 'unfolding volition, habituation, performance capacity, and environments through plots and metaphors that sum up and assign meaning to these elements. Both our identity and our competence are reflected and enacted in the stories which we make sense of and go about doing our occupational lives' (2002, p. 127). Our role, then, is to help individuals find their occupational identity. Here, we help them to make sense of their capacities and find satisfaction in the activities and roles that fill their lives.

In summary, narrative is both 'the meaning we assign to occupational life and the medium through which we enact it.' (Kielhofner *et al.*, 2002, p. 143).

---

### *Research example 2.2*

#### The use of narratives in occupational therapy

Over the last decade the use of narrative in occupational therapy practice has proliferated. Contributing to this growth have been the findings of the Clinical Reasoning Study funded by the American Association of Occupational Therapy and the American Occupational Therapy Foundation. This study explored how, and in what ways, occupational therapists reason. Mattingly and Fleming (1994) proposed that occupational therapists used narratives in their everyday practice reasoning to enhance their understanding of their own and their client's understanding of the client's situation.

To date, narratives have been used in occupational therapy to explore a range of issues. The body of literature encompasses work that illuminates clients' narratives (Clark, 1993; Fanchiang, 1996; Mostert *et al.*, 1996), student and educational issues (McKay and Ryan, 1995; Ryan and McKay, 1999; Fortune, 1999), therapeutic potential (Polkinghorne, 1996; Hughes, 2002) and narrative as a research method (Molineux and Rickard, 2003; Mallinson *et al.*, 1996; Frank, 1996, 2000).

---

## 2.5 CONCLUSION AND REFLECTIONS

Three ordinary, yet uniquely rich and powerful, stories give us a taste of what it means to experience mental illness. More than anything else, perhaps, they serve to remind us of how important it is to view individuals as whole persons within a wider social context. Every individual is involved with family, friends, and a wider community. Each has a life they are negotiating and trying to hang on to or reclaim. It is not enough to see the person in terms of their illness and problems, or even their occupations. Instead, to provide a properly 'needs-led' service, we need to see the person along with their hopes, dreams, interests, skills, values and strengths. Dealing with mental illness then becomes a challenge and an opportunity, rather than a process of containment. The difference is well illustrated by Linda Hart's assessment of her own condition as 'well with break-downs' in contrast to that of her psychiatrist, who is quick to write her off as 'ill with remissions' (Hart, 1994).

Both of us (Linda and Elizabeth) believe in the need to listen to, and really hear, the stories our service users tell. In our view, this is the way to become a better therapist. Ultimately, we would argue, it is not about instituting standards, protocols, audits or even increasing our evidence base, although these too play a part. First and foremost, we need to listen, understand, empathise and care. These stories remind us that, for all our knowledge and expertise as therapists, it is the service users who are the experts on themselves. Our role is to enable and encourage. Moreover, while we can make a difference as therapists, it is the wisdom and healing that the individuals give themselves that are the key. Their strengths are what have enabled them to survive and cope as well as they have.

It takes a lot of courage to tell such personal stories. The three individuals here wanted to tell their story, to share their experience towards helping others understand better. We appreciate their gift.

# 3 OCCUPATION AND ACTIVITY FOR THERAPY

*Meaningful occupation animates and extends the human spirit.*

Peloquin

Our belief in the centrality of occupations and the healing power of activities has defined our profession over the last century. Early pioneers emphasised how the health of individuals could be influenced by purposeful activities: by 'the use of muscles and mind together in games, exercise and handicraft, as well as in work' (Hopkins, 1983, p. 3). Contemporary literature identifies three basic assumptions underpinning occupational therapy:

- Humans have an occupational nature. We have a basic need to engage in occupations; they are essential to living.
- Illness/disability can interfere with our ability to do things which are important to us, and this diminishes our health and well-being.
- Occupations and activities can positively influence health and well-being (Research example 3.1).

Occupational therapists are thus concerned about individuals' daily life *occupations* and we use *purposeful activities* when we intervene therapeutically. Precisely how and why occupational therapists use occupations and purposeful activities is the focus of this chapter. First, I define the terms 'occupation' and 'purposeful activity' and explore the psychosocial nature of occupations. Second, through drawing on contemporary research, I examine different dimensions of occupation and how these impact on health. Third, I analyse some activities and explore how and why occupational therapists use purposeful activities therapeutically. A final section offers five contrasting case illustrations showing how occupation and activity have been used in practice. Throughout this chapter numerous research examples and references are offered to illustrate occupational therapy's growing evidence base.

---

### Research example 3.1

### The value of occupations

Three studies show the value of occupations:

- Laliberte-Rudman *et al.* (1997) studied the occupations of and meanings attached to occupations by elderly persons living in the community in Canada. Activity was perceived as:
  - A contributor to well-being
  - A means to express and manage identity

---

- A connector to people
- An organiser of time
- A connector between past, present and future.

Laliberte-Rudman *et al.* emphasised the importance of ensuring that individuals are given choice of occupations, enabling them to feel an enhanced sense of control.

- Rebeiro and Cook (1999) similarly explored the use of 'occupation-as-means to mental health' in a group of women attending a quilt-making group. The study demonstrated the benefits of this group occupation:

    - Members affirmed each other as worthy, cared for and important
    - The activity confirmed members' evolving sense of competence
    - It enabled new and positive self-definitions.

- Green (2003) studied the meaning of occupations to 12 vulnerable elderly people in the UK. All the participants valued occupational involvement as part of their quality of life. They all actively took steps to ensure ongoing engagement in chosen pastimes to fill their days. Occupations were seen as a core reason for 'being' and provided validation of self. Time was experienced as well spent.

## 3.1 PSYCHOSOCIAL DIMENSIONS OF OCCUPATION

### Defining occupation

Occupations are the everyday, meaningful activities we engage in, related to our work, leisure and self-care. They take place in the context of our material and social worlds. They are our 'daily living tasks that are part of an individual's lifestyle' (Golledge, 1998c, p. 102).

- **Work** – Our occupations related to work span the full range of productive activities/tasks, both paid and unpaid, where we provide goods or services. Our work occupations could include being a parent, student, volunteer worker, and so forth.
- **Leisure** – Our leisure occupations include the freely chosen activities and hobbies we engage in for enjoyment. These may be fun, creative, exciting, relaxing, stimulating or restful. Leisure involves play, imagination, personal exploration and/or making social connections.
- **Self-care** – Self-care occupations include the basic tasks necessary for self-maintenance such as personal care (e.g. dressing, bathing) and domestic activities of daily living (e.g. cooking, housework).

Of course, the different categories of work, leisure and self-care overlap considerably. A housewife 'works' at her domestic activities; someone who pursues a leisure hobby seriously (e.g. DIY, trainspotting, gardening) is probably simultaneously engaging in a form of work. Much depends on the **personal meanings** the individual brings to bear and the **social circumstances** involved. For instance, an unemployed person may regard their degree studies with the Open University as 'work', while someone else might choose to do the same degree for 'leisure'. One individual may paint for pleasure but this definition might change if they started to paint on commission.

Definitions of occupation have been contested, demonstrating just how complex and multidimensional the concept is. Some authors use the terms 'occupation' and 'purposeful activity' interchangeably (see Golledge, 1998b, c for a comprehensive review).* These authors emphasise the 'goal-directed' and 'active' quality of occupations. Others, for instance Christiansen and Baum (1997), distinguish between these terms, arguing that all occupation is purposeful activity, while not all purposeful activity is occupation. Simple acts may be purposeful but they only become occupations when they are meaningful, are done in combination with other acts and take place in the person's usual daily life context. For instance, polishing shoes can be a purposeful activity but it only becomes an occupation when combined with other acts of dressing. Putting a lead on a dog can be purposeful; walking the dog every morning is an occupation. An occupational therapy example is the use of purposeful activities like cooking in a departmental kitchen, as opposed to the cooking individuals do in their own homes, which can be viewed as occupation.

However we define and differentiate occupations, they are concerned with people's **use of time** and how daily activities structure our lives. The way we use time – in the past, in the present, and in our planning for the future – defines who we are in some ways. Ross (1997) studied 24 young adults living in the community who had serious mental disorders and found a correlation between higher numbers of life roles and life satisfaction. Occupational roles provided a framework for organising time and gave individuals a sense of meaning. In this way, our daily activities, habits and routines give us meaning and a degree of stability, together with a sense of coherence and continuity. They enable us to satisfy our needs and to realise hopes and aspirations (Wilcock, 1998). As Betty Hasselkus puts it:, occupations, and the experience of occupations, enhance health and well being across the life span 'propelling us along the journey of our lives as we strive daily to sort out and make choices about the actual and possible' (Hasselkus, 2002, p. 69).

## Occupations and personal meanings

Occupations need to be understood in terms of individuals' personal meanings. Individuals perceive and interpret their occupations in different ways. On experi-

---

*Controversy continues to surround the use of these concepts. I would recommend studying Mocellin's (1995, 1996) critique of the use of 'occupation' as a core concept for occupational therapy. For a deeper exploration of the ideas underlying the use of occupation and activity, see the American Occupational Therapy Association's position paper on occupation (American Occupational Therapy Association 1995); Predretti's (1996) distinction between 'adjunctive' and 'enabling' activities; and Chapter 1 of Christiansen and Baum, 1997.

encing occupations, we each have idiosyncratic emotional responses and the activities have particular symbolic and practical significance to us. As Crabtree puts it: 'The nature of humans is to make meaning through occupations' (Crabtree, 1998, p. 205). You only have to think about why and how you engage in your daily activities, and how others might react differently, to recognise that multiple personal meanings are often involved (Theory into practice 3.1).

---

***Theory into practice 3.1***

**Idiosyncratic personal meanings and motivations**

**Antonia** loves cooking her special lasagne for the family. In addition to valuing her role as 'provider', Antonia feels rewarded when people enjoy her meals. That the lasagne is based on a 'secret recipe' passed down to her from her great-grandmother adds a sense of specialness and occasion. She also enjoys the touch, taste and smell of the food as she works with it.

**Roy's** no. 1 work/leisure occupation is to 'hang out at the shopping mall and check out the talent'. For him, this is a productive activity as well as a social one.

**Gwyn** enjoys washing up and leaving a kitchen sparkling clean at the end of a day. He takes pride in his high standards and looks forward to walking into the 'sparkling clean' kitchen each morning.

**Karam** enjoys the peace and tranquillity that comes from his daily yoga and meditation session. In the midst of an otherwise busy life, he values this time of spiritual contemplation and bodily discipline.

**Lenny** loves to play football. He enjoys being outdoors and being energetic. He enjoys, and feels good about, his considerable ball skills. He likes the sense of his body working in a co-ordinated, flowing way. It is even more exciting for him when he can play competitively with others, and win.

---

Take a hobby that means different things to different people – for instance, photography. Some people carry their camera with them wherever they go as it is important to them to record events as they are happening. Others might take a few snaps once a year on holiday, when they remember. Similarly, there is the activity of organising photographs into albums – some of us enjoy doing this, others find it laborious. Although we all might enjoy riffling through our holiday snaps, we react differently to the photographs themselves. We see a particular photograph and it captures a particular moment. We remember a scene, special people, places, relationships, smells, tastes. The act of sorting photographs can be highly significant at a personal level as we remember our life, our friends and family, our history. Any one photograph will carry different meanings for different individuals.

Personal meanings and occupational choices are also revealed in our narratives

– the stories we tell ourselves and others about our lives (Mattingly, 1998). For instance, Antonia in Theory into practice 3.1 has a story about her Italian heritage and how she is positioned in generations of the women in her family who are 'special providers'. Research example 3.2 describes the story of a man with schizophrenia who moves beyond telling a story of being a victim of mental illness to telling a story about himself as a competent, productive member of society.

---

**Research example 3.2**

**The social construction of identity**

Rebeiro and Allen (1998) explored how one individual with schizophrenia experienced his voluntary work. During his interviews, he referred to social stigma, social identity and self-identity related to the experience of living with his condition. He perceived his voluntary work as a valuable socially acceptable occupation that allowed him to contribute to, and be a productive member of, society. His 'work' helped him to construct a socially acceptable identity as a competent individual.

---

## Occupations and culture

As well as being imbued with personal meanings, occupations are culturally embedded. Any occupation or activity needs to be understood as arising in a particular cultural context. This notion is such a important one for occupational therapists as we need to be careful not to impose our own values on others.

A clearcut example of imposing cultural values is when we think of the way people in other cultures carry out daily living activities in ways different from our own. Imagine the following situation. You are doing a kitchen assessment observing how a man makes tea. He proceeds to put tea leaves into the kettle on the hob. So you step in to assist. You (reasonably) deduce that he is confused and that possibly his visual perception/object recognition is somewhat impaired.

This is in fact a true story and it happened to a friend of mine. What the occupational therapist did not realise was that my friend had come from an African village where they boil tea in a kettle with milk and sugar. However, had the therapist given my friend the electric kettle, he would have made tea the Western way! (See Theory into practice 3.2 for another relevant example.)

---

**Theory into practice 3.2**

**Therapists should avoid imposing their own cultural values**

An example of a situation where a therapist unthinkingly imposed her own values occurred on a home visit with a Bangladeshi woman. She had been referred as she was suffering tearfulness and anxiety. During the interview the therapist discovered that her client did not have any 'leisure' occupations because she spent several hours every day cooking elaborate meals for her large family. The woman also cared for two children under the age of 5 and for an ageing, infirm uncle. The occupational therapist diagnosed stress and tried to encourage the woman to take some time off – for instance, by using convenience meals or getting her husband to cook. The point the therapist missed, however, was that the woman's caring activities were both valued and expected, and she enjoyed doing them! Furthermore, the shame/distress the woman would feel at not carrying out her 'role' properly could have been far more damaging than any benefit more leisure time might offer.

This example illustrates the need for us to be aware that people's attitudes and meanings about daily activities and how they should be performed depends on the cultural context. Needless to say, this idea doesn't apply only to people who have been brought up in other countries. It also applies to people who we might think are from the 'same' culture as ourselves.

We could go even further and recognise that our therapy practice and values are themselves culturally shaped. Take, for example, our concept of 'promoting independence' – a major value of occupational therapy. Independence is, as Kinebanian and Stomph (1992) remind us, a 'Western, white, middle-class value. It is associated with making one's own decisions, having freedom of choice, knowing what one wants to achieve in life, and accepting personal responsibility'. They go on to describe how in many non-Western societies values such as honouring the family and accepting other people's decisions are far more important than independence. As they say, 'dependency is a respectable choice' (Kinebanian and Stomph, 1992 p. 752).

If our interventions are to have a chance of being effective, we need to recognise the cultural biases and assumptions underpinning our professional practice, our ideas about occupation and our personal beliefs about values and standards.

## Social construction of occupation

People are occupational beings. We go through life being active. We adopt different roles and carry out different activities at different points in our life span. While individuals can be seen to play an active role in choosing these occupations, it can also be argued (particularly by social constructionists) that society shapes what and how activities are performed. Laliberte-Rudman (2002) picks up this point in her research. She explores how occupations influence one's sense of both personal and social identity and how they can be used to promote self-growth. She demonstrates how individuals' preferences for identity influences their choice of occupation, in that a person may choose an occupation because it carries with it certain social images/identities that he or she aspires to.

At a *macrosocial level*, we can see that occupations are influenced by society in that the very notions of what constitute work and play are a product of society's norms and ideas. Ideologies in our society carry images of what are appropriate occupations for different groups of people. For example, in our culture elderly people are supposed to retire from paid work and children are supposed to play. In other cultures, elders are the community leaders and children are required to work. In our culture, it is accepted that both men and women seek employment. In other cultures men may be expected to be the breadwinners while the women stay at home. At a microsocial level, occupational behaviour is shaped through social relationships and is negotiated through interactions. Every encounter potentially plays a part in producing and positioning the self. (See section 4.5 for a fuller discussion of the social constructionist position.)

Think of any situation where a person is involved in activity. Imagine a girl playing with a doll, for instance. Now develop the scene. She is playing on the floor in front of her parents. It is her birthday, she has just received this doll, her parents are smiling benignly, taking pleasure in her pleasure. The girl starts to play a bit roughly with the doll and is gently reprimanded: 'You must take care of the pretty baby doll!'

In this example, thinking at the macrosocial level, we could make several comments about how society defines what is appropriate children's activity (i.e. play), or what is an appropriate girl's toy (e.g. doll). Society even lays down how we do the activity (e.g. using a doll symbolically like a baby). Western culture is also relevant to this story in the sense that the celebration of birthdays by giving a person presents is a culture-specific practice. At a microsocial level, we can see that the girl's behaviour is being influenced by her parents – their choice of gift, their expectations of what she will do with it, their smiles, their reprimands. Their (and other people's) expectations and responses will similarly shape how the girl performs other activities and her attitudes to those activities.

## 3.2   OCCUPATION FOR HEALTH

Recent research, particularly in the field of occupational science, has demonstrated the link between occupation and health/well-being. For instance, in a review of literature on occupations and mental health in care homes for older people, Mozley (2001) provides evidence that opportunities for occupation and pleasure in homes contributes not only to mood state but to actual survival rates.

Wilcock's (1998) influential work on 'occupation for health' stresses the importance of being in tune with our occupational nature in terms of the dynamic balance of 'doing, being and becoming'. She shows how 'being' arises from 'doing' and becoming is dependent on doing and being. She argues how we are 'more susceptible to illness as a result of continuing occupational injustice, deprivation, alienation or balance' (Wilcock, 1999, p. 195).

These ideas are now briefly explored using two concepts that are particularly relevant for occupational therapists: occupational balance and occupational engagement.

## Occupational balance

Occupational balance is a key concept in our practice. Often misunderstood as the balance between work, play and rest, it is, in fact, a much more complex and holistic concept related to balance in life style and tasks. Balance is about the relationship between a person, their occupations and their worlds. It means being able to engage in a diverse range of appropriate occupations in order to meet our varied needs. We have needs for balance in activities that involve novelty/familiarity, stimulation/relaxation, solitude/sociability, attachment/independence, emotion/lightness, challenge/easy-achievement, physical exercise/mental work, and so on. Importantly, the needs and meanings that surround our occupations vary with each individual.

To give a concrete, personal example, some people suggest that my writing this book (which has entailed long hours over and above my normal working day) demonstrates considerable occupational imbalance. They say I am unduly focused on my work. The contrary feels right to me. I am enjoying the creativity, learning, variety, stimulation and mental challenge involved in this writing. My book-writing is as much leisure as it is work. My quiet times of writing provide a welcome contrast to my lecturing where I am busy relating to others and have other pressures. However, another person engaged in book-writing may subjectively experience a more problematic occupational imbalance.

Wilcock (1998) and others (e.g. Christiansen, 1996) have demonstrated that a lack of occupational balance is associated with ill health and stress. People with mental health problems are shown to lack occupational balance, while diminished, limited occupational experiences are likely to aggravate mental health problems. This problem can usefully be addressed in occupational therapy. The first step is to clarify the nature of the occupational imbalance.

First, lack of balance can occur when a person experiences either **boredom** (as a response to lack of occupation) or **burnout** (as a response to over-stimulation and too much occupation). Second, people can experience **occupational alienation,** for instance where employment is exhausting, boring, degrading, demeaning, dirty, deskilling and/or socially alienating. In such cases, their broader physical, emotional and social needs are not being met. Third, lack of balance can be seen when occupation leads to **preoccupation**. This occurs when individuals become so obsessed and overly focused on certain activities that other important needs and occupations are ignored or excluded. An example that comes to mind is excessive, habitual use of computer/Internet games, which can become a problem when the person stops attending to their regular work and self-care activities. Finally, an extreme form of imbalance is **occupational deprivation,** when a person is kept from acquiring or enjoying occupations as a result of poverty, lack of employment opportunities, ill health/disability, discrimination, abuse, being a prisoner or war refugee, and so on (Whiteford, 2000). Here, the cost can be high: individuals lose a sense of personal efficacy and their interaction with the world is diminished, often resulting in mental and physical deterioration (Research example 3.3)

---

*Research example 3.3*

**Occupational imbalance when unemployed**

- Nagle *et al.* (2002) studied the occupational choices made by persons with severe and persistent mental illness. They recognised the high unemployment rates of this group and asked how the individuals managed this lack of work. The authors found that these individuals still had occupational goals. While some were unable to modify the aspirations they had prior to falling ill, others had become less ambitious (e.g. aiming to become a cleaner instead of a teacher). All the participants recognised that occupational experience could both hinder and support their health. They knew that good health allowed them to be occupationally engaged, while not doing enough or doing too much exacerbated their symptoms. The study found that the individuals made active choices and that they aimed for **balance**. They worked hard to enjoy a broad range of leisure activities and consciously used opportunities to connect with others. They were not in paid employment but they worked hard on themselves and their lives.

- Shimitras *et al.* (2003) studied how 229 adults in London diagnosed with schizophrenia used their time. The findings indicate that people with schizophrenia tend not to be engaged in occupations that support active, meaningful life styles or social inclusion. Few of the participants engaged in active leisure, work, education or volunteer occupations. Their predominant occupations were sleeping, personal care and passive leisure. In terms of specific patterns: the women spent significantly more time in domestic occupations; younger participants engaged in more social occupations; older participants spent more time in passive leisure; and there were few differences found between inpatient and community dwelling subgroups.

---

## Occupational engagement

*The meaning of our daily lives lies in the experiencing ... in the consciousness of the moment . ... It is the experience – the dance – of the occupation that is important, not the occupation itself or the outcome.*

Hasselkus, 2002, p. 132

In this quote, Betty Hasselkus reminds us that while the type and variety of our occupations are important, it is the *quality of our experience* and the process of engaging in the occupation that is vital. It is important to appreciate how activities are experienced and to understand what motivates individuals to engage in them.

Many subjective accounts of occupational experiences have been published. Phenomenological research, for instance, is devoted to exploring consciousness and much of it relates to the experience of doing and being). One example is Csikszentmihalyi's (1999) exploration of 'flow' – the subjective psychological state that occurs when we are totally absorbed in an activity (see the section on the humanistic approach in Chapter 4). Csikszentmihalyi found that flow states involve feeling good, highly motivated and being 'in the zone'. During flow, concentration can be so intense that there is a loss of self-consciousness and a temporary reprieve from one's worries. Research by Csikszentmihalyi and others suggests that flow states relate to self-esteem, life satisfaction and the ability to cope with stress. Conversely, ill health and lack of well being are associated with being unable to enjoy activities and engage in flow (Research example 3.4).

In occupational therapy, our key aim is to enable individuals to engage in satisfying and meaningful occupations. Motivating individuals to become engaged in occupations or activities is a crucial part of this. This is a particular challenge for those of us working in the mental health field. The skill is to discover those factors that are going to be influential for engaging particular individuals. Our task is to be aware of individuals' meanings and occupational experience. The research outlined in Research example 3.5 identifies some key dimensions that impact on occupational engagement.

---

### Research example 3.4

**Flow and enjoyment experiences of persons with schizophrenia**

Emerson *et al.* (1998) studied the accounts of nine individuals with schizophrenia. In contrast to previous research by Csikszentmihalyi, which suggested that people with schizophrenia might not be able to experience 'flow', Emerson *et al.* found that their participants were able to describe many enjoyable experiences. Some experiences were seen as being 'exciting' and 'exhilarating' (e.g. the excitement felt while doing competitive, challenging sports/games). Others expressed feeling a sense of accomplishment and pride when they became focused during creative and intellectual activities. Other themes that emerged included feeling relaxed, socially connecting and being interested while being involved in activities.

This study suggests that individuals with schizophrenia can and do experience enjoyment through activity. A key lesson for occupational therapists is the need for us to ensure that a range of activities are offered to individuals so they choose which are going to be meaningful. Cueing into people's particular sense of interest and dimension of meaning helps promote occupational engagement (if not optimal flow experience).

---

### Research example 3.5

**Factors influencing occupational engagement**

Chugg and Craik (2002) studied the factors influencing occupational engagement in the case of eight individuals with schizophrenia living in the community. Four themes emerged:

- **The relevance of health** – Poor physical health and the impact of medication could limit occupational engagement
- **The importance of routines and structures** – Weekends, when there was less structure and fewer social contacts, were perceived as more difficult
- **The role of external factors** – Other people (and pets) were found to be important in encouraging and supporting the individuals to engage in occupations
- **The role of internal factors** – Poor self-concept seemed to result in individuals expecting little of themselves and performing fewer occupations.

The findings overall suggest that occupational therapists need to be open to hearing clients tell their 'stories' in order to build a picture of their meanings and identify the factors most likely to help them engage successfully in occupations (see Chapter 2).

## 3.3   THERAPEUTIC USE OF ACTIVITIES

In section 3.1, we distinguished between occupations and the purposeful activities that can be used as treatment. Having discussed the role of occupation, we now focus on the therapeutic benefit of purposeful activity. These purposeful activities might be used within structured activity programmes that take place in occupational therapy units. Alternatively, they might be the focus when encouraging clients to engage in such activities on their own (i.e. without the therapist present) in their local community.

First, the intrinsic value of activity in general is considered. Then the range and value of activities commonly used in occupational therapy practice are explored, with reference to relevant research evidence. A final subsection describes how occupational therapists analyse activities in order to strengthen their therapeutic content. (See section 8.3 for a discussion of factors influencing choice of therapeutic activity.)

### Intrinsic value of activities

Activity (in its widest sense) is fundamental to human existence. We have an innate, spontaneous tendency to be active and to explore our world. We also need to be active in order to survive and have some quality of life. Activities – both the process of doing them and their end product – have value at many different levels. We can see this applied both to ourselves and to therapy:

- We use activity as a **learning tool** to develop our skills and help us to explore ourselves, others and the environment. A child's use of activity, in the form of play, illustrates how play can be used to practise or learn skills and to test out knowledge and perceptions.

- Engaging in activity offers the opportunity to gain awareness of our capacity for **competence, control and mastery**. Through successfully engaging in activities we can gain a sense of self-esteem, self-efficacy and agency.
- Activity **stimulates our senses** and activates us. It motivates and energises us at both a physical and a mental level. Consider the times you have felt lethargic and sluggish but after some exercise have felt revitalised.
- The process of engaging in activity can be a form of play and has **social value**. It can be both pleasurable and diversional. It offers us the opportunity to interact and connect with others, to build relationships and to participate in community life.
- Activity can be a vehicle to **express and explore feelings**. For example, writing a diary has a projective function in that it can release tensions and be cathartic.
- Occupations provide us with social roles. Activity helps us to fill our time and **structure our day**, giving meaning and a sense of purpose to our lives.
- Finally, activity is **productive**. Both the process of doing and the end product can be gratifying. Being purposeful or creative meets our esteem needs and carries tangible rewards (Figure 3.1).

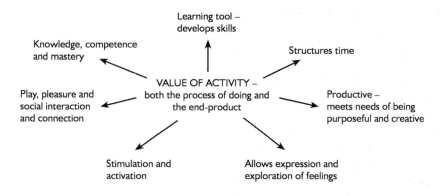

**Figure 3.1** Value of activity

Behind the notion of the value of activity is an acknowledgement that activity has the potential to meet different 'needs' (Research example 3.6). This can be illustrated by using Maslow's (1954) 'hierarchy of needs' as a reference. Cooking, for example, offers opportunities to satisfy physiological needs, if a person is hungry; esteem needs, if he or she receives praise; mastery needs, as the individual learns new skills; and self-actualisation needs, if he or she simply enjoys cooking. Group work, as another example, can offer individuals the opportunity to have their love and belonging needs met when they are accepted by the group, and their esteem needs met if they are recognised as having an useful contribution to make.

*Research example 3.6*

**Evaluating the benefits of an allotment group**

Fieldhouse (2003, p. 290) studied the subjective experience of nine people participating in a horticultural group. He shows how the plant–person relationship promotes interaction with the environment and so enhances people's health, functioning and subjective well being. That allotments are embedded within communities adds to their potential as a medium for occupational therapy and as mechanisms for social inclusion. He highlights three dimensions that demonstrate the complexity and value of this occupation:

'1. **Dimensions of the environment**

    1.1 *Dimensions of the physical environment*
        Outdoors, natural, green
        Peaceful and away from customary stressors
    1.2 *Dimensions of the occupational form*
        Destigmatising and 'normalising'
        Productive
    1.3 *Dimensions of the social milieu*
        Accepting, mutually supportive
        Ease of communication

2. **Dimensions of individuals' subjective experience**

    2.1 *Thinking or cognition*
        Improved concentration
        Fascination with growing plants
        Flow experiences
        Enhanced sense of personal agency
    2.2 *Emotional responses*
        Appreciating beauty
        Attachment to the group
        Relationships with plants
        'Feeling different' – enhanced mood, reduced arousal, feelings of spirituality
    2.3 *Aspects of 'being' or identity*
        Destigmatised identity
        Awareness of physical self and environment
        Temporal orientation
        Personal narrative

3. **Dimensions of occupational performance**

    3.1 *Becoming engaged*
    3.2 *Generating goals*
    3.3 *Social networking*'

Occupational therapists believe in activity and its inherent values (see Moll and Cook, 1997 for a more detailed examination of therapists' beliefs about the value of activity). However, we also place emphasis on activities being *structured, adapted and graded*. We analyse activities in order to understand their component parts and inherent demands, and carefully apply a particular activity to suit an individual or group and enhance their functioning. Generally occupational therapists modify, and therapeutically use, activities with the following aims in mind:

- To help people **acquire new skills** – to help the patient cope better in the present, (e.g. through learning relaxation techniques) or in the future (e.g. through the therapist suggesting a new hobby)
- To improve specific **areas of deficit,** e.g. cognitive skills being improved with extra training using quizzes or work tasks
- To **raise self-esteem** and promote a positive self-concept by helping a person gain awareness of his or her potential and develop confidence through achievement
- To provide an enjoyable **social outlet** through activities and to help develop social relationships
- To enable individuals to connect to valued occupational roles and tasks and develop healthy, **balanced routines**
- Lastly, **to assess** a person's occupational performance and measure future progress.

## Practical applications of activities

Many purposeful activities are potentially available to occupational therapists. However, their choice of activities is constrained by what the patients or clients themselves want to do as well as by practicalities and the resources available. Certain activities seem to turn up regularly within occupational therapy programmes (in hospital or day units). Some of these are briefly described and evaluated below to give a flavour of their aims and therapeutic use.

We can view purposeful activities along a spectrum, moving from those that aim to teach task skills to those that aim to explore feelings psychotherapeutically, with social-communication-type activities in the middle (Figure 3.2). These divisions should not, however, be see as rigid.

- Most activities can be adapted to fit into one or other category, depending on the desired aim. Art, for example, can be equally well used as a work task or projectively.
- Any one activity can simultaneously fit into several levels, e.g. a pottery work group may also be a social gathering.
- Each individual will respond differently to a given activity. Embroidery may be a relaxing social activity for a person skilled in it but a daunting challenge for the uninitiated.

The following four sections examine these activity groupings in more detail. The

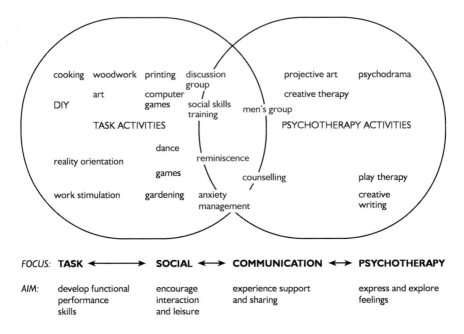

**Figure 3.2** Spectrum of occupational therapy activities

few descriptions of specific activities and their evidence base offered are necessarily brief but serve as examples to show the richness and variety of purposeful activities and how they can be used in occupational therapy.

## Task activities

Task activities aim to improve daily living, work or task performance skills. They can be run at different levels, from trying to improve concentration in a craft group to work simulation and training.

### Cookery

Cooking is a commonly used occupational therapy activity, mainly because it can be graded so easily while being almost universally practical. It offers opportunities for people to develop task performance skills (e.g. following instructions, problem solving) and can also be applied to later stages of treatment when individuals are practising their domestic role skills (e.g. when home management units use cookery as part of wider domestic rehabilitation). Cooking seems to be enjoyed by people of all age groups and abilities, not least because of its tasty end-products.

Research by Kremer *et al.* (1984) using a randomised post-test experimental design confirms the value of cooking as a therapeutic activity. They investigated the degree of meaning different activities held for chronic psychiatric patients. A total of 22 patients were randomly assigned to three groups: cooking, craft and sensory awareness groups. After their group activity, each patient rated its affective meaning. Results showed differences in meaning for each activity and cooking was found to be significantly more meaningful than the others. The authors concluded that possible reasons for this included the fact that it is a concrete activity with a consumable end-product, that it offers oral stimulation, and that it is age-appropriate and culturally meaningful.

Melton (1998) explored how five clients with learning disabilities evaluated their experience of cooking with the occupational therapist. The findings revealed that the clients had powerful individual routines and meanings that they associated with cooking (including perceiving it as a substitute for work, a survival task and a leisure activity). The study also highlighted the importance of the therapists' empowering, respectful approach in enabling the clients to benefit from the cooking activity.

*Work simulation*
Work in contemporary Western society has changed dramatically in the last decades. Extensive de-skilling and re-skilling has taken place as a result of the expansion of technology and automation. An increasing variety of work practices now exist, such as part-time, flexible work, job share and voluntary work (Steward, 1997). Occupational therapists need to be aware of the different work opportunities – and barriers to work – in their local areas.

Work rehabilitation in today's socioeconomic climate remains problematic. While the value of paid work is acknowledged, people with psychosocial disabilities experience many barriers to re-employment. The debilitating effects of mental health problems, discrimination, lack of appropriate training and few sheltered work opportunities are among the obstacles. For these reasons,

---

**Research example 3.7**

**Work therapy and the homeless: a randomised controlled trial**

Kashner *et al.* (2002) investigated the impact of compensated work therapy (CWT) – including vocational rehabilitation, sheltered workshops, job clubs and supportive employment – on the ability to homeless people in America to gain employment. The authors found that, compared to a control group (who also had access to medical, psychiatric, addiction and rehabilitation services), those on the CWT programme had better non-vocational outcomes. Although there were no effects on psychiatric status, those on the CWT programme:

- Were more likely to begin out-patient addiction treatment
- Had few substance misuse problems
- Avoided decline in physical functioning
- Had fewer periods of homelessness and imprisonment.

---

treatment is often geared towards developing more general productive occupations (e.g. voluntary work or DIY) rather than vocational resettlement.

Oxley (1995) argues that work rehabilitation programmes need to be flexible
and to cater for a wide range of clients – from those who need supported
sheltered employment to those able to progress to open employment. She recommends that rehabilitation starts with a thorough work skills assessment using a
range of standardised assessments. Following assessment there should be a period
of work adjustment and work skills training (e.g. in a workshop) before moving
on to sheltered employment. Transitional employment and training schemes may
also be helpful (e.g. local work experience and sponsored placements) in
preparing individuals for open employment.

Durham (1997) reviews the literature on the role and value of work-related
activities for people with long-term schizophrenia. She cites evidence from a
handful of outcome studies that structured activity programmes are beneficial in
reducing symptomatology and maintaining community tenure. The importance of
carefully evaluating optimal levels of stimulation is stressed.

### Social activities

The wide spectrum of social activities used within occupational therapy aims to
promote interaction and enjoyment and to develop new leisure/hobby interests
(Ravetz, 1964) See Pieris (2002) for an in-depth exploration of what leisure
means to clients with enduring mental health problems and how occupational
therapists might enable individuals to overcome barriers towards using leisure in
their recovery process.

### *Crafts*

A group of people sitting in a circle and engaged in a craft is still a common sight
in many day units. The range of crafts, from traditional activities such as basketry
to more recently introduced activities such as photography, offers something for
every age group and ability level. These activities are useful for task skills and
provide a focal point for social interaction. The most successful craft sessions
seem to be those where clear aims are pursued and products are attractively
displayed or sold (rather than thrown away or recycled).

The research base validating the use of activities/crafts is growing. McDermott
(1988) considered the effect of three types of group treatment (using pottery/art
group; activity based discussion group; verbal group without activity). She found
that craft activities produced more positive socio-emotional communications
(compliments, expressed satisfaction, joking), more interactions between
members and fewer uninvolved members than did the more strictly verbal
groups. Klyczek and Mann (1986) compared two different treatment
programmes, one offering a greater emphasis on activity and the other focused
on psychotherapy. The activity-oriented programme was found to be significantly
more effective with respect to a wide range of challenges including improving
decision making, developing use of leisure time, increasing self-esteem and
promoting vocational adjustment.

More recent research in the UK has also demonstrated the value of craftwork. Reynolds (1997) studied the role of a creative leisure pursuit in long-term coping with illness and disability. Studying the written narratives of 35 women, she found that creative needlecraft was commonly viewed as providing a means of managing pain and unstructured time, as well as facilitating self-esteem and reciprocal social roles. Slater (2000) measured and explored the benefits gained from four different photography groups as part of an overall day hospital programme. She concluded that these groups did indeed promote mental health through occupation.

*Sports and games*
The popularity of physical activity, from aerobics to skateboarding, finds reflection in the activities we promote in occupational therapy. We may encourage individuals to go swimming (perhaps at the local baths) or enjoy exercising in a gym or playing badminton. Activity programmes within units often offer games such as table-tennis, Trivial Pursuit, quizzes, computer games and group activities such as bingo. The way the activities are structured has a significant bearing on the results. Bingo, for example, can be used as a way of teaching number/letter recognition, to encourage interaction (through participants sharing a card), or simply for fun. Whether competitive or not, sports or games offer enjoyment, opportunities for challenge, group interaction and scope for enhanced leisure.

Much research attests to the link between physical exercise and mental health (Everett *et al.*, 2003). Moore and Bracegirdle (1994) examined the impact of a six-week exercise programme on 15 elderly community-dwelling women. The results indicated that the exercising women experienced significant improvements in happiness and well being. Fox (2000) provides a systematic review that identifies 36 randomised controlled trials dealing with physical activity and self-esteem. Positive changes were found in 76% of all trials. Lawlor and Hopker (2001) reviewed 14 studies and found that exercise produced a significant decrease in depression scores – a decrease similar to that achieved by cognitive therapy.

## Activities involving communication and sharing
Communication and sharing with others can be incorporated into almost any activity, though most often they fall under the guise of 'groupwork'. Group members are encouraged to share their experiences and provide each other with mutual support and encouragement. Often, the format of the activity is determined by the theoretical framework used: for instance, dramatherapy (based on psychodynamic ideas) contrasts with social skills training (based on cognitive–behavioural principles). For a more in-depth exploration of the application of groupwork in occupational therapy see Finlay (2002).

*Discussion groups*
Discussion groups can be handled in many different ways. The aims of discussion groups, their structure and format, and the role played by the therapist can all be

adapted. For example, a structured discussion can be a straightforward 'hat discussion' (hat passed round containing topic suggestions on slips of paper) or more personal (such as reading out and discussing the Problem Page/Agony Aunt letters in magazines).

The evidence base for the value of groupwork is considerable. For instance, Kanas (1996) reviews 46 controlled studies of groupwork for people with psychosis and 70% show significant improvements. Coupland *et al.* (2002) summarise the successful work of the Gloucestershire Hearing Voices user groups. Here, group members gain information about their psychosis and share ways to cope. Research by McDermott (1988) demonstrates that discussion-based activity groups and verbal groups are beneficial for personal growth and learning in that they promote greater discussion of feelings than do craft-focused groups.

*Communication skills training*
Communication skills training (also referred to as 'social skills training') is a cognitive–behavioural technique designed to teach, systematically, elements of social behaviour (verbal, non-verbal, assertion, etc.). People who benefit may never have acquired the skills (e.g. people with learning disabilities), may once have had the skills but have lost them (e.g. institutionalised patients) or may have the skills but lack the confidence to apply them (e.g. anxious individuals).

The practical emphasis on 'doing' and step-by-step learning of skills via role play, modelling, feedback, and so on makes communication skills training a particularly relevant technique to use in occupational therapy. Special sensitivity is needed, however, to tread the line between imposing one's own standards of behaviour and facilitating the development of new or different behaviours in someone who wants to change. A comprehensive account of the theory and practice of communication skills training, together with a survey of relevant research, is offered by Hargie (1997).

*Relaxation and anxiety management courses*
Anxiety management courses, based on cognitive–behavioural principles, commonly entail running a closed group over a set number of weeks (e.g. 10 sessions). During a course a number of purposeful activities, including education, group work, role play, relaxation exercises, etc., are offered. Table 3.1 summarises the different areas of focus and types of intervention. In-depth accounts of anxiety management programmes are offered in Keable (1996) and Rosier *et al.* (1998).

## Psychotherapy activities
These highly specialised activities arise mainly from the psychodynamic school and focus on facilitating the expression and exploration of feelings. The activities can be either analytically based (focused on the symbolic potential of activities and resolving unconscious conflict) or humanistically oriented towards making self-awareness and personal growth the main goals.

**Table 3.1** Anxiety management

| Focus – anxiety component | Treatment intervention |
| --- | --- |
| **Cognition** (e.g. negative thoughts) | 1. **Educating** the person about the nature of anxiety (how different components can be natural/positive and how to 'spot and stop' the anxiety spiral)<br>2. **Cognitive restructuring** to encourage the person to stop negative thoughts/talk/anticipatory anxiety and to think more positively |
| **Behaviour** (e.g. avoidance of anxiety provoking stimuli) | 3. **Systematic desensitisation** (or other structured and graded approaches) to unlearn avoidance behaviour<br>4. **Role play** to practise specific skills and coping strategies for particular situations (such as an interview) |
| **Physiology** (e.g. autonomic responses) | 5. **Relaxation** (e.g. Jacobson's Progressive Muscular method or Mitchell's (1977) specific muscle group focus) and applied relaxation (e.g. what to do when sitting in a public place)<br>6. **Relaxing activities** (e.g. going swimming, listening to music, doing yoga, playing squash). The individual is encouraged to find what works best for them and do it on a regular basis |

## Creative writing

Creative writing can be used in many different ways. 'Free writing', without regard for grammar/spelling, can encourage the spontaneous expression of emotion. The use of poetry and verse can similarly enable powerful emotions and conflicts to be expressed. Atkinson and Wells describe this eloquently: 'Words give the opportunity for release, for imagination of the most personal and creative kind, the fantasy world built around stories where the soul joins the self in journeying beyond the confines of the body' (Atkinson and Wells, 2000, p. 236).

Jensen and Blair (1997) explored the relationship between creative writing and mental well being with the co-operation of 14 adults who had been users of mental health services and were involved in a community creative writing group. The findings revealed a tension between the cathartic expression of thoughts/feelings and the production of quality writing. The theme of finding an identity and voice to combat the social stigma experienced also emerged. The authors suggested there might be a dynamic relationship between creative writing as a productive activity (rhyme) and its therapeutic by-product in terms of helping individuals to gain better command over their inner world (reason).

## Projective activities

Art, drama, pottery and music are creative activities all of which have been used in a psychotherapeutic way to help individuals gain insight into their inner conflicts and explore their feelings (Theory into practice 3.3). (For a comprehensive account of the theory and practice of projective activities, see Atkinson and Wells, 2000.) The key process underlying any projective activity involves individuals 'projecting' or externalising their inner feelings outwards on to a creative object (for instance, paper). As Waller puts it, 'image making in the

*Theory into practice 3.3*

**Example activity evaluation – projective art**

Value
1. Self-awareness, insight
2. Expression and exploration of emotions or catharsis
3. Group communication, sharing, cohesion, support
4. Enjoyable

Note that there are two different stages involved: doing the art work and then talking about it afterwards. The art process itself (for example, painting a picture on 'how I feel') can offer some cathartic release. Talking about it afterwards (discussion or psychotherapy format) can help individuals further explore their feelings and enables group members to give each other support. Different therapists place a different emphasis on the two stages – some prefer the doing, others the talk.

Ways of adapting
- Extend the time for either 'doing' or 'talking'
- Activity itself – free self-expression, fun games, painting to music, painting to a theme, interpretative analysis, and so on
- Vary themes and titles, e.g. 'How I see myself now . . . in five years', 'My family', 'Schizophrenia', 'Happiness', What I like/dislike', 'What alcohol means to me'
- Media used – clay, paint, finger-paint, collage, rollerbrushes, etc.

Considerations
- Emotional safety/trust within the group essential
- Emphasise the importance of free, spontaneous art as opposed to being concerned about the artistic quality of the end-product
- Contraindications:
  - Dangers of stirring up unmanageable or negative feelings, as such activities can be emotionally powerful
  - Over-interpretation can be offensive or simply wrong
  - Such activities may reinforce fantasy and/or confusion and would not be appropriate for use with individuals with thought disorder
- Decide between running a more analytical/psychodynamic art group, where interpretation is desirable, and one focused more humanistically on the goals of self-awareness and growth.

presence of the therapist may enable a client to get in touch with early repressed feelings . . . and . . . the ensuing art object may act as a container for powerful emotions that cannot be easily expressed' (Waller, 1993 p. 3).

When these projective activities take place in a group setting additional benefits can be gained, for instance mutual support.

## Activity analysis

One key skill used by occupational therapists is the ability to analyse the component parts of an activity in order to use it purposefully, meaningfully and therapeutically. Step-by-step analysis can be laborious but it is important and must be done until the therapist feels familiar with the nature of an activity and understands its potential as a treatment medium (see Research example 3.6 and Theory into practice 3.3 for examples of such analyses).

### What do we analyse?

Activity analysis usually occurs in two stages. First, we try to understand the **intrinsic** aspects of the activity itself. We then analyse how the activity can be used (i.e. graded and adapted) towards a **therapeutic** end (what Hagedorn (1995) refers to as 'applied analysis').

Young and Quinn (1992) suggest that activities can be analysed in terms of:

- The permanent, unchanging requirements intrinsic to the activity (e.g. sensori-motor and cognitive demands)
- Permanent, changing requirements (such as space, equipment, materials and cost)
- Social and cultural perceptions of the performances of an activity (e.g. expectations related to gender, age and ethnicity).

Occupational therapists probe activity in different ways, examining:

- The procedures, processes and steps involved
- The materials and tools required
- The motions and sequences involved
- The environmental context
- The results of the process
- The cultural and social meanings associated with the activity.

As we look at all these aspects, paying particular attention to how demanding the activity is in terms of a person's functioning, we might ask the following questions:

- **Physical** – What types of movement are required: fine? gross? repetitive? aggressive? What kind of tolerance and strength are needed?
- **Sensory/perceptual** – What visual, tactile, proprioceptive aspects are involved?
- **Cognitive** – How much concentration, memory, intellectual ability, abstract thought, etc. is needed?

- **Emotional** – Does the activity ease expression of feelings? Does it satisfy needs? Is it stimulating? Is it intrinsically/extrinsically motivating?
- **Social** – What level of communication skill is required? How much sharing and co-operative behaviour is expected?

In addition to analysing the demands of an activity on an individual, we build up a picture of the inherent nature of the activity. We may jot down notes on the demands made by the activity: 'This activity needs attention to detail', or 'Some amount of tolerance of dirt is required', or 'There are cultural assumptions behind this activity making it unsuitable for certain groups'. We then marry this information with the individual's needs, ability and motivation.

**Why analyse an activity?**
Having broken down an activity into its components, we are ready to think about how to utilise the activity's potential to restore or maintain function:

- We analyse an activity **to determine if a patient/client can do it.** For example, the apparently simple task of making a collage may not be so easily achieved if it takes place in a group setting and the individual concerned operates below a parallel group level in terms of Mosey's group interaction skill levels. Or we might feel more confident about encouraging a person to use a pottery wheel if we assess that he or she has some standing tolerance, co-ordination, familiarity with claywork and a degree of perseverance while learning a new skill. (Note that an *increase* in skill level can only be achieved if some aspect of the activity is slightly beyond the person's ability, thus creating a goal to strive towards.)
- We also break down activity into smaller steps and subtasks **for teaching purposes.** An accurate preliminary analysis allows us to consider if there is a logical progression or if any steps need to be simplified or eliminated. The process of teaching someone how to make a coil pot, for example, might involve the following step-by-step progression:

  1. Therapist demonstrates, showing basic idea and result
  2. Individual makes base after another demonstration and with physical and verbal promoting
  3. Individual practises making coils with advice
  4. Individual makes coils and applies to pot using slip, after instruction and demonstration
  5. Therapist demonstrates how to finish off coil pot
  6. Individual makes another pot with minimal instruction given.

  Each stage of the process contains its own skill levels and needs to be carried out in sequence if the end-product is to be successful. Throughout the teaching process, it is important to consider the individual's cognitive ability as well as his or her need for reward or encouragement.
- We also analyse activities in order **to identify what aspects need to be adapted or altered** to suit an individual's functional ability and meanings. A person who finds working in a group difficult and is therefore unable to join in a

group collage may be asked to make an individual collage that is later added to the larger one, offering a symbolic gesture of group connection. An individual who is unable to read and is learning to cook may need picture recipe cards instead of written ones.

- Lastly, we analyse activity **in order to grade it** so as to bring about change. For example, we can identify which components need to be made more demanding, thereby stretching the level of function required. In the case of woodwork, for example, treatment might move from simple sanding to making intricate sculpture puzzles, thus encouraging greater concentration or attention to detail.

## 3.4 OCCUPATION AND ACTIVITY IN TREATMENT

One mistake occupational therapists make when using activities is to *assume* their inherent therapeutic effect. An example of this is the person with poor eye contact who is encouraged to play a game of 'wink murder' because it uses eye contact. Or a person with poor concentration who is given the activity of dress-making because it requires a degree of mental application. On careful examination, though, it is clear that these activities will only prove beneficial as part of a graded programme. Wink murder is only useful for eye contact if the person concerned finds it slightly difficult to do, and this requires the occupational therapist to carefully adjust the demands of the game. Likewise, people with poor concentration who engage in dressmaking will need regular encouragement by the occupational therapist, enabling them to attend to the task. In other words, it is not the dressmaking itself that improves concentration, but *how it is applied*.

Consider the five case examples below of how activities may be applied as part of the occupational therapy problem-solving process. The examples show how the therapist's approach, combined with the process of structuring of the environment, are fundamentally linked to the grading of an activity.

## CASE STUDY 3.1    MICHAEL

- **Problem** – Poor task performance skills
- **Activity** – Woodwork
- **Grading** – Increasing the demands and complexity of the task.

Michael, aged 40, has had repeated admissions to hospital with schizophrenic episodes. His basic task performance is poor, probably resulting from a cognitive deficit stemming from his illness, passive behaviour due to institutionalisation, and the sedating effects of his medication. Woodwork is an activity in which Michael expresses an interest.

### Stage 1: Basic task and quick results

With his concentration being so poor initially, the occupational therapist encourages Michael to make something that can be completed fairly quickly and that requires a minimal amount of skill. Over the first week several tasks are completed – varnishing a ready-made stool and sanding/polishing a bookcase for the ward. These activities require the minimum of instruction and are repetitive enough to allow Michael's attention to wander. However, Michael can still feel pleasure and a sense of achievement: he has produced results.

### Stage 2: Increased task demands

As Michael settles into the routines of the new area, more complex tasks are introduced involving more complex instructions and absorbing longer amounts of time. First, he makes a plant trough out of pre-cut strips of wood, which he then paints. Later, with the occupational therapist's help, he makes an intricate chessboard requiring careful cutting and staining of the wood.

### Stage 3: Discharge

Michael pursues his new interest in woodwork when he is discharged to attend a day centre three times a week.

### Discussion point

Michael's progress can be clearly measured by outcomes in the form of the increasingly complex end-products. However, much of the value of his treatment lies in less measurable and intangible aspects to do with his sense of self and sense of competence/productivity. Michael's treatment is not just about improving his skills. Instead, the purposeful activity of woodwork has been used to enable Michael to feel productive and so strengthen his self-esteem. The activity has also been chosen for its long-term utility: the therapist knew that Michael could follow up this activity at a local day centre. Occupational therapists 'never do only one thing at a time' and 'never do anything for just one reason' (Mattingly and Fleming, 1994, p. 34). That our aims are multilayered, and at times tacit, makes them hard to measure and makes it difficult for others to appreciate the value of our interventions.

---

## CASE STUDY 3.2    JUNE

- **Problem** – Lack of self-confidence
- **Activity** – Jewellery making with metalwork
- **Grading** – Early success experience leading on to increased task demands and difficulty as therapist gradually reduces supportive assistance.

June, a 23-year-old unemployed woman, lacks confidence in her abilities. She has started several college courses but has either failed or given up. She feels 'useless'. However, she agrees to give occupational therapy a chance.

## Stage 1: Introducing the activity

June expresses an interest in jewellery making, while adding, 'I won't be able to make anything as nice as those samples'. The occupational therapist suggests she give it a week, and that she first learn the basic skills. This approach is adopted to avoid being overly praising (as June is not likely to take compliments on board) and also to encourage June to be realistic about her skills.

## Stage 2: Teach basic skills and provide success experience

The occupational therapist teaches June a simple and quick method of beading and bending a piece of wire to make an earring. June is provided with a range of examples and ideas and is encouraged to 'have a go'. The results are quick and successful, and provide an immediate reward. June is no longer able to deny that she can produce simple, attractive jewellery.

## Stage 3: Increase demands of activity

June's initial good feelings about her achievement soon diminish and she begins to put down her skill, saying 'the task was too easy'. The occupational therapist agrees, and shows her a much more complicated method requiring new welding and enamelling techniques. The occupational therapist is actively involved, encouraging June and supervising her closely in order to pre-empt any failure.

## Stage 4: Reduce therapist support

As June's ability and confidence grow, the occupational therapist scales down her help and encouragement. The occupational therapist begins to 'allow' June to use her own ideas and to make mistakes. Constructive criticism is made of June's work. Her confidence in her own ability grows.

## Discussion point

Lack of confidence is something most of us experience in some aspect of our lives. It is usually specific to a particular situation: for example, we may feel inadequate when it comes to competitive sports or DIY. Tackling our lack of confidence through activity, or 'doing' treatment, will only prove effective if the activity zeros in on the area in which we feel inadequate. For instance, cookery and dressmaking may be beneficial treatment activities for a housewife who feels inadequate in those particular areas. However, in the case of a housewife whose negative self-image results from abuse at the hands of her partner, dressmaking and cookery classes are unlikely to have a significant impact. Having said that, a tangible success experience can result in positive self-feelings and may be the start of some longer-term work.

A word of caution, though – if the activity is too easy or lacking in challenge, negative feelings may be confirmed and the activity can prove destructive. Care must be taken to grade both the activity and the therapist's role carefully.

## CASE STUDY 3.3 ▏ KATHY

- **Problem** – Compulsive behaviour interfering with daily occupations
- **Activity** – Anxiety management group
- **Grading** – Occurs through the course of 12 supportive cognitive–behavioural educational sessions where the therapist increasingly encourages group members to support each other and implement their own problem-solving as their knowledge and skill increases.

Kathy is a 32-year-old secretary. She has begun to feel extremely anxious at work, although she does not know why. She is finding it hard to manage at work and is concerned that she may make mistakes. As a result, she is tending to do tasks over and over again when this is not necessary. She worries that something bad will happen if she doesn't carry out her clerical tasks (e.g. filing) perfectly. She feels she is failing at everything and she lacks confidence in her judgements. Kathy becomes particularly frightened after experiencing a full-blown 'panic attack'. This was triggered when she was prevented from triple-checking a letter she had just typed. On assessment, the therapist discovers that Kathy lives with her unemployed husband and is possibly being physically abused by him. However, Kathy says she wants children 'before it is too late'.

### Stage 1: Education about anxiety and relaxation techniques

Kathy joins a newly formed anxiety management group. The emphasis in the first couple of sessions is on learning how to contain and cope with anxiety. She learns how her negative thoughts and anxiety about anxiety provoke an anxiety spiral. The therapist gets her to challenge her own negative thinking (e.g. that something bad will happen if she doesn't triple-check things). She practises different relaxation techniques in order to identify which works best for her.

### Stage 2: Support and sharing in the group

Kathy begins to sense that her anxiety is under control and that she can cope with it in her work environment. Through the support and sharing she experiences in the group she realises that her anxiety is probably linked to marital stress.

### Stage 3: Discharge planning

Kathy gains confidence in managing her own anxiety by teaching and supporting others. Her final 'homework' task is to begin marital counselling sessions with Relate. Once these sessions begin she is discharged from the group, with a follow-up appointment for three months later.

### Discussion point

The extent to which anxiety management is an appropriate occupational therapy activity (as opposed to being a generic therapeutic intervention) has been the subject of considerable debate. Surveys indicate it to be among the most frequently applied interventions in community mental health. Rosier *et al.* (1998) describe one successful group format. They view therapists as being educators who help individuals function more productively in their daily living activities. If the focus remains on occupations, the argument goes, then this intervention falls under the occupational therapy domain of concern. Anxiety management groups often use a range of group activities (e.g. relaxation and role play) and this lends weight to the argument that the occupational therapists' skills are well suited to such interventions.

---

## CASE STUDY 3.4    CLYDE

- **Problem** – Identity and work conflicts
- **Activity**– Counselling and groupwork
- **Grading** – Not particularly relevant – group process evolved over time.

Clyde is a 35-year-old accountant. He is under a great deal of stress at work and goes to his GP complaining of insomnia and palpitations. The GP refers him to a community mental health team and the occupational therapist picks up the referral. On assessment he discovers that Clyde's work is a problem area. At work, Clyde is irritable and is experiencing interpersonal difficulties. In particular, Clyde feels angry and upset because he has been repeatedly passed over for promotion. He believes his bosses are racist (Clyde has a white Scottish mother and a black African father).

### Stage 1: One-to-one supportive counselling

The therapist's main intervention is to see Clyde once a week for one-to-one counselling. The main focus is on exploring how Clyde could cope better with his tensions at work.

### Stage 2: Joining a men's group

After four weeks of these exploratory sessions, Clyde is encouraged to join a supportive men's group that the occupational therapist runs. The group consists of seven men (including the therapist) aged between 22 and 37. They use the opportunity to explore issues concerning work, relationships, gender, sexuality, power and racism. During one session, the group specifically helps Clyde by practising a role-play of how Clyde could tackle the racism/promotion issue with his boss.

### Discussion point

Much of this therapeutic intervention is based on 'talk' as opposed to 'activity'. The therapist, in this case, is content to work generically and use counselling and group work as needed. However, the intervention could also be seen as being particularly appropriate for the occupational therapist as the focus is on Clyde's occupations and occupational performance with regard to work. Recent research, for instance by Moll and Cook (1997) with reference to practice in North America, recognises the shift in community mental health practice towards valuing verbal-based groups over task ones. That the interventions are linked to 'doing' that occurs away from treatment sessions makes sense in an era of increasing community work.

## CASE STUDY 3.5 DARREN

- **Problem** – Hyperactivity and poor concentration
- **Activity** – Cooking
- **Grading** – Increase social distractions and demands of the task.

Darren, aged 12, has a history of being overactive. This state impairs both his concentration and his social skills. His behaviour tends to get out of control and this has resulted in him being excluded from school on several occasions. Twice-weekly remedial therapy sessions are implemented, utilising both structured learning activities and cooking.

### Stage 1: Quick cookery tasks

Initially the therapist works at a one-to-one level with Darren, doing quick cookery tasks. For instance, Darren bakes a small cake using a cake mix. He responds positively to these sessions and takes pleasure in consuming the products at the end.

### Stage 2: Longer cookery tasks

Once Darren can contain himself and concentrate on tasks lasting between 15 and 30 minutes, he begins to cook more complicated things. At his request he cooks a cake from 'scratch' and produces an entire lunch of fish fingers and baked beans.

### Stage 3: Group work

Darren agrees to let two other boys join him. Initially he finds having others in the group difficult, and this results in him being aggressive and letting his attention span weaken. As he begins to feel more comfortable, he is given the responsibility of 'being in charge'. He rises to the occasion, responding well to responsibility. The group celebrates their last session by cooking a special lunch for all the children in the unit (no mean feat!).

### Discussion point

Darren's treatment programme shifts from focusing on concentration in the short term to improving social interaction in the longer term. On the surface Darren is simply cooking – doing a nice activity with a tasty end product. However, the structure of the session and the way cooking has been used was varied. From Darren's perspective, the experience of cooking has been as important as the end-product. The skill of the occupational therapist lies in subtly structuring and modifying a given activity to meet therapeutic aims.

## 3.5  CONCLUSION AND REFLECTIONS

This chapter has examined how occupational therapists focus on occupation and use a variety of purposeful activities. Our belief is that the healing power of occupations comes from both their intrinsic value and from the skill with which they are therapeutically applied. In order to use activities effectively we need to appreciate their specific properties and limitations. The therapeutic potential of an occupation or activity only emerges when it is carefully analysed, structured and graded to suit the individuals concerned. It is this process that we need to communicate to both our service users and the wider interprofessional team.

In my experience, our most difficult challenge arises when we try to engage an individual in activity. Here we seek to interest a person and motivate them to be active when their impulse is to do the reverse. This is where we have to discover, and take into account, the special meanings particular occupations and activities have for the person. This is where we subtly use humour and encourage, even push, someone to grow through, and into, their occupations. This is where we need to develop a trusting therapeutic relationship. We then have to keep the individuals engaged, using all our skills and resources to keep their motivation alive as we ratchet up the activity in terms of the pressures it involves, the demands it makes – and the rewards it promises. Herein lies our art. As Creek (1998) puts it:

> *To provide an activity to pass time or to exercise a limb is not very difficult, but to enable an individual to engage in an activity that has purpose and meaning for her or him, and which will assist in the development of performance skills, is the highest art of the occupational therapist.*
>
> Creek, 1998, p. 27

# 4 OCCUPATIONAL THERAPY THEORY AND MODELS

*The challenge to OT is to identify a body of knowledge that reflects its scientific base and philosophical assumptions in order to organise this knowledge in ways that serve clinical practice.*

Williamson

When asked how you would treat a particular client, do you reply that it depends on how you analyse his or her problem, implying that a 'right' analysis will lead inevitably to a 'right' way to treat the person? Unfortunately, things are not so straightforward. Our treatments depend on many factors: the health-care context, team policy, practical constraints and, arguably most significantly, which theoretical perspective is adopted. That theoretical perspective (in the form of theory or model) gives us our 'spectacles' through which we view our patients or clients, their needs and problems and the occupational therapy process. It helps us know what to look for and how to intervene. It also gives us different thera-peutic tools we can used for assessment and treatment (Case example 4.1).

---

### Case example 4.1

**Using two alternative theoretical approaches**

Phil is a 42-year-old man who was made redundant two years ago. He has since remained unemployed. Phil has had several bouts of depression in the past couple of years: on the last occasion he was suicidal and needed to be hospitalised. He often feels that life is not worth living and that he will probably end up like his brother, who died of a drug overdose last year. Phil also has an alcohol problem, which results in periodic drinking binges that last several days. During these he becomes both morose, and unpredictably aggressive. In addition to these problems he has become overweight which worsens his already negative self-image. He used to enjoy physical activity and sports, but now lacks the drive to be active. Phil lives in a small bedsit with his girlfriend and a 1-year-old daughter whom he adores (and who he says is his main reason for living).

**Using a model of human occupation**

If we used the model of human occupation as our spectacles through which to view Phil, his problems would be understood in terms of loss of work role/work habits, which have resulted in volitional problems (reduced sense of competence and lack of valued activities/hobby interests). He is in a vicious cycle as he is not getting any positive feedback (whether internally or externally related to the environment) on his

---

occupational performance. Treatment interventions would be directed towards encouraging Phil to engage more in valued occupations.

### Using a cognitive–behavioural approach

A therapist using a cognitive–behavioural approach would focus on Phil's negative self-concept and how he seems locked in a pattern of negative thinking that results in spiralling destructive behaviours. The functions that alcohol serve might also be examined: for example, Phil may mistakenly feel that alcohol 'helps' him in some way. These different aspects could be explored in one-to-one counselling. A behavioural contract could also be drawn up for him to abstain from drinking during his treatment.

Theories and models give us a way to frame a person's problems and treatment. Case example 4.1 shows how Phil's treatment would change radically depending on which of the two theoretical approaches was adopted. Both approaches offer a positive way forward. Neither offers a comprehensive solution to *all* his problems – i.e. each deals with particular aspects related to its particular interest and focus. (It is often the case that if one or two problems are resolved, the others will unravel in their own way. If Phil can feel positive about one thing, or succeed in one area of his life, he may well be able to marshal his resources to cope with his other problems himself.)

Both this chapter and the next are designed to persuade therapists who eschew 'theory' that it is fundamental to, and even necessary for, effective practice. I will attempt to do this, in this chapter, by first drawing our **theoretical context** in broad brush strokes. Then, in subsequent sections, five of the more widely used **models** in occupational therapy practice* are discussed:

- Model of human occupation
- Canadian model of occupational performance
- Client-centred model of practice
- Adaptive skills model
- Occupational adaptation model.

---

* Side-stepping any debate about whether or not the five 'models' are in fact models at all(!), I have selected these five on pragmatic grounds. They are all models (in the sense that they offer some theory and/or are a guide to practice) that seem to capture the essence of occupational therapy and reflect our practice concerns. Not surprisingly, they overlap at points and contain similar elements. Also, the first four seem to be the main ones used by occupational therapists practising in the UK. Many UK readers will be less familiar with my fifth model – the Occupational Adaptation model. This has emerged in the last decade in the USA and its research/practice base is still developing. I include it here as it seems to have somewhat superseded the Adaptation for Occupation model (Reed, 1984) which is more familiar to British therapists.

In each of these sections, case illustrations demonstrate how the different models can be applied in practice. It is of course impossible to do justice to any of these models in just one chapter, so I strongly recommend that you return to the original source materials to gain a deeper understanding. Chapter 5 will continue the exploration of our use of theory by analysing how psychological theories and approaches are applied in occupational therapy.

## 4.1 THE THEORETICAL CONTEXT

### Why have theory?

Theory, models and frames of reference are our 'mental filing cabinets' (Yerxa, 1987). They help us organise our knowledge and allow us to communicate knowledge and understanding to others. While theory is often used unconsciously or implicitly, the value of applying some theoretical framework explicitly and self-consciously can be seen at a number of levels:

- **A guide to practice** – When we are faced with the daunting task of treating another human being with all his or her complexities, our theoretical framework gives us a place to start and a way of moving forward. Further, we need some theory base to encourage coherent and systematic treatment. Without it we risk 'synthesising a plan for therapy that contains contradictory assumptions and modes of practice' (Briggs *et al*, 1979, p. 2). An example here is the use of reward star charts (behavioural strategy) with a child, while using non-directive play therapy (humanistic strategy) simultaneously.
- **A tool to reflect and be critical about practice** – Different theories often define the problems differently and suggest alternative treatment strategies. Being aware of other theories/perspectives helps us to reflect on and evaluate our work and critique the approaches taken by others.
- **A vehicle to encourage team collaboration** – If we are ignorant of the theoretical biases within the team, our opportunities to blend treatment co-operatively and to communicate effectively are lessened. It follows both that any divisions between the team members may arise because they are subscribing to different theoretical frameworks and that if we want to challenge existing practice we need to understand the positions of others.
- **A way forward for professional development and unity** – A theoretical base provides both a rationale and method for documenting and researching our practice. This is vital, given increasing demands for accountability. 'A well-developed theoretical structure allows the therapist to meet questions from administrators, other professional, families, clients and perhaps most importantly, questions that may arise from oneself as a therapist' (Fidler, 1985, p. 292). Can we even call ourselves professional if we do not have coherent, logical, unifying theoretical frameworks within which to work?

---

*Theory into practice 4.1* _____

**Working definitions of key terms**

- **Paradigm** – Broad philosophical movement and explanatory framework
- **Philosophy** – Our fundamental beliefs, guiding precepts and values
- **Theory** – A system of assumptions and principles devised to analyse, predict or explain behaviour or experience (or other phenomena)
- **Model** – A simplified representation of a phenomenon that can account for certain data/relationships or a synthesised body of knowledge that links theory and practice
- **Approach** – Our orientation or way of putting a chosen theory/model into practice.

Having defined these terms, let me emphasise one point. Ultimately it is the content of these concepts/theories that is important. Rather than getting side-tracked into semantics and trying to define the terms, I would recommend that we acknowledge that they are 'contested concepts' and move on. Once we have a reasonable understanding about what is being expressed by the different ideas and theories, then we can engage in debates about definitions. Perhaps Kortman (1994) had the right idea when he declared, 'a model is an approach, is a theory, is a paradigm'!

---

## Our theoretical framework: defining terms and concepts

Theory, model, frame of reference, approach, philosophy and paradigm – all interact in practice. When amalgamated they can be called our theoretical framework or **frame of reference** (Figure 4.1).

Much confusion and corresponding debate surround definitions of these terms. Pick up any book concerned with occupational therapy theory and the author seems to present another view! We have Reed and Sanderson (1999) and Kielhofner (1992), who both focus on 'models' but disagree as to what the are. For instance, Reed and Sanderson attempt to place all our theory under the banner of models, whereas Kielhofner prefers to link them more specifically with occupational therapy practice. Kielhofner's conceptual practice model parallels what Mosey (1981) describes as a frame of reference (although she is largely referring to theories borrowed from other disciplines and applied to occupational therapy). In this country, Hagedorn (1995) and Mayers (1990), amongst others have entered into the fray with their own definitions. At the risk of muddying the water further, I would like to offer my simplified schema of how some of these concepts, theories and models fit together (see Theory into practice 4.1 for the working definitions I favour). For deeper, more sophisticated explorations I would strongly recommend you return to the references above.

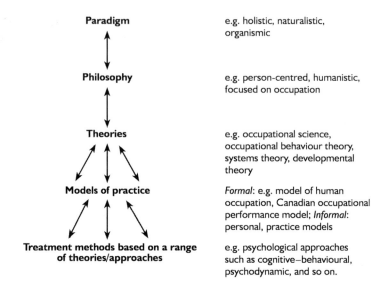

**Figure 4.1**   Theoretical framework

## Paradigm and philosophy

We start with our fundamental professional beliefs and values as arising out of the paradigm and philosophies we favour. Our paradigm is our profession's 'world view' (Creek and Feaver, 1993). In occupational therapy, we embrace a naturalistic, holistic, organismic paradigm. We strive to view humans as total organisms, rejecting the reductionism and positivism implied in mechanistic views of humans as being simply collections of parts (such as a person being represented in terms of their 'diseased limb').

Our philosophical base is essentially humanistic and person-centred. We strive to view individuals holistically, seeing them as active, autonomous, unique beings. Each individual has his/her own value and potential. We also believe in the value of activity and occupation. We believe that the drive to act is a basic human need. Moreover, we believe that an individual's health can be influenced by engaging in occupation, so we exploit this in therapy. (See Section 1.1 for our six core professional values.)

## Theories

Occupational therapy's theoretical base is broad and eclectic. A huge range of theories underpins, informs and guides our practice. Much of our current practice now draws on the ideas and research culled from occupational science theory (see Theory into practice 4.2 and Section 3.2). Also, different occupational therapy models draw on a range of other theories. For instance, the model of human occupation draws on ideas from the work of Mary Reilly, based on occupational behaviour theory and phenomenological philosophy. The adaptive skills model is largely based on psychological developmental and learning theories.

## Models

Our philosophy and different theories then feed into our model/s of practice – be they occupational therapy models or ones culled from other disciplines. These models act as our 'conceptual lenses' (Kielhofner, 1992) through which we can understand a person's function/dysfunction. They also can suggest a structure for clinical reasoning and how we might view the therapy process. Thus, models both generate theory about a phenomenon and can be used to develop tools and techniques for use in practice. At any point in time occupational therapy as a profession will have numerous models to draw upon. No single model is able to address all the multiple dimensions involved in health, occupation and therapy.

In the past decades, much debate has taken place (Creek and Feaver, 1993, Kielhofner, 1992) regarding definitions of our occupational therapy models of practice. Some occupational therapists say they operate with implicit, personal models (see Kortman, 1994). Other writers (e.g. Reed and Sanderson, 1999) distinguish between **conceptual models** (i.e. those that offer a theoretical framework, such as a model of human development) and **practice models** (i.e. those that provide practical guidance, such as a model of occupational therapy practice).

Four of the most widely applied models in practice in the UK are the model of human occupation (Kielhofner, 2002a), the Canadian model of occupational performance (Canadian Association of Occupational Therapists, 1997), the client-centred model of practice (Sumsion, 1999a) and the adaptive skills model (Mosey, 1986). Many other occupational therapy models are used in practice, including the person–environment occupational performance model (Christiansen and Baum, 1997), the occupational adaptation model (Schkade and Schultz, 1992), the cognitive disabilities model (Allen, 1985), Reed's adaptation through occupation model (1984) and Ayres's sensory integration model, to name a few. More recently, the newly evolving lifestyle performance model (Velde and Fidler, 2002) has stirred interest by focusing on how patterns of lifestyle activities can enhance a person's quality of life.

## Treatment methods and approaches

Once we have established our particular focus (using a model as our spectacles), we then implement treatment. Here we can draw on a whole range of other theories, models and approaches. For example, we can apply a psychodynamic approach or implement specific cognitive–behavioural treatment methods. We can even bring in other practice models – for instance Egan's (1986) counselling model of 'the skilled helper'. So the treatment methods we use can be based on other theories, but we draw on them as *therapeutic tools*. This use of psychology theory and approaches will be specifically explored in Chapter 5.

---

*Theory into practice 4.2*—————————————————————————

**Occupational science: the new theory for occupational therapy?**

The field of occupational science has grown out of the work of Larson, Clark, Yerxa and Wilcock amongst others. They see it as a new interdisciplinary 'social science' designed to study humans as occupational beings, the purpose of occupation in survival and health, and how humans realise a sense of meaning through activity. Its main ideas are encapsulated in the following quote :

> *Occupational science will study the person's experience of engagement in occupation recognising that observing behaviour is not sufficient for understanding occupation. The organisation and balance of occupations in daily life and how these relate to adaptation, life satisfaction and social expectations will be central issues as will timing, planning and anticipation. Occupational science will seek to learn more about intrinsic motivation and the drive for effectance. Finally it will need to be true to its humanistic roots by preserving human complexity, diversity and dignity.*

> Yerxa *et al.*, 1990, cited in Hagedorn, 1995, p. 91

Yerxa (1993) identifies certain assumptions underlying occupational science:

- That skills are an essential component of occupation
- That people need to perceive themselves as skilled in order to experience satisfaction in engaging in occupation
- That occupation is engaged in by the 'whole' and complex being.

Wilcock (1998) goes a step further, taking an evolutionary and biological perspective that argues for a three way link between survival, health and occupation.

The field of occupational science has witnessed some heated debate (e.g. in the letters pages of the *American Journal of Occupational Therapy* and *British Journal of Occupational Therapy*). There has been argument between those who feel that it is a distinct science separate from occupational therapy, those who feel it is part of our professional theoretical base and those who see it as an irrelevant discipline (arguing that we already have a comprehensive knowledge base). The fact that many contemporary occupational therapy models now privilege occupation rather than functional skills suggests that the profession is increasingly accepting a role for occupational science.

---

A final point to bear in mind about having the type of theoretical framework I have described is that it is not static. Different occupational therapists employ different versions at different times. While I would say the majority of occupational therapists would subscribe to the philosophy outlined above, everything else is open for negotiation. Some therapists will use a range of occupational therapy models and treatment approaches; others prefer to work within one consistent theoretical framework; for instance, using the model of human occupation or taking a psychodynamic approach or being client-centred.

## 4.2 A MODEL OF HUMAN OCCUPATION

### Key concepts

The model of human occupation (MOHO; Kielhofner, 2002a) emphasises the circumstances – both within the person and in the environment – that contribute to the person's *motivation, patterns of behaviour and occupational performance*. It aims to:

- Understand people's occupational nature and lives
- Guide interventions towards enabling occupational performance
- Offer a range of practical tools and strategies for occupational therapy intervention.

The model offers a broad view of human occupation that attempts to intertwine the self and the world. Here, physical–mental components of individual's performance are holistically integrated and understood in their environmental context (which acts as both an enabler of and a barrier to occupation).

Individuals are conceptualised as being made up of three interrelated *components* – volition, habituation and performance capacity – that occur within the broader (physical, social, cultural) environment.

**Volition** refers to the motivation for occupation and concerns:

- A person's sense of effectiveness and ability
- The importance or worth attached to occupations/activities
- The enjoyment or satisfaction experienced in doing.

(Previously these dimensions were conceptualised as personal causation, values and interests.)

Volition is seen to occur over time as people experience, understand, anticipate and choose their occupations. In concrete terms, this means that if people experience themselves as competent in a particular occupation they will tend to view that occupation positively and, in turn, this will make them want to choose to do it again.

**Habituation** refers to our internalised, automatic and familiar patterns of behaviour. It is guided by our roles and habits set within temporal (i.e. use of time and biological rhythms), physical and social environments. Habituation is responsible for our daily routines – how we go about doing things from getting up in the morning and doing our work to how we interact with others.

**Performance** focuses on our ability and experience of doing. It is approached from the point of view of both our physical and mental capacity and our lived, embodied experience. MOHO stresses that to learn any performance, we need to have the skill *and* to find the experience of it – how it feels. Disability, for instance, is understood in terms of what a person is able to do, as well as their sense of subjective experience of doing. For instance, a person with a paralysed limb may well feel a sense of bodily alienation in that the limb is no longer experienced as fully a part of him or herself. Coming to terms with this alienation is an important task towards regaining functional capacity.

**Environment** – MOHO emphasises the inseparability of environment and occupation, and how much we depend on context for our experience and actions. 'Occupation is, after all, action that occupies a particular social and physical space' (Kielhofner, 2002b, p. 111). The environment is seen to provide the resources for our performance, impacting on what we do and how we do it. Humans are also seen to seek out certain types of environment for the impacts, challenges, stimulations and comfort they offer. When the demands of an environment (from others or the physical space) are experienced as beyond our capacity, we can feel overwhelmed, anxious or hopeless.

Experiences of disability thus relate to the degree a person can cope, and how much support there is, in their physical and social environment. Disability can be prevented – or at least reduced – by offering an environment free from physical barriers and with appropriate emotional and practical support.

## Application in occupational therapy

The model of human occupation has been applied extensively over the last 20 years. First published in 1980 as four articles, it has evolved through the cumulative contributions of many academics and practitioners around the world, through successive versions in 1985, 1995 and 2002. The model can currently boast of over 250 journal articles exploring its research and practice base and numerous influential published assessment tools (Table 4.1). (For further details of these go to the MOHO Clearinghouse website: http://www.uic.edu/ahp/OT/MOHOC/Reference_List/reference_list.html and http://www.uic.edu/ahp/OT/MOHOC/assessments.html.)

In MOHO terms, occupational dysfunction is seen to occur when an individual has difficulty *choosing, organising or performing* his or her occupations. It is also a problem when occupations fail to provide quality of life or is insufficient to meet the demands of the environment. Kielhofner spells this out thus:

*When an individual's life demonstrates such loss, disruption of direction, lack of meaning or purpose that the person is unable to place himself or herself in a personal narrative which has possibilities and hope ... then it may be said that the person is experiencing an occupational dysfunction. Moreover, society has a right to expect its members do their best to care for themselves and make reasonable contributions to the collective. When persons do not use their capacities in a reasonable way ... we can also recognise occupational dysfunction.*

Kielhofner, 1995, p. 183

***Table 4.1*** Assessment tools and the areas they assess based on a model of human occupation (adapted from Kielhofner and Forsyth, 2002, p. 288)

| Assessment tools | Volition | Habituation | Performance | Environment |
|---|---|---|---|---|
| Assessment of Communication and Interaction Skills | | | ✓ | |
| Assessment of Motor and Process Skills | | | ✓ | |
| Assessment of Occupational Functioning | ✓ | ✓ | ✓ | |
| Child Occupational Self Assessment | ✓ | ✓ | ✓ | |
| Interest Checklist | ✓ | | | |
| Model of Human Occupation Screening Tool | ✓ | ✓ | ✓ | ✓ |
| NIH Activity Record | ✓ | ✓ | | |
| Occupational Circumstances Assessment – Interview and Rating Scale | ✓ | ✓ | ✓ | ✓ |
| Occupational Performance History Interview II | ✓ | ✓ | ✓ | ✓ |
| Occupational Questionnaire | ✓ | ✓ | | |
| Occupational Self-Assessment | ✓ | ✓ | ✓ | ✓ |
| Occupational Therapy Psychosocial Assessment of Learning | ✓ | ✓ | | ✓ |
| Pediatric Volitional Questionnaire | ✓ | | | |
| Pediatric Interest Profiles | ✓ | | | |
| Role Checklist | ✓ | ✓ | | |
| School Setting Interview | | | | ✓ |
| Volitional Questionnaire | ✓ | | | ✓ |
| Work Environment Impact Scale | | | ✓ | ✓ |
| Worker Role Interview | ✓ | ✓ | | ✓ |

The model of human occupation emphasises the way people 'craft', and make meaning out of, their occupational lives. Here, we are seen as locating ourselves in an unfolding **occupational narrative**. The stories we tell integrate our past, present and future selves and give meaning to our lives. Kielhofner *et al.* (2002) argue that, as each person lives life, they develop an occupational identity and competence that represents ongoing patterns of doing/feeling/thinking. 'Occupational identity is reflected in the relative success the person has in formulating a vision of life that carries him or her forward. Occupational competence is reflected in each person's relative success in putting that vision into effect.' (Kielhofner *et al.*, 2002, p. 143).

The occupational therapist's role involves attempting to understand how circumstances (mental and physical components within the person and related to the environment) contribute to our occupational lives and any dysfunction. To this end an enormous range of assessment tools and clinical reasoning protocols have been researched and developed (see Table 4.1).

The goal of treatment is to facilitate *change* through engaging the individual in action. For instance, we might enable someone to cope with a loss of a role and develop new occupations by introducing them to a new leisure pursuit. Kielhofner explains that, when therapy is successful it enables people to engage in occupational behaviour that continues their lives in a positive direction: 'The crux of all therapy is to get the patient to do something anew ... the onset of action begins the process of change' (Kielhofner, 1995, p. 256). This process of change is complex and involves a dynamic interaction. For instance, if a person develops their work skills (performance capacity), that person's knowledge of his or her capacity is increased and confidence rises (volition). The person could then opt to change his or her occupational choices (volition), which results in new roles and work patterns (habituation). As the individual engages in the new work performance, skills increase (performance capacity) and others around might comment positively (environment), which in turn encourages the person to take more risks (volition).

## Evaluation

The model of human occupation has many strengths. It offers a sophisticated theoretical and holistic approach to understanding occupational performance and the nature of occupational identity. It also is underpinned, tested and validated by an extensive research and practice base. Being relatively easy to apply practically (through using simple and relevant assessment tools), the model has many converts who appreciate its use as a generic occupational therapy model suited to practice in many areas. Therapists seem to value it as a framework or checklist towards understanding occupational experience. A particular strength of the model is its in-depth exploration of the nature of occupational narratives and the role of volition in initiating occupations. That MOHO has been elaborated and refined over time ensures that it has kept up to date with current professional thinking and concerns.

This model is the most well developed occupational therapy model, with a substantial and evolving research base. The research has occurred at three levels:

- Theoretical arguments have been validated or developed (as seen in the successive revisions)
- Numerous published assessment tools have been developed (Table 4.1)
- Many clinical application studies have been described (see the selection of 80 research abstracts in Kielhofner, 2002a, pp. 536–545).

One of the main criticisms levelled at the model in the past was that its 'jargon' and dense abstract ideas were too difficult to follow. Also, some of its conceptualisations were challenged as being problematic, insufficiently developed or overly focused on the individual. The 1995 and 2002 revisions to the model have answered many, if not all, of these criticisms. The new emphasis on disability studies and occupational narratives (rather than on more mechanical, distant accounts of 'interacting sub-subsystems') have been positively received. Kielhofner and others have worked hard to emphasise the role of the environment and social/cultural meanings to balance the accent on the individual. The 2002 version, particularly, has drawn on many international contributions, offering greater breadth of cross-cultural and clinical understandings.

The 2002 version of MOHO is both simpler and more complex. It is simpler as it uses a lot less jargon and the concepts emphasised, such as client-centred occupational narratives, are already widely accepted within our professional discourse. The model is more complex as it is more explicitly underpinned by a sophisticated philosophy (in particular, phenomenological understandings of embodied, lived experience). The aim to provide a fully integrated account of our mind–body experience of occupations within a broader environment is ambitious and adds to the complexity. Practitioners learning MOHO may find it difficult to appreciate and integrate the different dimensions. Accordingly, Kielhofner suggests that learning MOHO needs to be an ongoing process in which we need to work actively and continually with the concepts in reflection, practice and discussion.

## CASE STUDY 4.1    USING A MODEL OF HUMAN OCCUPATION

- **Problem focus** – Anxiety and limited meaningful occupations to structure each day.

Jack, a 40-year-old man with a mild learning disability, is referred to an outpatient psychiatric service as he is having 'fits'/seizures, which appeared to be anxiety-related. The problem has become particularly severe over the last year, during which he has regularly suffered severe shaking and has passed out unconscious. He has been hospitalised on several occasions but no organic cause has been found.

Jack has a wife and three teenage daughters. He used to work in a tannery as a general dogsbody – a job that he enjoyed and that gave him a sense of purpose. He became unemployed two years ago. He is now highly anxious about his fits and this results in him sitting in a chair all day long, doing nothing except waiting for the next fit to occur. For this reason, the psychiatrist refers Jack to the occupational therapist.

### Occupational therapy assessment

On the basis of her impressions on interview and from findings using the Occupational Questionnaire, the occupational therapist gives the following verbal report:

*Jack is a shy, warm, responsive man who is slightly slow in his understanding. He is overweight, unhealthy in appearance, rather sweaty and clearly anxious. Emotionally he is confused about everything: the interviews, investigations, hospitals, his fits and what is happening to his life. He dimly understands the fact that he has been referred to a psychiatric unit but finds it hard to understand that his fits are an emotional problem.*

*He describes his typical day as 'doing nothing'. He has little in his life – no interests, little family involvement, no work – just a fear of when his next fit will occur when he will be required to go into hospital again. Jack's wife seems supportive in that she takes care of his basic self-care needs (keeping his house, feeding him, doing his laundry). His daughters tend to ignore him. Overall he appears to function at home like a lodger.*

Applying the model of human occupation, the therapist makes the following formulation:

- **Volition** – Poor level of: interests, meaning in life, doesn't feel competent; feels out of control (related to his fits and loss of work)
- **Habituation** – No productive roles or routines; sick role and passive habits adopted
- **Performance –** Low level of skill in all areas; some process skills problems related to using knowledge and transfer of learning
- **Environment** – Wife seems supportive; hospital services now activated that are probably going to be positive, although care needs to be taken not to reinforce a sick role.

## Treatment plan

The occupational therapist invites Jack to attend the occupational therapy department as an outpatient four mornings a week. This daily attendance aims to provide Jack with a structured, meaningful and active day in an effort to break the vicious cycle of his anxiety and inactivity. The daily contact also allows the therapist to assess Jack's potential further.

Jack completes a Modified Activity Checklist and an Interest Checklist self-rating scale in discussion with the therapist. On the basis of the information revealed, Jack and the therapist plan an activity programme that includes a pottery session (with the focus on improving performance skills) and a sports group (including football and swimming at the local swimming pool).

| Problem area/treatment aims | Treatment method |
| --- | --- |
| **Short term**<br>*Habituation*: Break passive habits/routines<br>*Volition*: Re-activate meaningful activities and interests | *Environment* = day patient attendance for four mornings a week to give a meaningful structure to day<br>*Treatment activities*   a) Pottery group<br>     b) Sports group<br>     c) Newspaper group |
| **Middle term**<br>*Volition*: Develop sense of competence, control and confidence in skills<br>*Habituation/performance*: Increase task performance skills and social interaction | *Therapist approach* = allow more autonomy and decision making. Give feedback (positive and constructively critical)<br>*Activity*   a) daily activity programme and gradually encourage the use of community facilities (such as local swimming baths)<br>     b) Cooking classes |
| **Long term**<br>*Habituation:* Develop new productive roles (home work and reduce sick role)<br>Introduce new community-oriented habits<br>Resettlement to day centre for continued daily structure/stimulation | *Therapist approach* = reduce dependence giving less support and expecting more from him<br>*Activity* = cooking classes with 'homework'<br>*Environment* = more community activities and graded settlement to day centre |

## Progress/evaluation

Jack attends the department conscientiously each morning and appears to value his activity sessions. He particularly enjoys the pottery as he is learning new skills and he can give his end-products to his family. It is also an activity he will be able to continue long-term at a day centre. He also values the swimming session as he has always wanted to learn to swim. After a few weeks of being accompanied Jack begins to go to the pool independently and/or with his family. The activity of cooking is introduced at a later stage at Jack's request. He learns how to make three simple, tasty meals. He pleasantly surprises his family, who gives him much praise and encouragement. He takes on the role of cooking the dinner for his family once a week.

Over the course of six months Jack's condition improves considerably. He no longer has any fits – and importantly, when a fit occurs, he does not let it overtake his life. He no longer fears having a fit and feels, even if he had one, he would be all right. In terms of his daily life roles, his situation has been dramatically altered through his occupational therapy programme. By the end of his treatment he has a much more active and satisfying life. His family relationships improve as he begins to contribute to home life.

The one significant problem that occurred during his treatment was his reluctance to leave occupational therapy. The therapists recognised their error in encouraging too much dependence on their programme. Extra effort needed to be put into reducing his time and grading a discharge to the day centre.

---

## CASE STUDY 4.2 — USING A MODEL OF HUMAN OCCUPATION

- **Problem focus** – Occupational narrative: volition and replacing lost roles.

Edna, 63 years old, was admitted to hospital with depression. It was triggered in part by the death of her husband, Vincent, last year. She felt she no longer had any meaning in her life. In hospital she was not motivated to engage in treatment as she felt that nothing could change. However, the environment was supportive and she began to respond positively to the social contact around the ward.

### Occupational therapy assessment

During the interview (using OPHI) Edna told the following story:

She was born 63 years ago, the youngest child in a family of six children. Although they were poor, she had a happy childhood. Throughout her childhood she had one dream – to be a professional dancer. She loved dancing and with much determination she put in many hours of gruelling exercises and lessons in order to achieve her aim. When she was 17, she went to train in London and eventually joined a company. She was utterly committed to her profession and she remembers it as a very special time.

She gave up her dancing career to marry Vincent when she was 27 years old. Although she missed her dancing life dreadfully she felt she had to give it up in order to be a 'proper wife'. She maintained her routines of exercising and dancing for several hours each day, but this became something she did only for her own pleasure. Vincent and Edna had a full life together. They worked together managing their pet shop business. Socially, they were active theatre-goers and played bridge and golf with friends. They had one son, Martin, whom they both adored.

Edna's middle years were basically happy and productive with the exception of two difficult periods of depression that occurred after the death of her mother and when Martin left home to go to university.

Then, 15 years ago, Vincent suffered two severe strokes. He was left partially paralysed down his right side, with speech and perceptual problems and an unsteady, wide-based gait. They sold their business, took early retirement and Edna devoted herself full-time to caring for her husband. Their leisure activities of golf and bridge playing were curtailed as Edna felt it was unfair to her husband for her to carry on doing these activities without him.

Over the years Vincent deteriorated in his functioning and Edna worked harder to care for him. She began to feel guilty/anxious every time she left him as Vincent played up in order to keep Edna by his side. Sometimes she arrived home from shopping or being with her friends to find Vincent balanced precariously on ladders or using dangerous power tools. Edna became more tired because of the demands of caring for her husband and within a few years stopped having any sort of social life. Although she walked their dog daily, she was often too tired to carry out her dance exercises. She was stressed and exhausted but she was unable to attend to her own needs.

Edna was devastated when Vincent died. Not only had she lost her husband of 36 years, she had lost her main 'work' role. She also could not let go of a deep feeling of guilt that somehow she had failed him as his carer.

Edna felt unable to cope alone and moved into a small granny flat attached to her son Martin's house. She became increasingly dependent on him and the practical and emotional support he offered. When he had to go away on a month long business trip, Edna was unable to cope and, 11 months after Vincent's death, she was admitted to hospital with a severe depression. She felt she was a burden on her son and no longer wished to go on living.

## Treatment Plan

| Problem area/treatment aims | Treatment method |
|---|---|
| **Short term** | |
| *Habituation:* break passive habits/routines and activate new roles | *Environment* = OT department as outpatient |
| *Volition:* develop self awareness and knowledge of her competence and capacity | *Treatment activities*  a) 1:1 supportive counselling<br>b) Movement to music class<br>c) Photography group<br>d) Creative group |
| **Middle term** | *Goal setting in the community* |
| *Volition:* develop sense of efficacy/control over self and outcomes | a) At least 1 hour exercise dance each day |
| *Habituation:* increase social contacts | b) One productive outing daily e.g. theatre, trip out, evening dance class, golf lessons, walk into town<br>c) Reactivate one social contact each week |

**Long term**

| | |
|---|---|
| *Habituation*: develop new productive work and leisure roles | a) 1:1 counselling tailed off |
| | b) Co-lead beginner's dance evening class |
| | c) Rejoin golf course |

## Progress/Evaluation

The focus of treatment was helping Edna to craft (reconstruct) a *new* story for herself (occupational narrative): not as a dancer, not as a 'proper wife', not even as a 'carer' but as an active person with lots of friends and hobbies. The climax of the treatment came in one session where she insisted she had nothing to give. The therapist suggested she work out what she had to give as a homework task. Edna came back the following session saying she could teach a beginner's dance class. She eventually achieved this. At the end of treatment she was able to reclaim enough of her previous self to construct a new future life story.

# 4.3  CANADIAN MODEL OF OCCUPATIONAL PERFORMANCE

## Key concepts

The Canadian Model of Occupational Performance (CMOP) was initially developed in the 1980s and then revised in 1997 (Canadian Association of Occupational Therapists, 1991, 1997). Both versions are discussed here as both are in use in current practice.

The *original model* developed in tandem with ideas about client-centred practice. Here the interdependent, collaborative relationship between client and therapist is stressed. Client-centred therapists attempt to view their clients holistically. They strive to value clients' individuality, respect their autonomy and allow them to make their own decisions (Law *et al.*, 1995). Drawing on Reed's Adaptation Through Occupation Model, the Model of Occupational Performance (as it was then called) depicted three concentric circles containing factors that are seen to influence occupational performance. The inner circle represents the **individual** (with associated physical, mental, sociocultural and spiritual performance components that make the individual unique). The second circle comprises a person's **occupations** (productivity, leisure, self-care). The third circle represents the physical, cultural and social **environments** in which the person engages their occupational performance.

The 1997 version (now called the Canadian Model of Occupational Performance) has retained its **client-centred** approach to practice while developing a number of new concepts. The model emphasises the interactive nature of **person–**

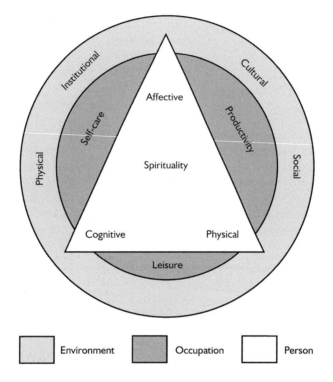

**Figure 4.2**   Interaction of person–occupation–environment (Canadian Association of Occupational Therapists, 1997). Reproduced with the permission of CAOT Publications ACE.

occupation–environment,* placing the person within their environment rather than the environment outside the person (Figure 4.2).

- The person is now represented as a central triangle with affective, cognitive and physical components at each corner and spirituality at the core. The new central position for spirituality (defined broadly as experience of personal meaning, spirit, hope, dignity and worth) emphasises the importance of this dimension. As Sumsion (1999a, p. 10) notes: 'Therapists should be concerned about the inner strength that allows clients to keep functioning in the face of great challenges and adversity'.
- Occupation, comprising productivity, leisure and self-care, is retained as the middle circle but its component concepts have been developed: Productivity covers the occupations that make a social or economic contribution or that

---

* The Person–Environment–Occupation Model builds on the concepts presented in CMOP. Three components, conceptualised as three overlapping circles, are: the individual's skills, environmental supports and barriers, and occupational demands. Optimum occupational performance occurs when these three components overlap or fit well.

provide for economic sustenance. Leisure is now seen as the occupations engaged in for enjoyment. Self-care comprises all the activities a person does to look after themselves and carry out personal responsibilities.

- The environment circle retains its recognition of the impact of physical, social and cultural environments while adding a fourth – the institutional environment (i.e. comprising legal, political and economic aspects).

## Application in occupational therapy

The application of the model of occupational performance is best seen in the practical use of the Canadian Occupational Performance Measure (COPM) – an assessment that acts as a clinical measure of the client's self-perception of occupational performance. The COPM is a client-centred semi-structured interview and self-rating assessment whereby the client identifies significant issues in daily activities that are causing difficulty. Clients consider their full range of daily activities (self-care, productivity and leisure) and rate their *importance*, their perception of their *performance* and their *level of satisfaction* (on a scale of 1–10). After the occupational therapy intervention, the assessment is repeated. The process allows client and therapist to have a numeric indication of changes perceived by the client. Research carried out on applications of the model and COPM is steadily accumulating (e.g. Cresswell, 1997; Bodium, 1999).

Sumsion (1999a) suggests that the Canadian Model of Occupational Performance can also be used alongside other models and approaches. The use of a cognitive approach, for instance, where the focus is on memory, attention, emotions and problem-solving ability, fits in with the performance components of CMOP. As another example, the compensatory focus of the rehabilitative approach which focuses on environmental adaptations is consistent with detailed information about environments offered by CMOP.

## Evaluation

The strength of this model is its client-centred approach and clearly articulated focus on occupation and occupational performance. As such, it is well in tune with our professional philosophy and describes both the therapy process and our unique occupational therapy focus. The revisions to the model have highlighted some key dimensions such as spirituality and the relevance of the institutional environment to occupational performance.

The COPM assessment has generated much interest in the UK (helped by having been piloted beyond Canadian borders in the UK, New Zealand and Greece). The assessment is relatively straightforward to apply. It has the additional benefit that it can be used to explain occupational therapy to both clients and team members. Useful validating research on the application of the model and the COPM assessment has been conducted (Law *et al.*, 1994; Toomey *et al.*, 1995; Waters, 1995; Chesworth *et al.*, 2002).

However, various criticisms have been levelled at the model. Some critics argue that the theoretical rational underlying the model needs to be developed further. While the concept of client-centred practice has been well described, the interaction of different elements of the model could do with deeper exploration (rather than simply asserting concepts and their relationship). Other practitioners critique the limited focus of the model. For example, COPM is more useful for clients with practical rather than emotional problems. With the emphasis so strongly on occupation, important psychodynamic and interactive aspects may tend to get overlooked.

## CASE STUDY 4.3   USING THE CANADIAN MODEL OF OCCUPATIONAL PERFORMANCE

- **Problem focus** – Resettlement in the community, emphasis on productivity.

Sharon, aged 29, has a long history of abusing drugs (e.g. heroin and crack cocaine), self-mutilation and crime (theft, shoplifting, making fraudulent social security claims). She has had several relationships with men who have abused her physically and has often lived rough (the first time when she ran away from home). She has spent the last two years being treated in a secure unit and is now preparing for discharge feeling motivated to begin a different life. The team have been closely involved with helping Sharon come off drugs and manage her 'out of control' feelings and behaviour. The team decided it was now time for a heavier occupational therapy input looking towards Sharon's reintegration into the community. As this was a new stage of treatment, it was decided that a new therapist should be involved who could relate to Sharon as she was now (as opposed to someone who had shared her negative history).

### Occupational therapy assessment

Over the course of several sessions the occupational therapist observed that Sharon presented inconsistently. At times she was full of bravado, saying things like 'I can't wait to get out of here away from all you screws' or 'I don't need your help, I can look after myself'. At other times she seemed young and vulnerable, uncertain of how she was going to manage and scared she would return to her past life. As she once recognised, 'I only know how to be my 'past-me'. I don't know the 'future me'. She's a stranger and she scares me.'

In order to enable Sharon take control of her own life the therapist decided to use the COPM (gaining a shared view of problems/strengths and values/interests regarding future performance). In terms of **self care**, Sharon described being unsure about how to make decisions and structure her day. She admitted to not taking care of her body before, but now she was trying to eat healthily and look after her appearance. In terms of **productivity**, Sharon's dream was to have a 'proper job' but she knew this was not going to happen easily as she had never worked before. Sharon thought her aunt might give her some work at her seaside cafe, which would supplement her social security benefit money. In terms of **leisure**, Sharon described having few hobbies outside her social life with her friends in the drug culture. In fact, without the drug connection, she found social contact difficult and rather meaningless. She enjoyed the solitary pursuits of watching videos and listening to music and she expressed an interest in learning to use the computer and play computer games.

## Treatment planning

| Aims/outcomes | Treatment method |
|---|---|
| **Short term** | |
| *Leisure:* To explore her interest in computer games and develop both skills and confidence in this area. *Productivity:* To practise a range of domestic activities towards independent living | Daily practice on the computer in the OT department Accompanied shopping in town; plus cooking, budgeting, laundry, DIY sessions in the unit |
| **Long term** | |
| *Productivity:* To investigate the possibility of computer classes To investigate what computer games were available on the market and recommend three for the unit to buy To approach Aunt Jean about the possibility of living and working with her | Goals negotiated and written down during a weekly one to one session |

## Progress /Evaluation

Sharon's rehabilitation took place over several months. Although she slipped back a number of times, she made good progress. She learned that she functioned best when busy and acknowledged the value of structuring her time. She quickly gained skill and confidence with computer work and took on the role of teaching others (including the occupational therapist!). She was also successful in researching and buying some new computer games for the unit. Sharon resolved to get a job and save up to buy her own computer.

On the **domestic** side, Sharon was not motivated to carry out any of the ordinary domestic rehabilitation activities. In these sessions she proved difficult and tended to be destructive, stirring up trouble with other group members. The occupational therapist recognised that she might have imposed her own values on Sharon. On review, the domestic programme was cancelled, although Sharon expressed an interest in learning how to cook Chinese food with a wok. This she did once a week in a one-to-one lunch cookery session with the occupational therapist that included shopping for the ingredients.

When Sharon eventually got the courage to contact her aunt, she was offered **part-time work** at the cafe on a trial basis. This coincided with her discharge. She decided to move to temporary bed and breakfast accommodation at the seaside town. She agreed that moving to this new area would be quite difficult in that she knew only her aunt. On the other hand it would allow her a chance to start a completely new life – it gave her hope that she might be able to change.

Overall this treatment demonstrated the value of taking a **client-centred** approach where activities were chosen to be meaningful for Sharon. The occupational therapist would have liked her to become more involved with the domestic rehabilitation programme and with more social/group activities. However, the therapist recognised that the spiritual dimension – for Sharon's sense of self worth and motivation – was crucial and that it was important to respond to Sharon's expressed preferences. Had the occupational therapist not done this Sharon might well have disengaged from treatment and not faced the challenge of changing her life.

## 4.4   CLIENT-CENTRED MODEL OF PRACTICE

### Key concepts

First coined by Carl Rogers in the 1930s, the expression 'client-centred' came into the occupational therapy literature in the 1980s through a document published by the Canadian Association of Occupational Therapists (Canadian Association of Occupational Therapists, 1983) entitled *Guidelines for the Client-Centred Practice of Occupational Therapy*. Today, Canadian Association of Occupational Therapists, 1997 characterises client-centred practice as:

- A collaborative and partnership approach between therapist and client
- Therapist demonstrates respect for clients' experience and knowledge
- Client is actively involved in own decision making
- Therapist acts as advocate with, and for, client.

Sumsion (1999a) offers a provisional definition of client-centred practice as it relates to British occupational therapy practice:

> *Client-centred occupational therapy is a partnership between the therapist and client. The client's occupational goals are given priority and are at the centre of assessment and treatment. The therapist listens to and respects the client's standards and adapts the intervention to meet the client's needs. The client actively participates in negotiating goals for intervention and is empowered to make decisions through training and education. The therapist and client work together to address the issues presented by a variety of environments to enable the client to fulfil his/her role expectations.*
>
> Sumsion 1999, p. 5

### Application

Over the last 20 years, client-centred models of practice have been used extensively in practice and they have been the topic of much research. They have also spawned a number of valuable therapeutic tools – notably the Canadian Occupational Performance Measure, among other self-rating tools. Tools such as these enable therapists to maintain a client-centred focus.

A number of authors have described client-centred practice with different client groups, for instance, elderly people and individuals with cognitive impairment (Hobson, 1999), individuals with mental health needs (Kuszir and Scott, 1999) and individuals with physical disabilities (Gage, 1999). Mayers

(2000, 2003) promotes client-focused practice when interviewing people with enduring mental health problems based on her Quality of Life Questionnaire.

The degree to which these therapists are able to apply, rather than simply strive towards, a client-centred model in practice varies. Examples of what adopting a client-centred model actually means in practice include the following:

- With partnership and collaboration in mind, the client-centred therapist 'hands over' **power** and responsibility to the client. For instance, clients identify their own priorities/problems and take responsibility for identifying their own treatment goals. Client-centred therapists aim to enable clients by working with them to achieve goals they have set for themselves.
- Client-centred therapists **respect** the specialness, values and dignity of each individual. They strive to provide individualised assessment and intervention. The use of standardised assessment procedures and set protocols for intervention, for instance, is not consistent with client-centred philosophy.
- Respecting clients' capacity to make their own choices, therapists aim to provide the **opportunity** and enough information to enable this to occur. Therapists need to ensure they use language that is understood by clients while truly listening to, and learning from, clients' experiences.
- When clients choose to act in a way that places them at some risk (e.g. risk of failure), client-centred therapists may need to **accept** and respect that choice (within the bounds of being ethical and taking professional responsibility). Firstly, the clients are regarded as knowing their own needs better than the therapists. Secondly, therapists recognise that taking such risks and coping with the consequences can provide an important learning experience.

The idea of client-centred practice is widely valued in health and social care. Implementing client-centred practice, however, is not without challenges and barriers. Wilkins *et al.* (2001) identify three broad challenges at the levels of the system, the therapist and the client. At the level of the *system*, therapists are constrained by their organisations in terms of the priorities set for them and the time/resources they have at their disposal. At the level of the *therapist*, Wilkins *et al.* suggest that some therapists are confused about what client-centred actually means and some lack the enhanced negotiation and collaboration skills necessary. At the level of the *client*, some clients may not be suitable for, or benefit from, client-centred approaches – particularly clients with cognitive problems, poor insight, depression or language barriers. That the majority of our clients tend not to be cognitively intact nor to have good problem-solving skills is problematic and limits the usefulness of the model.

## Evaluation

Client-centred models of practice are consistent with our holistic, person-centred philosophy. Practising therapists are drawn to such models. Moreover, the literature suggests that the development of client–therapist partnerships can lead to increased client participation, satisfaction and a sense of self-efficacy (Corring and Cook, 1999; Parker, 1999). That client-centred models can also be used in combination with other models demonstrates their utility and flexibility. Case study 4.5 (p. 93), for example, shows the combined use of a client-centred model and the Canadian Model of Occupational Performance. MOHO similarly can be used in conjunction with a client-centred approach providing a theoretical under-pinning, which would otherwise be missing, towards conceptualising a client's situation.

On the negative side, findings such as those by Corring and Cook (1999) and Wilkins *et al.* (2001) mentioned above demonstrate the continuing struggle thera-pists have to translate client-centred ideals into day-to-day practice. Some critics argue that the model is unrealistic and that therapists need to be more critical and to probe the nature of the client–therapist relationship more deeply. For instance, when a therapist directs a client to be involved in his/her own decision making, is this client-centred? What happens when the client prefers to be directed and guided by the therapist? If the therapist 'hands over' power to the client, then is it not the therapist who really has the power? Such questions about who actually has (or should have) power and control make implementing a client-centred model problematic. That the rhetoric of 'client-centred' is sometimes used to justify practice that is anything but client-centred (i.e. the model is abused or misunderstood) adds a further problematic dimension.

Others point to a need to explore further what is meant by 'client-centred' and to match this with how therapists act in practice. Falardeau and Durand (2002), for instance, argue that we should focus on the idea of 'negotiation-centred' rather than client-centred practice, where the emphasis is on collaboration, partnership and interdependence.

## CASE STUDY 4.4   CLIENT-CENTRED MODEL OF PRACTICE

- **Problem** – Lack of skills to cope independently at home.

Jean is an 85-year-old widowed woman who lives alone in a one-bedroomed ground floor flat. After suffering a stroke she was admitted to hospital and then discharged to a residential home. Jean's doctor and the nursing staff were convinced that she would be better off staying in the residential home permanently and that she would be at consid-erable risk if she went home. She was referred to the community occupational therapist for full assessment.

### Occupational therapy assessment

The occupational therapist observes that Jean's capacity for independent living is clearly impaired. She cannot dress, bath or cook for herself without assistance. She walks unsteadily with a frame and her mobility around the flat is compromised by the numerous obstacles (tables, wires, small rugs) that litter every room. She is sometimes incontinent at night. Despite these problems, Jean is insistent that she wants to stay in (and eventually die in) her own special flat – whatever the risk or cost.

### Intervention

Persuaded that Jean is resolute in her wishes, the occupational therapist takes on the role of advocate on Jean's behalf. Together they discuss and work through how to handle each problem in turn. The first step they both agree is to move Jean's bed into the main living room to be nearer the bathroom. It also contains the television and telephone and has the benefits of a nicer view. Jean accepts that she may have to spend most of her days in her night clothes, providing that these can be changed each day if soiled and she is helped to have a bath twice a week. Jean is clear that she can exist on cereal, sandwiches and cups of hot soup or tea. She just requires some daily help for her personal care: to clean her sheets and commode and do her laundry. Both the therapist and Jean recognise that she is at risk of having falls and may not be able to manage on her own in the long term.

The occupational therapist provides several items of equipment, including a commode, an electric bath seat and a kettle tipper, to ease Jean's life. The therapist then organises for Jean to have a daily home care visit (half an hour) and supplies an alarm system linked to the phone that can be activated in case of falls or emergencies. While the therapist remains concerned about Jean's social isolation, Jean insists that her television provides sufficient human contact.

The end result is that Jean has been enabled to stay in her own home. Although her quality of life does not reflect the occupational therapist's or the team's ideas of what she could have in a care home, Jean has her priorities and has made her choices.

---

| CASE STUDY 4.5 | APPLYING THE CLIENT-CENTRED MODEL IN COMBINATION WITH THE CANADIAN MODEL OF OCCUPATIONAL PERFORMANCE |

- **Problem focus** – Antisocial behaviour at school

Rick (a 15-year-old young man with newly diagnosed ADHD) and his mother (who is a single parent) are referred to a child and family unit. He has been excluded from school a number of times in the last three years as a result of his anti-social behaviour (e.g. being disruptive in class, rude to his teachers and not doing his homework). The occupational therapist is invited to investigate the problems Rick is having at school.

### Occupational therapy assessment

On first speaking to the occupational therapist, Rick expresses his anger at the teachers and how much he hates school. He says he does not value his school work and instead enjoys socialising with his friends. His dream for the future is to earn 'plenty of money' so that he can buy 'loads of cool gear' (primarily related to his interest in music and burning CDs).

The occupational therapist then separately interviews Rick, his mother and his main school teacher using COPM and focusing on Rick's school performance. The results shows how all three of them seem to have different priorities and ideas. Rick's priorities lie with enjoying the social aspects of school while his mother and teacher are more work-focused (see the table below, in which performance is rated in terms of importance, performance, satisfaction). All three acknowledge Rick's capacity to be a friend and the fact that his sociability is a great strength. It emerges that much of his rudeness to teachers is Rick's way of gaining status and 'sticking up for' his friends.

| Person | Occupational performance | Importance | Performance | Satisfaction |
|--------|--------------------------|------------|-------------|--------------|
| Rick | Being popular | 8 | 3 | 3 |
| | Supporting friends | 10 | 8 | 8 |
| | Coping with school work | 6 | 5 | 5 |
| Mother | Passing school work | 10 | 4 | 2 |
| | Doing homework | 9 | 3 | 2 |
| | Making friends | 8 | 8 | 8 |
| Teacher | Learning in the classroom | 10 | 3 | 1 |
| | Interacting positively with teachers | 10 | 2 | 1 |
| | Doing homework | 8 | 5 | 4 |

## Intervention

The therapist, acting in the role of Rick's advocate, brings all three people together for a conference to negotiate a compromise. The therapist's main role is to help Rick communicate his priorities and needs. In particular, he strongly expresses a dislike of school and looks forward to the time when he can work (and 'earn lots of money'). His mother expresses some shock and dismay at this, as she has assumed and hoped Rick would go on to college. The therapist directs their attention to the more immediate concern – to find a way for Rick to complete his schooling (just seven months left) without getting expelled.

Eventually, a contract is mutually agreed:

1.  Rick will not have to attend school every day. Some work will be provided for him at home where he will be guided by his mother and a private tutor. (Both Rick and his mother feel that he would concentrate better in his less stimulating/distracting home environment anyway.)
2.  Rick's mother will allow him extra socialising time at weekends if he works well during the week at his school work.
3.  When Rick is required to be in school, he will moderate his behaviour in class and try to work constructively. If he has a problem with a teacher he is to deal with it outside class time.
4.  If Rick manages to get through the next seven months (and his exams) satisfactorily,

he will be allowed to take a year out of school and get a job. (After that point plans would be reviewed.)

**Progress and evaluation**

The programme of limited school attendance worked well. Rick's work at home proved to be relatively successful and his self-esteem improved accordingly. He was generally happier, calmer and more relaxed in his behaviour, which resulted in more positive interactions with his teachers. He managed to complete his seven months and (to everyone's surprise) he passed four of his exams. He happily went to work at a local fast food restaurant. After a month he expressed an interest in trying for a college course.

## 4.5 ADAPTIVE SKILLS MODEL

Mosey's ideas about adaptive skills were first developed in the 1960s and 1970s and later incorporated into her 1986 volume *Psychosocial Components of Occupational Therapy*. While Mosey does not describe a specific model of practice (as this is a term she equates to paradigm), portions of her work can be represented as different models.

In 1974 she proposed the '**biopsychosocial model**' as an alternative to medical and health models. This model recognised that individuals are biological and thinking/feelings beings who are members of a wider social community. The strength of this model lies in its recognition that health is more than an absence of disease. However, its chief limitation is the lack of attention it pays to occupations and activity.

Taking a different direction, Mosey then articulated her 'three frames of reference' (1970, 1986) – analytical, acquisitional and developmental – for the practice of occupational therapy in psychiatry. The **analytical** frame of reference recognises how individuals strive to get their needs (often unconscious) met and is largely located in the psychodynamic tradition. The **acquisitional** frame of reference stems from a cognitive–behavioural tradition and emphasises the acquisition of skills. The **developmental** frame (based on the work of Ayres and other developmental theorists) focuses on how adaptive skills are learned in a sequence.

In common with other developmental theorists, Mosey describes some basic principles, which can be summarised in five points:

- Development is the orderly progression of an individual through a series of complex, interacting stages
- An individual grows and learns in a sequential way – each gain provides the base for the next stage
- Qualitatively different problems and opportunities emerge at each stage – each of which need to be mastered
- Under stress or illness, individuals can regress to previous stages
- Treatment involves identifying the particular functioning level and providing

experiences to facilitate step-by-step learning and adaptation (applied learning).

## Occupational therapy application

Mosey emphasises how occupational therapists are concerned with all aspects of *development* and that we should apply our knowledge of 'normal' expectations to facilitate development in individuals who have developmental aspects that are impaired. She sees this being achieved by applying a *teaching–learning process* that includes:

- Providing success experience that confirms stage learning
- Encouraging safe exploration while practising skills
- Providing opportunities for challenge.

Mosey (1986) outlines six (previously seven) areas of functioning or adaptive skills, which are further divided into subskills. These subskills give us the specific ladder rungs or goals to use in the teaching/learning process.

The six adaptive skills can be summarised as:

- **Sensory integration skill** – the ability to co-ordinate vestibular, proprioceptive and tactile information for functional use
- **Cognitive skill** – the ability to organise sensory information for problem solving
- **Dyadic interaction skill** – the ability to engage in a variety of one-to-one relationships
- **Group interaction skill** – the ability to participate in a variety of groups
- **Self-identity skill** – the ability to perceive self as a relatively autonomous, acceptable person who has continuity over time
- **Sexual identity skill** – the ability to perceive one's sexual nature as good and participate in mutually enjoyable, long-term sexual relationships (Mosey, 1986, p. 416–42).

When treating a patient or client, it is not possible to work on all these areas at once, although a focus on one area usually prompts growth in another. Some occupational therapy units organise their programme offering learning experiences related to one adaptive skill such as group interaction skill (Table 4.2). In such a case, the process involves:

- Identifying a newly referred individual's skills level
- Slotting them in the appropriate level group (one that is both safe and offers challenges)
- Facilitating 'higher' behaviours.

## Evaluation

Mosey's ideas have been applied widely, in different ways, since the 1980s. Her notion of 'adaptive skills' offers us an account of the sequence of development and indicates how to intervene therapeutically (and therefore this can be viewed

**Table 4.2**  Summary of group interaction subskills

| Associated age | Group level | Criterion |
|---|---|---|
| 18 months–2 years | Parallel group level | Able to work alongside others in a group |
| 2–4 years | Project group level | Minimally shares, competes and co-operates with prompting from the therapist |
| 5–7 years | Egocentric-co-operative group level | Co-operative and competitive, experiments with group roles |
| 9–12 years | Co-operative group level | Meets needs of other members and expresses both positive and negative thoughts |
| 15–18 years | Mature group level | Flexibility in taking on various roles within a heterogeneous group |

as a 'practice model'). Her recognition that the environment (human and non-human) powerfully structures behaviour has continued to have a significant place in occupational therapy theory.

Different aspects of Mosey's work have been criticised. At a general level, given the profession's current focus on occupation, her ideas can be critiqued for being dated – too-skills focused and insufficiently client-centred and concerned about occupational performance.

In a specific critique of Mosey's hierarchy of group interaction skills, Donohue (1999) points out some gaps in its assumptions and theory. She argues, for instance, that most people function at two levels of interaction (e.g. adults frequently operate at both co-operative and mature levels depending on the type of group). She also highlights the relationship between the nature of activity and level of function. Here, individuals may well operate at a parallel level when activities are structured that way, such as when people watch a movie. The same individuals may then be able to cooperage when playing a team sport. Such ideas have important implications for the way we structure activities in occupational therapy and warrant further investigation.

## CASE STUDY 4.6   APPLYING THE ADAPTIVE SKILLS MODEL

- **Problem focus** – Process of teaching and learning group interaction skills

Willis, aged 30, was an inpatient in a psychiatric hospital with a diagnosis of schizophrenia. His disorder resulted in him being withdrawn and self-absorbed, and he occasionally made bizarre comments, which affected his ability to relate to others.

### Occupational therapy assessment

The occupational therapist assessed Willis's task performance and group interaction skills during a cooking group and in other task activities. The therapist observed that Willis seemed unaware of other people's needs and appeared to find it difficult to share (for instance, he took over the cooker area and only moved out of others' way when prompted). He only interacted with the therapist when a direct question was asked, otherwise he remained withdrawn. The occupational therapist considered that he was functioning developmentally at a low project group level.

### Treatment plan

Willis's difficulty in group interaction prompted a referral to the Project Group. The Project Group was a group that was already established and consisted of seven other patients functioning at or marginally below project group interaction level. The group met daily for an hour to engage in a mixture of activities. The treatment programme described below shows how the art activity of using collage was graded and adapted.

### Progress/evaluation

**Stage 1: Early-level project group experience:** Willis was introduced to the group and joined their activity, which took place around one table. Each patient was asked to make an individual collage by cutting out pictures of food from magazines and sticking them on to a sheet of paper. At the end the occupational therapist encouraged the group members to be aware of each other and work together more by asking them to arrange each individual's sheet with the others on a larger poster. Willis found the latter task of working with the whole group more difficult, so he remained relatively passive.

**Stage 2: Medium-level project group experience:** After a few sessions similar to the above, the occupational therapist encouraged Willis and the others to make a collage in pairs, requiring them to minimally share and interact with at least one other person. Willis enjoyed this, and was also able to work a bit with the group as a whole, as they discussed how to arrange the pictures.

**Stage 3: Advanced-level project group experience:** On a later occasion the occupational therapist encouraged the group to make a collage as a whole. Individuals first collected their own pile of 'rubbish', such as leaves or empty matchboxes. These were then placed all together in a pile. The group then stuck the bits randomly on to a large card. Willis was given the responsibility at the end to spray the collage an attractive gold colour. At this level of group working the therapist attempted to further group sharing and awareness of others by promoting discussion and also by reducing the quantity of glue and number of pairs of scissors available.

## 4.6   OCCUPATIONAL ADAPTATION MODEL

### Key concepts

The occupational adaptation model (Schkade and Schultz, 1992; Schultz and Schkade, 1992) focuses on how occupation and adaptation become integrated within a person. Occupational adaptation is the process through which the 'person and the occupational environment interact when the person is faced with an occupational challenge that calls for an occupational response reflecting an experience of relative mastery' (Schkade and Schultz, 1992, p. 831). It is seen as both a state of function and the process through which competence in occupational functioning develops. Its theoretical foundations draw on the work of Reed's adaptation through occupation model, a MOHO and general systems theory, among other theories.

The model defines several key concepts and assumptions:

- The satisfying performance of occupational roles is seen to be a vital component of successful occupational functioning throughout the lifespan.
- The person is seen to be made up of sensorimotor, cognitive and psychosocial systems (and underlying subsystems).
- Occupational environments are viewed as the contexts in which occupations (work, leisure, self-maintenance) occur and which demand occupational performance (of life roles).
- As the environment and persons interact, both demand a level of occupational mastery and role expectations.
- Occupations are activities characterised by active participation, meaning and output/product.

## Application in occupational therapy

The model guides therapists to view a person holistically in terms of their functioning within the environment. A close, collaborative therapist–client relationship is seen as being important. The model is client-centred in that the person is seen as the agent of their own change and the primary evaluator of the effectiveness of any intervention. The therapist's role is to provide the opportunity and the challenges in the environment that will demand an adaptive response. In a specific *Guide to Practice* (Schultz and Schkade, 1992), key questions that the therapist needs to answer when preparing an intervention are offered for assessment, programming and evaluation of occupational adaptation.

The aim and expected outcome of therapy is competency and mastery in occupational functioning (i.e. occupational adaptation rather than functional independence), concentrating on both the client's condition and the environment. This is measured in terms of the individual's perceptions of the degree to which they can self-initiate activities, their relative mastery in performing necessary roles and how spontaneously skills are transferred to novel situations. Treatment is directed to improving the person's internal ability to generate, evaluate and integrate adaptive responses where a sense of relative mastery is experienced. Treatment activities/techniques focus on occupational activity that promotes satisfaction.

The model holds that problems in mental health affect an individual's ability to tackle problems and that their occupational functioning is hindered by both internal and environmental constraints. This eventually results in an adaptive, but unhelpful, response of not engaging in occupations. Intervention therefore focuses on developing meaningful and satisfying occupational adaptation through the experience of doing. The activities offered must be personally meaningful to the individual and relevant to their occupational roles.

## Evaluation

The strength of this model is its generic and holistic focus on occupational demands/responses, activity and the therapeutic relationship, which nicely reflects occupational therapy concerns and values. While many theories/models explore the importance of occupation and adaptation, this one recognises their complex interaction. Further, it offers detailed operational definitions of key concepts and useful questions to guide practice.

The model is still being developed so lacks the associated tools and the extensive research and practice base enjoyed by the other models. Initial responses to the model suggest that it looks promising, although some people might find the language and abstract concepts difficult to understand and apply in practice.

---

| CASE STUDY 4.7 | APPLYING THE OCCUPATIONAL ADAPTATION MODEL |
| --- | --- |

- **Problem focus** – Unrealistic occupational role expectations; dysfunctional occupational adaptation

Bill, aged 78, is an ex-army Major. After the war, he became a property developer, specialising in large-scale developments (e.g. old manor houses). Bill retired 10 years ago, intending to travel with his wife, but this proved impossible when she developed dementia. Bill eventually took on a full-time carer role as his wife became dependent on him for all aspects of her activities of daily living. Lately Bill has become exhausted and stressed with his caring role and has developed angina. He has been referred to a community occupational therapist for advice on conserving his resources and managing his stress.

### Occupational therapy assessment

Bill presents as a 'gentleman' who is very concerned and anxious about his wife. He tends to do everything for her – both personal care and taking over all domestic responsibilities – and he constantly worries whether he is doing things correctly. The interview reveals that he has taken these roles so much to heart that he no longer has any time for himself. When an activities of daily living assessment is carried out on his wife, it emerges that she is more able than Bill imagines.

The occupational therapist poses the following questions and then seeks to answer them:

1. **What are Bill's occupational environment and roles that are of most concern?** Bill feels pressured by his desire to help and his wife's actual physical needs.

His caring role, however, takes up all of his time/energy, depleting his own resources. His occupational adaptation is poor and he has problems in his psychosocial functioning since he has stopped engaging in leisure and self-care activities.

2.  **What are Bill's performance and role expectations?** Bill needs to be able to care for his wife but his ability to do so suffers if he does not care for himself. He also expects himself to carry out daily living tasks to a very high standard (for instance, cooking elaborate meals and bleaching all surfaces every day).

3.  **What is Bill's level of relative mastery and what enables/limits these?** Bill's belief that he needs to do everything for his wife means that he is over-involved in her care. Although he gains some satisfaction from being caring it is also stressful and this is creating further problems. His own occupational adaptation is deteriorating as he has disengaged from other leisure/self-care pursuits. That he tries to do everything to the highest standard is unrealistic in terms of day-to-day functioning and creates pressures.

4.  **What occupational activity is necessary to promote adaptation?**

    - With advice and opportunities to practise, he needs to learn to manage his wife's daily care better (namely allowing her to do more for herself and feeling satisfied when this happens).
    - With practice and feedback, he needs to learn to prioritise and accept less than perfect performance in domestic activities.
    - With extra nursing care and support, Bill should be able to engage in more leisure/self-care activities (e.g. re-engaging with old hobbies and meeting up with friends).

The therapist and Bill agree that Bill needs to reduce the pressures on himself by modifying his role expectations for himself. He also needs to be encouraged to engage in more satisfying leisure/self-care activities. To help him achieve this, extra nursing and domestic support needs to be arranged for his wife.

### Progress/evaluation

Initially Bill is reluctant to ease off on his domestic/caring roles as he is anxious about how his wife will manage. With the help of the occupational therapist he begins to see the link between his angina, stress and lack of balance in occupations. He eventually sees the logic of bringing in some outside domestic and nursing help. The occupational therapist also advises him on how to manage his wife's activities of daily living. Bill learns to stand back a bit more, although this is difficult for him and he often lapses into doing things for his wife. Slowly Bill learns to feel more satisfied when she does things for herself. He also learns that he can afford to be more easy-going about some domestic chores and not feel pressured to do everything to the highest standards all the time (e.g. buying in convenience meals is acceptable, he doesn't need to cook a whole roast three times a week).

Bill is encouraged to take up some old hobbies and meet up with some friends at a club. With the therapist's prompting, he makes it a goal to take one trip abroad each year without his wife. On the day of his discharge, Bill proudly shows the therapist a return air ticket for a holiday in Cyprus that he has just bought for himself.

## 4.7 CONCLUSION AND REFLECTIONS

The models and theory explored in this chapter give us our unique occupational therapy 'gaze'. The chapter has shown how models can act as our spectacles through which we view both the client and the treatment process. While the models differ slightly in how they conceptualise function/dysfunction, it is no accident that the models share a preoccupation with occupation, activity, adaptation, performance skills and life roles. Without such a unified theoretical base, we cannot call ourselves a profession.

I hope I have shown how important theories/models can be in that they help us to define problems and give us tools to use in practice. They can also form the basis of working collaboratively with others, where the specific occupational therapy identity and contribution is clarified.

Personally speaking, I love theory and find the evolution of different occupational therapy models fascinating. While I appreciate that others may not share my enthusiasm, I feel concerned when I hear therapists assert that they don't use or need theory and models. More probably, these therapists are using versions of theory – they are just unaware of what these might be. This seems to me to be a recipe for confused and potentially contradictory practice.

I have tried to remain impartial in my judgements about which model is 'the best'. All the models have strengths and limitations – something that even the authors of the models would accept. I would argue that all occupational therapists should spend time thinking about and trying to use the different models *in practice* in order to better appreciate both their values and their problems when it comes to applying them. In my view it is important to remain both open to, and critical about, *all* our theories and models. Sometimes we can be too quick to reject models unthinkingly, effectively throwing out their potential and strengths with the criticisms. At other times, we may be inclined to embrace models unquestioningly when being more aware of their limitations would help us to avoid those traps.

I am hesitant that having focused on these particular models in some way gives them the status of 'tablets of stone'. This is not my intention, as models come and go – as we have seen when they are revised and/or replaced by other newer models that suit the current climate better. These five simply reflect our professional development, preoccupations and practice at the moment. In principle, I believe it is a healthy sign that our profession can draw on several models, i.e. that we can select whichever appears to be most appropriate at any one time or offers the most relevant therapeutic tools. As Creek puts it, 'Occupational therapy is a dynamic profession in a rapidly changing world; therefore it does not have a fixed, universally agreed model' (Creek, 1997, p. 43). I would go further and say that if we are to remain a dynamic profession, our models must develop, evolve and change, and what is more, we must be ready to change with them.

# 5 PSYCHOLOGICAL THEORIES AND APPROACHES

*To practise without theory is to sail in an uncharted sea; theory without practice is not to sail at all.*

Susser

The previous chapter made the point that theories act rather like spectacles through which we can view the world. The same sort of process applies when we select from different psychological theories. The psychological theory we choose will determine what we focus on, and so how we understand an individual's behaviour/experience. This, in turn, will influence how we view an individual's problems and it will set the template for offering particular problem-solving interventions rather than others.

Take, for example, Betty's problem. She has agoraphobia (fear of going outside). For Betty, the problem has now become so severe that she is unable to function in her daily life. Just stepping outside her front door precipitates a panic attack in her. How does such a crippling disorder come about? What can be done to help her? Here is where different theories come in.

Betty's treatment depends entirely on which theoretical approach is taken by her therapist. For instance, a cognitive–behavioural approach would see her problem in terms of a 'habit' of negative thinking and avoidance behaviour, which becomes exacerbated as she enters an 'anxiety spiral'. The treatment of choice would be to get Betty, very gradually, to go outside, using a technique called 'systematic desensitisation'. Betty would also be encouraged to control her negative thinking.

A psychodynamic approach, on the other hand, would seek to look behind Betty's fear and explore what is happening in her life generally. Is she having any difficulties in her marriage? What unconscious needs are being expressed? Might the threats she experiences around going outside represent something deeper? Does she feel insecure in herself? How does she feel being so dependent on others? Betty's behaviour would be seen as a symptom of unexpressed, underlying conflicts and needs. Therapists of this persuasion would ask these sorts of question and aim to enable Betty to express and explore her emotions through psychotherapy or other types of projective/creative activities.

In these ways, different psychological approaches offer us **analytical tools** to understand individuals' behaviour/experience and also ideas for different treatment **techniques or interventions**. Occupational therapists draw on these different tools and techniques to help us understand and work with particular problem areas. Psychological theories thus act as adjuncts to our overarching occupational therapy models.

In this chapter, we review five different psychological approaches commonly employed in psychosocial practice: the psychodynamic, behavioural, cognitive, humanistic and social constructionist approaches. I briefly outline the key ideas and techniques associated with each approach and, in turn, examine how occupational therapists apply these. A final section discusses the use and value of these different approaches more generally.

## 5.1   THE PSYCHODYNAMIC APPROACH

### Key concepts

The psychodynamic approach (consisting of different theories) arises out of psychoanalytic theory founded by Sigmund Freud and developed by others. These theories all emphasise how our emotional/personality or **ego** development is determined by both unconscious processes and past experiences. You'll be familiar with many of these ideas as they have come into our everyday language: for instance, when we say someone is 'needy' or 'looking for a father figure' or that they have 'repressed a bad experience', or when we talk of making a 'Freudian slip'.

Freud's (1936) most radical achievement was the uncovering of the dynamic **unconscious** mind – believed to be a repository (of which we are unaware) of powerful impulses, needs and fantasies at war with each other. These unconscious conflicts and anxieties are unconsciously 'handled' by developing defence mechanisms (Theory into practice 5.1). Freud also theorised that a child goes through a sequence of **psychosexual developmental stages** (oral, anal, phallic) that impact on adult personality. For example, a person who is dependent and 'needy' as an adult may have unresolved issues stemming back to trauma or insufficient nurturing experienced during the oral phase as an infant.

---

*Theory into practice 5.1* ————————————————————————

**Some common unconscious defence mechanisms**

- **Repression** – Blocking disturbing thoughts or desires. This is seen, for example, in the way we can 'forget' a traumatic incident.
- **Regression** – Returning to an earlier stage of development where needs (such as, security and love) were met. Psychodynamic therapists would say regression can be seen when a distressed individual curls up in a 'foetal position' for comfort, for instance.
- **Displacement** – Negative feelings are directed elsewhere. Here, we say we 'kick the cat' when really we are angry with someone else.
- **Denial** – Keeping unpleasant realities at bay. An example of this is how we might react to bad news by saying 'I don't believe it!'
- **Projection** – When a feeling that belongs to oneself is first brought out (externalised) and then directed on to another person or object, e.g. when we express our negative emotions on paper in art therapy.

---

- **Projective identification** – Unmanageable feelings are disowned by eliciting them in others. For instance, this occurs when we generate a sense of anger in someone else when really we are the ones who are angry. Then we unconsciously 'help' the other person to cope when really we are just trying to help ourselves.

Different psychodynamic theorists have different conceptions of the nature of development. Melanie Klein (1975), one of the first psychoanalysts to work with children, pioneered interpretation of their play. For her, critical development occurs in the first year of life where the child 'introjects' (i.e. internalises) a mother's love and/or rejection. Modern psychodynamic theory such as this argues that our minds are created from infancy, by **internally represented versions** of other people (objects) and their relations (object relations) with ourselves and each other, i.e. we are made up of symbolic parts of other people.

Klein, and theorists from what is known as the Object Relations School, developed these ideas focusing on the way we relate to others and how we use others to manage our emotions and meet our needs (such as our need for love). Their work was important in developing the notion that adult interactions/relationships often reflect **patterns laid down in childhood**. For instance, a child's early relationships are seen as playing a critical role in developing the child's ability to relate to others. This is where the child is seen to learn to love, trust and interact mutually with others. When early positive bonding is missing or relationships are distorted in some way, psychodynamic theorists say, the child is likely to have problematic relationships in the future. Bowlby (1988), for example, was a psychoanalyst who studied this topic in terms of attachment theory and separation anxiety. Other psychologists took up these ideas and showed that difficulties in relating to others seem to follow from early institutionalisation, lack of consistent care and/or distorted, abusive family relationships.

Other theorists have developed Freud's original psychodynamic ideas by introducing a stronger social dimension. Erikson (1977), for instance, argues that the identity/ego of an individual develops and changes throughout life. He identifies eight **life cycle stages**, characterising each stage in terms of a developmental conflict that needs to be resolved. Once worked through, the ego is strengthened and a special quality related to each stage develops. Importantly, each life-cycle stage is set in both a biological and a social/cultural context. For instance, the combination of physical ageing and society's negative attitudes to old age may precipitate 'despair' in later years.

Taking a different direction, Bion (1961) applied psychodynamic ideas to **group therapy** situations. He was important in initiating the idea that a group could be seen as a whole and was not simply a collection of individuals. He considered that two agendas tend to operate in groups: one is the overt, conscious, work-level agenda; the other is a hidden agenda, what he calls 'basic assumption' group. This consists of the unconscious intra-group tensions and emotions that unknowingly influence our behaviours. (Case example 5.1).

---

**Case example 5.1   Defensive manoeuvres – the application of psychodynamic ideas to a group context**

Bion's ideas of overt and hidden agendas can be illustrated by the following example of what occurred in one ward group. The group was experiencing a fair amount of interpersonal tension – much of it unexpressed (it felt unsafe to be honest). Mostly, the group members tended to avoid painful personal disclosure and group discussion by talking about issues outside the ward. At one meeting, a couple of members were allowed to pontificate at length about the quality of food offered in the canteen. Another member, Paul, attempted to challenge the way they were monopolising the discussion, but he was roundly criticised by the other members. They accused him of being insufficiently involved in, and committed to, ward concerns.

Some possible interpretations of the group's hidden unconscious agenda are as follows.

- The group avoided dealing with their personal problems and interpersonal conflicts by colluding with the discussion about outside issues (i.e. the discussion was a defensive manoeuvre).
- The group turned against and scapegoated Paul. This carried two pay-offs: it united the group and ensured that defensive avoidance was maintained, thus enabling individuals in the group to continue to avoid looking at their own material.
- The criticism levelled at Paul about insufficient commitment may well have been a product of the members' own 'projections' (i.e. they were insufficiently committed themselves but transferred their own emotions unconsciously on to Paul).

---

## The psychodynamic treatment approach

Classical psychoanalysis usually involves years of 'being on the couch', where the analyst listens to the client's stories and tries to uncover unconscious meanings through techniques such as dream interpretation and word association. Psychodynamically oriented therapists draw more loosely on psychoanalytic concepts. They tend to adopt a broader range of treatment methods under the banner of 'psychotherapy'. Here they might use either one-to-one or group situations and offer either talking-based or activity-centred treatments (e.g. the psychodrama described in Case example 5.2). Psychodynamic therapists aim to foster healthy ego functioning by encouraging an individual to express, explore and work through their unconscious needs and emotions. The key aim is to gain insight. In becoming aware of the unconscious needs driving their behaviours individuals can begin to make choices and try out new ways of behaving.

---

**Case example 5.2    Insights and healing through a psychodrama**

Carole used a psychodynamically orientated psychodrama session to explore her ambivalent feelings about becoming a mother. She was frightened that she was going to abuse her baby. In a psychodramatic construction – with the support of group members – she acted out her worst nightmare: she threw the baby against a wall. The 'Director' guided her to become 'the baby' and had someone else role-play Carole, 'the mother'. Carole then had to dialogue with this mother. Through this role reversal Carole was able for the first time to acknowledge feelings towards her own mother, who had abused her. With the group's help she realised that it was not inevitable that she would recreate what happened to her with her own children. The session ended with the group holding and rocking Carole. She began to explore what it meant to be nurtured and nurturing. The overall psychodrama experience was intense, emotional and deeply moving.

---

The **therapeutic relationship** is considered to be hugely significant. The therapist is seen as meeting a range of needs in the client, for instance offering some nurturing. Also, clients are thought to reveal unconscious conflicts in the way they 'transfer' on to the therapist emotions and patterns of relating from their early childhood relationships (a process known as 'transference'). For example, a female client reacting negatively to her therapist from seeing him as an 'authority figure' might be doing so because she is unconsciously transferring her emotions about her critical father to the therapist.

## Psychodynamic approach applied to occupational therapy

In common with other psychodynamic therapists, occupational therapists choosing this approach recognise the power of unconscious dynamics and individuals' use of defence mechanisms when they are in pain and conflict. Therapists would also focus on interpersonal relationships (between therapist and client and between clients). Exploring these different dynamics and transferences within therapy can help us become sensitive to the underlying needs of individuals and may help us understand them better.

What is unique about psychodynamic occupational therapists is the way they make use of the symbolic and projective **potential of activities**. For instance, we might use projective art to help a client express, explore and work through various unconscious needs and feelings. The emphasis on such activities is more on the process than on the end product. 'In creative therapy', say Atkinson and Wells (2000, p. 295), 'the product is implicit, achieved through a process of self-discovery, self-exploration and self-help'.

In the 1960s, Gail and Jay Fidler (1963) were influential in bringing this psychodynamic approach into occupational therapy. Like other psychoanalytical therapists, they stressed the role of the unconscious and *object relations* in influencing behaviour. Their theory and practice emphasised three other key processes:

- They argued that **communication** is the essence of occupational therapy. They saw the inability to communicate effectively as the key psychiatric disability. In occupational therapy, the process and end-product of activities are designed to facilitate individuals to communicate thoughts/feelings that they cannot at a verbal level. A cooking (and eating!) session, for example, can represent and communicate nurturing towards gratifying infantile needs.
- They then stressed the importance of **interpersonal relationships** in therapy. In the treatment process both the patient–therapist relationship and the patients' interactions in a group are considered of central significance for strengthening the ego and for reality testing. For instance, where an individual is consumed by fantasies that she might lose control and 'destroy everything', the therapist might take the opportunity in a session to reassure her, saying, 'I am not going to let you hurt yourself or me'.
- They further emphasised the **symbolic potential of activities** to allow the exploration of conflicts. Activities are seen as useful in dealing with self-concept; sexual identity; infantile, oral and anal needs; dependency; hostility and reality testing. Playing around with wet clay, for example, can provide an opportunity to regress symbolically. It also provides a safe environment to experience being both constructive and destructive (Case example 5.3)

---

### Case example 5.3   *Projective use of clay and play*

**Aim**

Clay work was used projectively in a psychotherapy-playtherapy session with an emotionally and behaviourally disturbed 9-year-old girl called Tracy. The aim of the session was to offer Tracy an opportunity to express and explore her feelings (in particular, anger) towards her family. First, Tracy created each family member in clay. She was then asked to show, through her play, 'how her family is' and 'how she wishes it could be'.

**The session**

Here the therapist describes what happened:

*Tracy started by creating her father – a special, much loved figure; then stepmother (loathed 'wicked witch'), and then the new baby (loathed interloper). Using the figure of herself she 'kicked' her stepmother around and tore the baby to bits. She then had her father apologise to her for marrying 'that awful woman' and the two of them settled down to 'live happily ever after'. After encouraging some exploration of this need I challenged Tracy's claim that that was how she wanted it to be. She then slowly remade the stepmother piece and placed her parents and herself into a close idealised family (without the baby!).*

---

**Therapist's analysis of significant themes**

Sibling rivalry and competition with the stepmother for her father's love are evident. Tracy has used the play session powerfully to express and act out her needs. By expressing the conflicts Tracy is beginning to understand her own 'bad' behaviour at home.

## 5.2 THE BEHAVIOURAL APPROACH

### Key concepts

The behavioural approach focuses on **learning** as the key to development and socialisation. This perspective maintains that children are born a 'blank slate' and are required to learn virtually everything – to talk, read, be toilet trained, study, play, socialise, and so on.

According to behaviourists such as John Watson and B. F. Skinner, learning occurs through the stimulation and rewards available in the **environment**. We routinely praise, encourage, reward, punish and even ignore children to change or develop their behaviour. Take for example how Colin's father taught 6-year-old Colin how to ride a bicycle. Colin had had a bad accident when he first tried to ride a two-wheeler – now he was frightened of it, saying he did not want to learn and he would stick to his tricycle. Colin's father set out to teach him. First he helped Colin associate bicycling with fun and safety by holding on to him while playfully wheeling him around. He gradually introduced the idea of letting go for a few seconds and using a lot of praise when Colin successfully rode by himself. Once Colin could ride by himself, his father rode another bicycle alongside to act as both a model and as an encourager. These teaching strategies are all based on scientifically researched, behavioural techniques – classical conditioning, operant conditioning, social learning and cognitive–behavioural theory.

**Classical conditioning** consists of learning by *association*. For instance, it is a common experience to suddenly experience tooth pain on hearing a drill. As another example, consider the case of Bill, who is no longer able to bear the smell of whiskey since he associates it with a previous occasion when he overindulged and was sick.

With **operant conditioning** learning occurs in three ways. First, we repeat behaviours when they are rewarded (*positive reinforcement*). Second, learning can occur by removing aversive stimuli (*negative reinforcement*). Third, learning can occur by applying a negative or removing a positive stimulus (*punishment*). However, while punishment can be effective for a while, research has shown that the undesired behaviour will come back if nothing more positive replaces it. If a parent criticises a child (punishment) for interrupting a conversation, the child may well stop interrupting for a while. Unless children are taught what else to do, they will return to interrupting (not least because criticism may be better than no attention at all!). In other words, operant conditioning states that, if we want to change the way someone behaves, we reinforce new, desired behaviours.

**Social learning theory** proposes that learning occurs in a social context through imitation and modelling on others. The best way to learn to ski, for example, is to model on the instructor's demonstration. Moreover, we not only copy but also select what we want to model on and we can learn vicariously through others – be it friends, parents, off the TV, etc. We don't copy all the behaviour we observe, so there must be an element of thinking and selecting behaviours we wish to reproduce. Bandura (1977) suggests that the behaviours we choose to imitate will be ones where we anticipate a positive consequence.

**Cognitive–behaviourism** attempts to redress the tendency of traditional behaviourism to focus on observable behaviour and processes (stimulus-response) while ignoring or downplaying internal processes such as thinking/emotions. By recognising *thinking* and *motivation*, cognitive–behaviourism is better able to explain complex learning such as learning how to talk. It also explains how we pick up beliefs and attitudes (such as prejudice) more convincingly than do more traditional models.

Cognitive–behaviourism emphasises the point that thinking, motivation and social context all play a significant role in learning. Take, for example, the situation where you are trying to teach Dorothy how to use a video camera. If she is going to learn effectively, she needs first to want to learn, then to respect your ability as a teacher. In terms of teaching the skill, it would not be sufficient to teach her by rewarding her each time she accidentally touches the correct button. Instead, you would need to teach the logic of each operation and ensure that Dorothy fully understands that logic.

## The behavioural treatment approach

Behavioural methods of treatment have been widely applied, particularly in work with children and in the field of learning disabilities – any time, in fact, where the focus is on learning and teaching skills. Some commonly used behavioural techniques are listed below.

- **Systematic desensitisation** – Here, a person is gradually introduced to a feared stimulus while trying to relax. For example, to work on agoraphobia, the person has progressive goals of walking to the front gate, then down the road 50 metres, 100 metres, and so forth.
- **Token economy** – This is where tangible rewards (e.g. sweets, tokens, stars) are systematically given to encourage positive behaviours. This technique is used most commonly with children/adolescents. For instance, Billy is given a 'gold star' for every half-hour period when he behaves well. At the end of the week he can then trade in his gold star collection for an appropriate prize.
- **Chaining or backward chaining** – Here, skills are taught in a linked sequence. This technique is commonly used when teaching individuals who have a learning disability such daily living skills as how to dress and eat independently. For instance, if teaching a person how to put on socks, we would need

to break down the learning into components, first teaching the step of pulling up the socks, then how to put the sock on the foot, then how to line up the sock to the foot.

- **Shaping** – This is where approximations to the desired behaviour are reinforced, gradually raising the standard until the desired behaviour is achieved. This is akin to rewarding the child who says 'ma-ma' *en route* to 'mummy'.
- **Contracts** – Contracts involve people agreeing, in writing, to change their behaviour. In return, they receive something they appreciate or value. An example from marital therapy is where a wife agrees to be 'more sociable' if her husband helps out in the house more. The exact behaviours required would be specified in the contract.
- **Time out** – This involves removing the person from sources of positive reinforcement. For instance, if a child is getting reinforced by attention while having a tantrum, time out would involve moving them to a mundane, attention-free zone until the tantrum ended.

## The behavioural approach applied to occupational therapy

Occupational therapists draw widely on behavioural principles (see, for instance, Yakobina *et al.*, 1997). We routinely apply them unconsciously/automatically – for example, in our use of rewarding with praise or when we give someone 'feedback'. We consciously and systematically **apply behavioural principles** when teaching patients/clients new skills and behaviours. Here, for instance, we might employ 'backward chaining methods' to teach a child to dress or we might use systematic desensitisation as part of an anxiety management programme. We might also employ cognitive–behavioural techniques such as 'dialectical behaviour therapy' (see Research example 5.1) or 'social skills training'. Salo-Chydenius (1996), for example, describes a successful social skills training programme for people with longer term mental health problems (Theory into practice 5.2).

---

*Theory into practice 5.2*————————————————————————

**Social skills training**

Social skills training (Ellis and Whittington, 1981) is a cognitive–behavioural technique designed to teach systematically elements of social behaviour (verbal, non-verbal, assertion, etc.). People who benefit may never have acquired the skills (because of learning disabilities), had the skills once and lost them (e.g. by becoming institutionalised), or have the skills but lack the confidence to apply them (prone to anxiety).

Social skills training typically starts with a 'contract' that requires the individual to attend and contribute to the group for a set number of weeks. Then, through a series of practical rehearsal and 'homework' exercises,

---

specific social skills are learned in sequence. For instance, in a 10-session programme the following skills might be taught:

- Session 1: 'Saying hello'
- Session 2: Making requests (in a shop or café context)
- Session 3: Appropriate body space and non-verbal communication
- Session 4: 'Making conversation', and so forth.

The practical emphasis on 'doing' and step-by-step learning of skills via role play, modelling, feedback and so on make social skills training a particularly relevant technique to use in occupational therapy. Special sensitivity is needed, however, to avoid overstepping the line between imposing one's own standards of behaviour and facilitating the development of new or different behaviours in someone who wants to change.

When applying behavioural techniques, it is possible to lose the 'person' through focusing in a reductionist way on small bits of behaviour. Used within a broader team strategy or programme that retains a holistic, person-centred approach, these methods can be invaluable. We would, for example, be likely to see occupational therapists exploiting group treatment situations (such as assertiveness training or anxiety management) that offer opportunities for social learning, rather than using mechanistic token economy programmes.

Mosey's work on 'adaptive skills' and the **teaching-learning process**, described in the last chapter, offer positive examples of how behavioural principles are applied in a broader context. She reminds us of the need to take into account broader motivational and social factors – especially the relationships between the teacher and the learner when she argues that 'A therapist can only help a client want to learn through the design of appropriate learning situations' (Mosey, 1986, p. 218).


## 5.3   THE COGNITIVE APPROACH

### Key concepts

Cognitive approaches aim to understand the structure and process of the mind. While a variety of theories come under this umbrella, all share the view that cognitions – i.e. our ability to think, attend, perceive, remember, problem-solve and reason – underlie all our behaviour and human activities.

Cognitive dysfunction manifests in different ways:

- In **organic disorders** (such as those resulting from dementia or head injury), cognitive impairment can be diffuse and damage can occur at different levels. This damage commonly shows itself in the way that individuals may have perceptual problems and memory loss or be confused and disorientated.

- Individuals who suffer from **major psychoses** such as schizophrenia show a different pattern of damage. In acute psychotic stages, thought disorder (with confused and irrational thinking) may be marked. People who have enduring mental health disorders are likely to exhibit cognitive disability in the form of poor task performance (where they find it difficult to concentrate, and to organise and carry out tasks independently).
- People who have **neurotic and affective disorders** (such as anxiety and depression) experience a different type of cognitive dysfunction. In addition to poor concentration and possible odd perceptions (such as the experience of depersonalisation), unrealistic, negative, self-defeating, repetitive thoughts often dominate (see Case example 5.4).

---

### Case example 5.4    Post-traumatic stress syndrome

Dalgleish (2002) describes the case of Arnold – a successful businessman happy about his imminent retirement. Then one of Arnold's old wartime friends, John, dies. Devastated by John's death, Arnold begins to have vivid and disturbing nightmares about his wartime experiences. During the day he thinks increasingly about the terrible things he did and witnessed during the war. He feels both guilt and shame. He becomes anxious and irritable and wonders if he is going mad. According to Dalgleish, Arnold is displaying 'normal' emotions and is exhibiting the symptoms of post-traumatic stress disorder.

---

## Cognitive treatment approaches

The diverse range of cognitive disorders described above makes it difficult to pinpoint any one psychological approach to treatment. Two specific approaches can be contrasted to show something of the range.

### Cognitive rehabilitation approach

Here, the focus is on treating individuals who have sustained some organic damage. The basic approach is one of problem-solving. For instance, when working with people who have memory impairment, a number of techniques and strategies could be used.

- Reality orientation – to regularly offer cues reminding the individual of the time, where they are, what they are doing and why
- To give advice on how to store information in easily retrievable ways
- To rebuild long-term memory through repetition and association
- To teach and develop compensatory strategies, such as writing lists, leaving note reminders around a room, using technology to give reminder prompts or sound an alarm, and so forth.

## Cognitive therapy

Cognitive therapy (also called cognitive–behavioural therapy, see Section 4.2) has been used with people who have negative, self-defeating or unrealistic thinking patterns. Cognitive therapists believe that the way an event is appraised determines the person's emotions. Further, they consider that the extreme and distressing emotions that characterise disorders such as anxiety and depression are the result of unrealistic beliefs (Research example 5.1).

---

*Research example 5.1*

**The proven efficacy of cognitive–behavioural therapy**

- Cognitive–behavioural therapy is commonly used in anxiety management programmes. Clark (1986) proposed a cognitive approach to panic that involved the following sequence of events. First the individual becomes apprehensive, which results in autonomic nervous system responses such as increased heart rate and hyperventilation. These are in turn interpreted as 'catastrophic', which increases the panic. Cognitive therapists advocate various strategies that focus on the anxious individual's beliefs. These strategies include trying to get him or her to realise that:

  – Attending to bodily sensations can lead to greater anxiety
  – Bodily symptoms can be controlled
  – Catastrophic consequences (like a heart attack) do not occur.

  In researching the effectiveness of such an approach, Clark *et al.* (1994) compared the outcomes of cognitive therapy, relaxation training and the use of the drug imipramine. Cognitive therapy emerged as most effective (both immediately after the therapy and 15 months later).

- Telch *et al.* (2001) evaluated the use of dialectical behaviour therapy (DBT) adapted for binge-eating disorder. A total of 44 women with binge-eating disorder were randomly assigned to DBT or the waiting list control condition. Treated women showed significant improvement on measures of binge eating and eating pathology compared to controls and 89% of the women receiving DBT had stopped binge eating by the end of treatment. Abstinence rates were reduced to 56% at the six-month follow-up.

---

Beck (1976), in his version of cognitive therapy, recommends that:

- The individual is first helped to become aware of their thoughts
- Therapy then focuses firstly, on stopping the negative spiral of thoughts (for instance, explicitly saying 'STOP!'); then searching for evidence to disprove these thoughts.
- The person is then ready to try to replace the negative thoughts with positive (but realistic) ones, using the technique of 'cognitive restructuring'.

Ellis (2000) offers his version of cognitive therapy which he calls 'rational emotive therapy'. This form of psychotherapy similarly focuses on disputing irrational beliefs. For instance, it is common to hear women with eating disorders say things like, 'Once I'm slim, I'll be happy' or 'I'm fat so I'm an awful person'. Therapy here would be geared to challenging these unrealistic expectations.

## Cognitive approaches applied to occupational therapy

Occupational therapists employ a wide range of cognitive and cognitive–behavioural techniques. Three contrasting approaches are particularly relevant:

### Cognitive rehabilitation

When we are involved with cognitive rehabilitation, we are particularly concerned to assess a person's cognitive and process skills in the context of their everyday functioning and occupations. From our perspective, the fact that a person has a memory deficit is not particularly a problem. It only becomes a problem if the memory deficit interferes with their functioning. To give an example, a person's memory may be so poor that they are unsafe to cook unsupervised. If that person is content to go out for their hot meals and otherwise live on sandwiches, then the cooking 'problem' diminishes. Cognitive rehabilitation therapists seek to offer a range of problem-solving strategies to suit the needs of the individual concerned.

### Cognitive disabilities model

In the USA, Claudia Allen (1985) devised what she called the 'cognitive disabil-ities model', a specific form of cognitive rehabilitation. The model was originally developed as an approach to treating chronic psychiatric patients but has since been developed for use with other groups (such as people with learning disabil-ities or head injuries and those suffering from dementia). The model proposes a continuum of function and dysfunction divided into six cognitive levels:

- Level 1 – Individuals display profound cognitive disability when they are barely conscious and unaware of other people/environment
- Level 2 – Individuals can follow very simple instructions; they often wander or pace aimlessly and are only partially aware of the environment
- Level 3 – Individuals can begin to carry out manual actions and use physical objects (e.g. they can carry out repetitive self-care tasks)
- Level 4 – Individuals are beginning to be purposeful and goal-directed; with help they can complete simple, concrete tasks
- Level 5 – Individuals show more flexibility and can attend to all elements in their environment; new learning can occur but problems are still apparent – e.g. anticipating or planning events and abstract thinking are still difficult
- Level 6 – Individuals function well: they can pre-plan actions, follow instruc-tions, consider hypothetical possibilities and understand abstract concepts.

The model provides detailed procedures for assessing patients (by observing their task performance using the Allen Cognitive Level test amongst other assessments). It also offers in-depth guidelines for analysing and structuring activities that are matched to the relevant level of cognitive function. Allen stresses the need to acknowledge and work within the permanent limitations of the patient's capacity.

### Cognitive therapy and cognitive–behavioural techniques

Occupational therapists who use counselling may well employ the cognitive therapy and cognitive–behavioural techniques described above (Case example 5.5).

---

**Case example 5.5  Cognitive–behavioural strategies to cope with exam phobia**

Susan is phobic about exams. This is a particular problem as she is in the third year of a university course and her finals are looming. On having to face an exam, she gets trapped in a negative spiral of thinking. She starts by thinking, 'I can't cope with exams …. I'm no good at them …. I always fail …. I'm going to fail this one …. I can feel myself getting panicky …. I won't be able to control it ….' She soon talks herself into a full blown panic attack. Cognitive–behavioural therapists would say that Susan's behaviour will only change if she changes the pattern of her negative thoughts, e.g. in the following ways:

**Stage 1 – Education**

Susan is advised about the nature of anxiety and how a certain amount is necessary for 'peak performance'.

**Stage 2 – Cognitive restructuring**

First Susan is taught to think differently about her anxiety, i.e. to look on it as 'a potentially helpful friend' and not 'an out of control enemy'. Second, she rehearses a new sequence of more positive thinking: 'I am not going to fail, I know I can do it, I have done it in practice. I have worked hard and I want to demonstrate my knowledge.' Susan is then given some homework, which involves chanting this sequence every time she catches herself thinking about exams negatively.

**Stage 3 – Relaxation**

Susan learns a range of relaxation techniques. She has to think through which would be most suitable for her in different situations. One particular strategy she is encouraged to use is to draw on humour. She learns to laugh at herself and to enjoy various antics (such as going to the toilet at intervals to do some fast 'running on the spot' – a strategy she finds helpful in relieving tension).

**Stage 4 – Systematic desensitisation**

Susan eventually has to face up to the practical side of actually sitting in an exam room under exam conditions. In order to prepare for this, with the help of her

---

therapist, Susan draws up a plan of action – breaking down the task into more manageable chunks (which includes built-in rewards and the application of relaxation techniques).

1.  Susan first sits down in her empty college exam hall comfortably.
2.  She then manages (successfully) a prepared mock exam question her tutor supplies.
3.  She then moves on to complete (successfully) a full mock exam.

## 5.4 THE HUMANISTIC APPROACH

### Key concepts

> As we face the severest threat in history to human survival, I find the possibilities of *being* [my emphasis] made more prominent by their contrast with our possible annihilation. The individual human is still the creature who can wonder, who can be enchanted by a sonata, who can place symbols together to make poetry to gladden our hearts, who can view a sunrise with a sense of majesty and awe.
>
> May, 1983, p. 10.

This quotation nicely captures the positive view of human experience held by humanistic psychologists – an approach that developed in the 1950s as a reaction to the determinism of the psychodynamic approach and the reductionism of the behaviourism. It operates both as an existential philosophy and as an approach to therapy.

While different humanistic theorists and therapists offer different accounts of human development, they all focus on:

- the unique individual who is seen to have personal autonomy and a sense of agency and self-concept
- our subjective, conscious, here-and-now experience
- our capacity to be self-aware and reflective
- the existential assumption that people can create themselves and make their own choices as they search for meaning in their lives.

Central to the humanistic approach is the development of **self-concept**. Humanists assert that each of us is unique and made up of our own individual feelings, thoughts and embodied experiences. Thus we have a self-awareness, a self-identity, a sense of our-self as continuing: there is only one of us. We have a sense of 'I'. Carl Rogers (1961), arguably the most famous humanistic therapist, has written much about self-concept. He argues that the way we perceive ourselves affects the way we experience and respond to events. The greater the congruence between what he called our 'actual self' (how we are) and our 'ideal self' (how we'd like to be), the better adjusted we are.

Importantly, we also have the capacity to reflect on our experience of being that individual – who I am now; whom I want to become. We have a sense of our own power and **agency**. We can do things to, and produce an effect on, others and our environment. I can cook a meal. I can make someone else feel happy. I can put out a fire. Along with the capacity to do, I can choose to do. I can even choose to die. To a greater or lesser degree, according to this approach, we are active, free agents – we have freedom of choice. For Abraham Maslow (1954), all human beings drive towards **personal growth** and self-fulfilment. We are motivated by a hierarchy of needs: physiological, safety, love/belonging, esteem, cognitive/aesthetic and finally self-actualisation.

While both psychodynamic and humanistic psychologists work with subjective meanings (feelings, needs, motivation), they differ in how they understand and view consciousness. Whereas psychodynamic therapists work with unconscious needs, humanistic therapists home in on here-and-now **lived experience** and subjective meanings (beliefs, feelings, needs, motivations). Stevens describes their focus thus:

> *At the core of our experience of being is the flow of conscious awareness. Moving inexorably through time, sometimes lagging, sometimes so fleeting that we are aware of awareness only in retrospect, the ever-changing kaleidoscope of consciousness is marked by changes in quality – from drowsiness to the freshness of waking, from the grey mists of depression to the excitement of expectation.*

Stevens, 2002, p. 195.

Maslow (1973) describes a particular type of conscious awareness that he calls 'peak experience'. This is when we experience a moment of delight, when our attention is completely focused and in the moment. It's as if we are 'high' – there is a sense of fusion with life, we forget our worries and anything seems possible. (Research example 5.2 gives a description of 'flow' – an analogous concept.)

---

**Research example 5.2**

**Flow experience**

'Flow' experience during activities

Csikszentmihalyi (a Hungarian named pronounced '*Chik*shentmeehai') (1993, 1999) devised the concept of 'flow' – the intrinsically rewarding experience that occurs when people are happily absorbed, even enraptured, in the moment of doing an activity. He cites a dancer's description of how it feels when a performance is going well: 'Your concentration is complete you are totally involved your energy is flowing very smoothly' (Csikszentmihalyi, 1992, p. 53). The sense of 'effortless performance' is often only possible because of well practised skills and techniques. As Csikszentmihalyi

---

notes, this is one of the 'paradoxes of flow: One has to be in control of the activity to experience it, yet one should not try to consciously control what one is doing' (Csikszentmihalyi, 1999, p. 825).

Such research has important implications for occupational therapy, particularly as Csikszentmihalyi suggests that happiness and well-being depends, at least in part, on a person being able to derive 'flow' from what activities they do and how they do them. See Research example 3.4, p. 49.

George Kelly (1955) argues that we derive our ideas about ourselves and the world from our experiences and interactions. Specifically, he describes consciousness in terms of us having 'bi-constructs' – a way of thinking/feeling/ perceiving – that help us make sense of the world. For instance, one of my core constructs, which seems to influence how I see people, is in terms of them being 'friendly/warm' or 'cold/unresponsive'. Kelly developed a technique called the 'repertory grid', which was designed to uncover a person's constructs patterns. This technique has also been used in therapy to raise **self-awareness**.

## Humanistic treatment approaches

Two particular forms of humanistic therapy are: client-centred counselling and gestalt therapy.

### Client-centred therapy

This approach to counselling aims to help clients develop self-awareness and to express their feelings. Rogers (1970) believed that every person has within themselves a vast resource for self-understanding but that these resources can only be tapped in a facilitative climate where the therapist offers non-judgemental, *unconditional positive regard*. The therapist aims to show warmth and empathy for clients, listening carefully without attempting to interpret what they're saying. Rogers argued that an over-controlling, directive therapist is giving a message that he or she can control events better than the client. Once clients realise that they can say anything and still be accepted, they are better able to open themselves up to what they really feel. Crucial to this approach to counselling is the therapist's avoidance of directing the action/conversation while maintaining a profound respect for the client's ability to solve their own situation.

Virginia Axline has applied these principles to her work doing play therapy with children. She writes that **non-directive counselling** or psychotherapy is 'one means of freeing the individual so that he can become a more spontaneous, creative, and happy individual...' (Axline, 1989 p. 26). The non-directive therapist is client-centred because 'to him, the client is the source of living power that directs the growth from within himself ...' (Axline, 1989 p. 22).

### Gestalt therapy

This therapy, developed by Fritz Perls (1973), is used in one-to-one and group situations. It encourages clients to become aware of and 'own' the actual bodily and perceptual sensations they are experiencing in the here-and-now, rather than talking about their problems in an intellectualised way. Various role-play and dramatherapy techniques are used to release blocked emotions and to encourage spontaneous expression of emotion (e.g. shouting and beating a pillow, or the therapist and the client reversing roles). A typical exercise is 'to have a conversation between your different selves' (i.e. making explicit conflicting voices in your head). In these ways, clients are stimulated to gain self-awareness and work through their inner conflicts and needs.

### Humanistic approach applied to occupational therapy

Occupational therapy is imbued with humanistic understandings and approaches. These emerge in our philosophy, in the way we relate to service users, and in our use of activities in treatment.

Yerxa has written widely about what she sees as the essentially **humanistic values** underpinning occupational therapy: our optimism, holism and approach to seeing the patient/client as active, autonomous and with a right to life satisfaction (Yerxa, 1983a). As she puts it, 'by increasing the client's capacity to be independent we help him perceive himself as possessing worth. He is not a "thing" to be manipulated helplessly by others but is a human being who can exercise some control over his environment' (Yerxa, 1967, p. 3).

Humanistic therapists place much emphasis on establishing a person-centred, empowering, **therapeutic relationship**. Relationships are seen as crucial to developing a person's self-esteem as well as fulfilling needs. The therapists believe that a non-judgemental approach allows a person to express, and thus examine, his or her less desirable feelings or behaviour without fearing censure. Also, having another person accept and value you helps you do the same for yourself.

When occupational therapists exploit the **healing potential of activities**, they are drawing on humanistic ideals. When therapists prescribe activities (any activity, from baking to typing to art), we do so in order to enable individuals to express themselves, to help them reach their potential, to excite their creativity, to experience 'flow' – all humanistic concerns. Our concern to enable people to discover meaningful, purposeful occupations and make conscious life choices derives from humanistic assumptions that such things are both possible and desirable. That we are particularly interested in individuals having a healthy self-concept and that we aim to develop their self-esteem expresses a fundamentally humanistic idea.

## 5.5 THE SOCIAL CONSTRUCTIONIST APPROACH

### Key concepts

Over the last century, people with learning disabilities have been labelled variously as 'imbeciles', 'cretins', 'moral defectives', 'the mentally handicapped'. Today we talk of them as 'people who have difficulty learning'. Imbeciles and cretins were kept in substandard, even subhuman, conditions as 'they didn't know any better'. Moral defectives were locked away 'to protect society'. The handicapped were 'cared for' in special institutions. Now, people with learning disabilities are seen as having full rights to live 'normal' lives and are seen just to have 'special needs' such as for additional education. The critical point here is that *the language reflects social attitudes and carries with it important consequences* – such as the way people are understood and treated.

This short examination of changing language use highlights a central concern of social constructionism: the role of **language and discourse** in understanding both human behaviour and society at large. Social constructionists (e.g. Potter and Wetherell, 1995) believe that our individual identities – i.e. our sense of self, our emotions, values, needs – do not originate within ourselves but are the product of our language, narratives and relationships set within a social context. 'The self', Bruner argues, 'is best understood not as a pure and enduring core but as "the sum and swarm" of participations in social life' (Bruner, 1990, p. 107). Bruner sees that we have *multiple social identities*, which emerge in, and are created through, interactions within different social contexts.

Underpinning this idea of **contextual selves** is the argument that our identities are *negotiated* through our relationships and interactions. In the terms of Goffman (1959), the contexts we find ourselves in offer us roles with associated 'scripts', unwritten codes and routines for saying and doing things. It is through the use of cultural references (social categories, narrative forms, metaphors, scripts and clichés) that we construct our version of the world – a version that we seek to persuade others to share. Put another way, every encounter has a role to play in *producing* the self and there is a purpose behind the language we use. As we saw in the discussion on language use related to learning disability, language is not neutral: it is impregnated with values and meanings.

Social constructionists try to take a systematic approach to the study of people's talk, focusing on the ways in which people use words to make meaning and present themselves. Specifically, they use a *qualitative research method* called 'discourse analysis' (Wetherell *et al.*, 2001). (Other methods commonly linked under the umbrella of social constructionism include ethnomethodology, conversation analysis, ethnography, feminist studies, symbolic interactionism and narrative analysis.) Consider, for instance, the following brief dialogue between an elderly person and a care manager. (Note that in both conversation and discourse analysis dialogues are usually carefully annotated to indicate pauses, timings, tone, changes of gear and emphasis. These have been omitted here for ease of reference.) Then see Theory into practice 5.3 for some ideas of how this discourse might be analysed.

**Mrs B**: I need to have more of the carers' time. Twenty minutes every day is no good. I need more. The carers hardly have time to do anything. All they can do is get me out of bed, washed and dressed and give me a cup of tea. But how do I cope the rest of the day? I can't manage. Do you expect me to do all my cooking and cleaning? I can't cope.

**Care Manager**: I know you would like more time with the carers. I'm really very sorry. If it were in my power I'd give it to you. But we just don't have the resources available. There are too many people needing care and a lot of them are in much more difficulty than you are. Some people can't even get out of bed themselves. There are just not enough carers to go round. Twenty minutes is all that I can offer you.

---

*Theory into practice 5.3*_____

**A discourse analysis**

Discourse analysts would pick up a number of points from the dialogue above, related to:

a) How the individuals are presenting themselves as part of a negotiation process
b) What cultural assumptions are being made and how these link to broader ideologies.

a) In this brief interaction, Mrs B seems to construct herself as powerless in terms of being dependent on others and having to ask for more help. The care manager clearly has the power to define and control access to resources. But the care manager, too, is constrained by her organisation and the fact that resources are limited. We might also view this communication as a complex negotiation, where Mrs B is actively positioning herself as someone 'in need' who can't manage while almost accusing the care manager of some negligence in not appreciating her difficulties! The care manager, in response, is presenting herself as sympathetic and on Mrs B's side, while also being 'powerless' herself in not being able to grant any further resources. Whatever way we view this interaction, we need to be careful not to assume either individual is making factual statements – **truth can be seen as being relative.** Mrs. B. may be able to cope better than she is letting on. The care manager might actually have the resources to allocate, providing she feels that it is justified. They are simply (well, not so simply!) presenting particular versions of themselves and their world, for a particular purpose, in a given context.

b) While Mrs B and the care manager seem to disagree about what represents an acceptable level of coping and care, they show a remarkable agreement, sharing understandings derived from our culture. They both accept our mixed-market system of health and social care and the role played by Social Services. They have both defined Mrs B's problems at an 'individual level' rather than seeing the wider pattern of the problem (that there are many isolated, elderly people who find it difficult to manage independently) at a 'social level'. There is some assumption that disability makes individuals a 'burden' or a 'victim' – that these individuals should be relatively acquiescent and grateful for help. They both seem to subscribe to the idea that 'help/caring' entails performing functional tasks such as helping the person to get out of bed (instead of other ways of caring such as providing company or attending to leisure needs). A linked point is that understandings of 'degree of need' relate primarily to a person's capacity to perform daily living tasks (and is not related to pain, anxiety, depression, loneliness, and so forth).

### Social constructionist treatment approach

While social constructionism has not had the same impact in terms of producing therapy techniques as the other psychological approaches, this more sociological approach has made a significant contribution to the health and social care literature. Two particular applications are the practice of narrative therapy and the use of discourse analysis as an analytical tool:

- Strands of the **narrative therapy** movement (Morgan, 2000; see also www. dulwichcentre.com.au) have arisen from social constructionist ideas. Here, individuals' personal stories are also viewed as cultural/social stories. Their identities are seen as being constructed through history and culture. Therapists working in this tradition examine a person's cultural scripts and encourage their clients to 're-author' their own lives towards preferred narratives. In reference to narrative work and occupational therapy, Mattingly (1998) discusses what she calls 'therapeutic emplotment', which attends to action and experience as being both personal and socially constructed. Healing, for instance, is viewed as a shifting process influenced, at least in part, by structural conditions and cultural meanings. (For other works on narrative, see Research example 2.2 in Chapter 2.)
- Social constructionism offers us an **analytical tool** to help us think clearly and critically about our language, in the context of our everyday assumptions and practices. In drawing attention to discourse, social constructionists also highlight the ways institutions and *structures of society* create inequalities. As such, social constructionists offer a strong critical voice against social divisions and inequalities of power based on class, gender, race, disability, and so forth. These theorists' critique of the use and abuse of 'professional power' underpins much of the development of *anti-oppressive practice* and the rise in popularity of 'social models of disability'.

At a more personal level, social constructionist research pushes us to become aware of, and challenge, elements in our own practice that may be discriminatory or disempowering. They remind us to be critical of the way we position ourselves and our service users. As Opie (1997) recommends, we should be *reflexive* in our interprofessional teams and acknowledge the inevitability of differential power relations between health professionals and service users (see Research example 6.3 in Chapter 6).

---

*Research example 5.3*

**Discursive analysis of a narrative of a sufferer from obsessive–compulsive disorder**

O'Neill (1999) provides an example of how a discursive reflexive approach can be used to explore, and work with, a person's sense of identity. She offers a discursive analysis of the narrative of a woman (Emma) about her life with obsessive–compulsive disorder (OCD). One finding was the association Emma experienced between her experience of OCD and religion. Analysis suggest that different 'voices' in Emma's narrative represented the power relations involved in her life. The controlling nature of Emma's experience of OCD was revealed through the 'controlling OCD voice', which seemed to be in control of her thoughts and actions. By distinguishing the controlling OCD voice, Emma was able to separate off the part of her that she saw was linked to her disorder. This allowed her to feel an increased sense of control and self-efficacy.

## Social constructionist approach applied to occupational therapy

One example of social constructionism applied to occupational therapy is the work of Claire Ballinger (2003). Ballinger offers a reflexive analysis of her research on the construction of falls by older people (Research example 5.4). Using **discourse analysis** she studied the way in which both therapists and service users account for falls. She found that the therapists she interviewed gave accounts which were broadly similar to her own – a finding that was not surprising given the fact that she is herself an occupational therapist. Surprisingly, however, service user accounts were notably different. Ballinger explains that the accounts had a 'protective function, designed to avert possible attributions of carelessness, forgetfulness and frailty' (2003, pp. 72–73). She recognised that the information she was getting, from both therapists and service users, related to her own role in the research as a 'researcher-therapist' and her institutional positioning.

---

*Research example 5.4*

**How falls in older people are constructed**

Ballinger and Payne (2000) studied how the falls of older people were constructed. Eight older people with fractured hips and 20 therapists were interviewed about the reasons for, the predictability of and the consequences of falls.

Discourse analytic findings suggested that the therapists constructed falls as predictable events in which personal characteristics of the older people were implicated, e.g. in terms of physical problems, senility, blood pressure and personal habits such as wearing inappropriate shoes. Problems concerning the older person's chosen home environment were also mentioned. The responses of the service users themselves focused on their commendable personal attributes and they refuted negative assessments of their mental state, character and capacity to take care of themselves. Accidents were often attributed to the carelessness of others or events external to themselves.

An important finding of this research is recognising how, for many older people, falling is an emotive topic. Many people are anxious to distance themselves from such events to avoid being negatively stereotyped. In this research, Ballinger and Payne also hope to encourage therapists to question assumptions underpinning biomedical research into falls so as to not unthinkingly reproduce these ideas in their own practice.

## 5.6 CHOOSING BETWEEN APPROACHES

### A case example

So far in this chapter, we have seen how occupational therapists' views of individuals' problems and needs (and thus our therapeutic interventions) *depend on* which theoretical approach we adopt.

The contrasts between the approaches emerges with particular sharpness if we compare the way adherents of each would understand and treat Katie, a person with a mental health problem described below. Different therapists' responses are illustrated in Case examples 5.6–5.9.

Katie, aged 22, has bulimia nervosa (an eating disorder that involves bingeing on huge quantities of food, resulting in overwhelming guilt and a compulsion to get rid of it by vomiting or purging). She is attractive, slim, intelligent and studying medicine successfully at university. On the face of it she seems to have a lot going for her but beneath the surface she is deeply unhappy and burdened by the dark secret of her condition.

In common with many of her friends, she wants to be slimmer and is invariably 'on a diet'. She believes, and hopes, that once she can control her food intake and diet successfully, she will 'become slim and happy'. Currently she is in a vicious cycle of crash dieting half the week and intensively bingeing and vomiting the other half. Usually her binges are associated with times of high emotion and stress, for instance when she has had an argument with her parents and feels unable to assert her needs.

Katie's course is very stressful and she feels pressured by her parents' high expectations of her. She describes always feeling 'a failure' and that she is 'somehow never good enough' for her parents. She has always had a tense relationship (anger is never directly expressed) with both her parents. She perceives her father as critical and abusive and her mother as distant. As a young girl Katie often took the responsibility of caring for her younger brothers, as her parents were involved with their careers/social life.

---

### Case example 5.6   Applying a psychodynamic approach

Here is what one psychodynamic therapist suggests:

I'd need to work with Katie more to understand what is going on in her inner world. However, I could suggest what some of her unconscious issues might be. Katie's food craving could be symbolic of her craving for love. She binges to fill a need – to fill her emptiness. At the same time, it is as if stuffing food down pushes her feelings down. Bingeing is a comfort and a way to stop feeling. Alternatively, I could suggest a whole package of dynamic unconscious processes around the idea that Katie's ego is 'split' – fragmented into parts. She feels that she is 'bad' (fat, ugly, unworthy) and this is a part of her which has emerged through her 'introjecting' her parents' critical, rejecting behaviour. To handle these negative aspects (of herself/her parents) she both projects them outward (as anger) on to her 'bad' parents while she continues to punish and abuse her 'bad' self. In these ways she is trying to 'get rid of' her bad bits.

   My recommended intervention would be psychotherapy (perhaps combined with projective activities) to help her express, explore and work through her unconscious needs. She is in a depressive position, which is a result of her conflicting feelings of both love and hate for her parents. She needs to work through her sadness and grief that her parents have let her down (by 'rejecting' her).

---

### Case example 5.7   Applying a cognitive–behavioural approach

Here is what one cognitive–behavioural therapist suggests:

Katie's main problem is the bingeing-vomiting behaviour. This vicious cycle is aggravated by her distorted attitudes to weight, diet and dieting. It is important to consider the antecedents of her bingeing, i.e. what sets it off? Are there any particular associations that are relevant? It seems that she is in the habit of handling her stress by bingeing. What then are the pay-offs to her behaviour? She wouldn't continue with such destructive behaviour unless it was rewarding at some level. The fact that the bingeing is likely to have a tranquillising effect (biochemically) will be effective in distracting her from other worries and this must be considered a potential reward. Also, her weight control is clearly a big factor in her vomiting. Her fears of gaining weight become a possible negative reinforcer when combined with her distorted understanding of diet.

My recommended intervention would be some cognitive–behavioural counselling around a three-pronged strategy:

- Help Katie to examine and modify her attitudes towards food, dieting, her body, i.e. help her see that she is not fat and that she will not gain weight if she sticks to three well-balanced daily meals
- Encourage her to recognise the antecedents and pay-offs of behaviour
- Re-train new dietary habits though using a diary in which she records everything that she eats and her associated thoughts/feelings at the time. These will then be discussed weekly with her therapist. Through this exercise Katie should become more aware of triggers and the way she is using her bingeing. In the process the therapist can positively reinforce (praise) any reduction in bulimic behaviour and Katie will want to avoid publicly failing (negative reinforcement).

---

### Case example 5.8 Applying a humanistic approach

Here is what one humanistic therapist suggests:

I'm struck by the relationship Katie has with her body and with herself generally. Katie needs to 'own' her body; to accept and appreciate both her body and who she is. Firstly, in terms of her relationship with her body, I have sense that she dislikes her body partly as it doesn't fit the way she wants to be – the way she feels inside. The gap between her 'real' and 'ideal' body may also mirror the gap between the person she feels she is and the person she wants to be. Secondly, her abusive relationship with herself seems to be linked to her angry feelings, which she is turning inwards. At the same time, she seems to have a successful, attractive outer self. She needs to connect these two personas and embrace them both as being her. She feels a 'failure', yet is very successful in some ways. Perhaps she doesn't value the areas where she has been a success? So, who does she want to be? Is she simply trying to please (however unsuccessfully) her parents?

My own valuing of Katie would be an important intervention as a first stage to helping her see herself more positively. Beyond this, Katie would need to take the lead in choosing the focus and type of therapeutic intervention. It would probably involve some counselling and/or creative activities to help to encourage her to explore her sense of self and her potential. We'd start by talking through some different options. In general, I'd suggest that Katie needs to be focused on developing self-awareness about who she is and who she wants to be. It could be useful to explore her negative self-concept and the disconnection between her inner and outer selves. I could work with her using some Gestalt and/or body work techniques. A good exercise could be for her to have conversations with her different inner and outer selves. Bringing out some of the negative and critical voices in her head may help her find a way of negotiating some peace with them.

---

### Case example 5.9   Applying a social constructionist approach

Here is what one social constructionist therapist suggests:

Katie's problem needs to be seen as a society-wide, not just individual, problem. It is not a coincidence that bulimia nervosa tends to occur in women, given the impossible ideological pressures they face from media images exhorting them to be slim and attractive or else feel a failure. Katie demonstrates her positioning within a 'discourse of femininity' that privileges being slim and encourages practices related to dieting, binge eating and vomiting. The idealisation of slenderness in our society produces problematic body images in women and Katie is constituted by these discourses and discursive practices, which derogate fatness.

I'm also struck by the relationship Katie has with her parents. She seems to have taken on board her parents' critical, judgemental discourses, which say she is 'not good enough'. I wonder what stories she tells herself about this – what narratives are being embraced and acted through? How are they positioning her and how is she positioning herself? What does medical training mean to her? She seems caught between enacting the family 'success story' and being 'the failure'.

Because I see that Katie's problem is mostly related to a problem with society, I would like to see more consciousness-raising in women generally. Speaking as a feminist, I would encourage women to 'come out' about their secret and then work together to challenge the pressures of these pernicious feminine ideals. Joining a supportive women's group in general could be helpful for Katie in terms of exploring issues around being a woman, sexuality, gender roles and the pressure of expectations. On a more individual level, as a therapist, I would recommend that Katie takes part in a group for women with eating disorders. In addition to sharing and giving each other support, they could help challenge each other to look at what they are doing.

---

### Comparing and contrasting the approaches

The case study above highlights the radically different contributions the alternative approaches make, given their distinctive focus on different dimensions and their use of different therapy/research techniques. It is difficult to compare the approaches – we're not comparing like with like.

In practice, sometimes the differences between the approaches are not so clear-cut and therapists may work **eclectically and pragmatically**, dipping into the different approaches. For a start, humanistic principles underpin much of our professional philosophy while at the same time we draw on techniques from other approaches. As we can see from the case study, behavioural and cognitive–behavioural techniques often mesh well together. Similarly, a number of therapists involved in counselling would position themselves between psychodynamic and humanistic approaches, focusing on trying to understand subjective experience and relationship needs. In general terms, therapists are likely to benefit from a social constructionist awareness of language and power and an understanding of the need to be reflexive about the use and abuse of professional power.

However, there are also clear contrasts between the approaches and simply meshing them together may well result in incoherent and **contradictory interventions** in practice. For instance, a behavioural approach designed to reward 'good' behaviour is explicitly judgemental and incompatible with a therapeutic approach that seeks to be humanistically person-centred and non-judgemental. The psychodynamic preoccupation with past experience and unconscious dynamics is at odds with a humanistic focus on conscious experience and the here-and-now. The humanistic insistence on agency and choice sits uncomfortably alongside the more determinist account of social constructionism. Behaviourism developed partly as a reaction against the focus on unconscious, unobservable motives found in psychodynamic approaches, and turned attention on to behaviour that could be observed and scientifically studied. Humanistic approaches rose in reaction to both behaviourist and psychodynamic approaches, which were seen as respectively too mechanistic and too determinist. Social constructionism tends to be critical of all other approaches for being overly individualistic and also overly universalist in not attending sufficiently to the particular social contexts involved.

At some point, we need to make a choice about which approach/es (and associated assumptions and techniques) we are going to subscribe to. I'm often asked which is the best approach. Unfortunately, the answer is not that simple! Each approach has specific strengths and offers useful insights into some aspects of human development. Each has limitations in terms of its assumptions and the way it omits certain factors in its analysis. The answer to this question depends, in part, on the criteria we bring to bear. By looking closely at what each approach has to say, we can begin to work out where we ourselves stand in relation to them. They solve different problems in different ways and one may be more appropriate than another at particular times.

**The psychodynamic approach** is based on a rich, comprehensive theory that encompasses biological, psychological and social aspects of development. Later theorists sought to tackle criticisms levelled against Freud by placing people's interpersonal relationships in a broader social context. Psychodynamic interventions offer much scope for exploring inner feelings and 'buried' motivations. The dynamics underlying mental illness (e.g. traumatic childhood experience and relationships) are well described. Its abstract, unobservable, unproven assumptions, however, make the validity of psychodynamic ideas difficult to establish. Also, much of the theory and practice is based on subjective interpretation. Critics say these often reveal more about the psychoanalyst than about the client!

**The behavioural and cognitive approaches**, in contrast, offer more objective accounts of human behaviour and rely on proven, 'scientific' research evidence. Behavioural methods of treatment are effective and produce tangible results such as clear behavioural change. However, the methods can be seen as superficial as they do not tackle the underlying cause of a problem behaviour and problem behaviours often re-emerge. An unhappy/angry child may continue to be naughty (although perhaps in a different way) if one behaviour is stopped. Behaviourism is inclined to be mechanistic and focuses narrowly on small elements of behaviour, losing sight of the 'whole' person. You can teach a child a new skill, but what of his/her thoughts, feelings, motivations, to say nothing of wider social aspects? While cognitive processes have recently been given attention, the approach is still criticised for insufficiently recognising a person's lived experience and the impact of the broader social context.

**The humanistic approach** takes ideas of the lived experience and the 'whole' person very much on board. It allows for our active, reflexive capacity and our ability consciously to choose a course of action: humans are not viewed as being at the mercy of internal or external drives. However, all the other perspectives would hotly debate the notion that humans are completely free agents. The humanistic approach remains vague and excessively individualistic. While occupational therapists tend to embrace its philosophy, its therapy methods (e.g. unconditional positive regard) can be unrealistic and insufficiently focused.

The strength of **social constructionism** is as an analytical tool. It offers an analysis of both macro-social forces (attending to social structure and ideology) and micro-social interactions (dialogue between individuals). It provides a strong, critical argument about the role of language shaping both individuals and society. While social constructionism can identify wider social processes at work (e.g. racial and gender divisions in society), their precise influence on individuals cannot be predicted. Although discourse analysis offers us a valuable qualitative research tool, it is primarily a tool for academic analysis rather than a specific therapeutic tool/technique we can apply in practice.

## Deciding which approach to use

In practice our choice of approach is guided by many factors including:

- **The team** – Some units work eclectically (combining approaches), while others have an explicit bias. For instance, a psychotherapy unit will privilege psychodynamic approaches. While it might be useful to offer a contrasting approach within the team, it may be important to be consistent. Suppose, for example, we work in a children's unit that operates on cognitive–behavioural lines. It could be very confusing for the child to receive mixed messages if some team members tolerate a certain behaviour and others don't. To some extent, this could be resolved if the team were explicit that certain treatment sessions (perhaps their free play session) were exempt. But everyone would need to be clear about this arrangement so they could reinforce this message to the child.
- **Practical constraints** – The environment, staffing resources and time available all constrain and determine what interventions are possible. For instance, if we are only going to be able to see a service user a few times, a cognitive–behavioural approach would probably be the appropriate choice.
- **Our own competence** – While we have the training to loosely apply the ideas from all the approaches, there are certain specific approaches and techniques

that are possibly beyond our professional competence without extra training, experience and support.

- **Personal preference** – It is important that we believe in our chosen approach. A half-hearted attempt to apply an approach will be unconvincing and probably ineffective. Our confidence in an approach or technique will communicate itself to our service users and should help inspire their own confidence that they will be helped.
- **Service user's needs** – Ultimately, we must choose an approach to suit individual service users. It needs to be one that the person will accept and one that suits their problem area and needs. Where a problem looks to have a relatively straightforward behaviour or skill element (e.g. managing anxiety or learning how to cook), a cognitive–behavioural approach may be best. Where a problem appears to be more long-standing and resists easy solutions, then a longer-term psychodynamic intervention might be more effective. Where the problem seems related to low self esteem, lack of confidence and confused feelings generally, then the humanistic approach comes into its own. In practice, we select the approach that appears to be most useful and effective given our resources, the particular situation, the person, their problems and their needs.

## 5.7 CONCLUSION AND REFLECTIONS

In this chapter, we have discussed the key concepts and practical applications of five psychological approaches: psychodynamic, behavioural, cognitive, humanistic and social constructionist (Table 5.1). I have tried to show the profound influence of theory – in terms both of how we understand problems and of how we apply theory in our interventions. I hope, too, that I have revealed something of the challenges, as well as pleasures, of theoretical debate. Some people find it frustrating that there is no clear-cut answer to the question of which approach is best. But the uncertainty and rich possibilities that we face every time we engage someone in treatment based on a particular theory is something that I, for my part, find endlessly fascinating.

Our awareness of *competing* perspectives – that there are alternative approaches even – acts as a continuing challenge to the approaches and practice we favour. Whatever choice of approach we make as therapists, it must be an informed one. We have a professional responsibility to try to grasp the logic, strengths and weaknesses of different theoretical approaches if we are to develop, and implement, a coherent treatment programme. If such a programme proves unworkable, or ineffective, our understanding of theory places us in a better position to make the necessary changes. And having an overall grasp of theory – with all the contrasts as well as similarities involved – helps us communicate more effectively with our team colleagues. A good grasp of theory enables us to evaluate, and challenge, every aspect of our therapeutic practice.

*Table 5.1*  Summary of five psychological approaches and their application

| Theory | Key concepts | Focus of assessment | Treatment/intervention |
|---|---|---|---|
| **Psychodynamic** | Dynamic, defensive unconscious; ways of relating linked to patterns laid down in childhood; internally represented version of others | Person's inner world of unconscious needs, drives and emotions; use of defence mechanisms | Projective activities; psychotherapy; use of transference within the therapeutic relationship |
| **Behavioural** | Learning and skills; the role of reinforcement | Observable behaviour including habits, interactions and skill levels | Behavioural modification (shaping, contracts, rewards); systematic desensitisation |
| **Cognitive** | Skills; patterns of thinking; cognitive development | Cognitive-perceptual functioning; distortions of thinking | Cognitive–behavioural techniques, e.g. cognitive restructuring; cognitive therapy; rational emotive therapy |
| **Humanistic** | Personal growth; agency; lived experience; flow; self-concept and awareness | Consciousness; subjective feelings, needs and experience; embodied self-identity and relations with others | Creative activities; gestalt therapy; non-directive, client-centred counselling; unconditional positive regard |
| **Social constructionist** | The role of language and discourse; the role played by power relations; multiple and negotiated identities | Critically analysing everyday discourses, discursive practices and narratives | Discourse analysis; reflexive approach examining power and inequalities |

# PART TWO

# OCCUPATIONAL THERAPY PROCESS

# 6 THE THERAPEUTIC RELATIONSHIP

*In the beginning was the relationship.*

Martin Buber

Our brand of healing is not to be equated with merely aiming to increase a person's skills. Instead, patients and clients 'must be addressed, reached, even changed in some inner way' (Mattingly, 1998, p. 168). That change is enabled through the relationship we build with the individual. The process of negotiating such therapeutic alliances is the biggest, and most important, challenge we face. Experiencing such relationships, particularly when they unfold positively, makes therapy meaningful and rewarding – both for our service users and for ourselves. The therapist–client relationship is fundamental to, and at the core of, occupational therapy practice (Peloquin,1993; Schwartzberg, 2002).

Case example 6.1 shows the impact of a therapist's approach on the course of treatment. In this case, the therapist takes a simple, natural and sympathetic approach to Les, encouraging him to participate in an open evaluation of his position. She remains open to the possibility, too, that Les might indeed be able to stay at home – at least for the time being. She is sensitive to Les's needs. Through her empathetic presence, she enables Les to feel a little safer. Clarifying and validating his position, she is able to build his trust and to begin engaging him in a more extended treatment process. By respecting his capacity to make appropriate decisions in his own time, she invites him to collaborate in a therapeutic partnership. Without such care, Les is unlikely to want to acknowledge his difficulties, let alone do anything about them.

---

### Case example 6.1   Impact of the therapist's approach

Les is a 66-year-old obese man who has been admitted to a Cardiac Intensive Care Unit. He is belligerent and aggressive in his behaviour. He has been referred to the occupational therapist as there are concerns about his ability to take care of himself once he is home. His family would like him to move to sheltered accommodation but he is resistant, asserting that he wants to live his own life and to be independent in his own home.

Adopting a person-centred approach, the occupational therapist acknowledges his need to feel independent and to stay in his own home. She agrees that the starting point is to look at his home situation and environment and at all the different options for what can be done to ensure he can stay there. 'Once you are clear about the different options,' she says, 'you'll be able to make an informed decision about what

---

you want to do.' Les is mollified and appreciates the logic of this approach. He agrees to work further with the occupational therapist.

Having established a degree of trust with Les, the occupational therapist goes a bit deeper. She empathises with how 'scary' it must feel to have his heart problems and not to feel in control of what is happening to him now and in the future. Her treatment approach explicitly aims to try to give him back some sense of control. She believes that Les will eventually decide that sheltered accommodation may be the best solution. He needs, however, to come to this conclusion in his own time.

This chapter aims to explore something of the many profound, subtle and complex elements that comprise the therapeutic relationship. I approach the topic from four different angles, exploring in turn:

- The evolving relationship
- Relationship skills
- Conscious use of self
- Care, power, collaboration.

The first section recognises that relationships evolve over time and vary in their degree of intensity. Different stages are outlined, from 'engaging the person in therapy', to 'negotiating and collaborating' and finally to 'letting go'. The second section describes ten dimensions of relationship skills that therapists aim to develop and apply in their work. The third section examines ways in which we are strategic in our interactions and consciously use ourselves as therapeutic tools. The final section offers a review of research that highlights the ways in which we enact care, power and collaboration in therapeutic relationships. The four sections approach the topic of therapeutic relationships in such different ways that I recommend that you 'dip in' where your impulse takes you.

## 6.1   THE EVOLVING RELATIONSHIP

Relationships develop during a process of mutual interaction which occurs over time and in particular contexts. Relationships evolve as we *engage* service users in treatment, *negotiate and collaborate* with them, and then *let go*.

### Engaging a person in therapy

The most important moments in the course of therapy are often those fragile first steps we take in the early stages of negotiating interventions. Here, the individual – potentially distressed, disturbed or damaged – has to take the challenging step to actively work with the therapist and in their own therapy. This process is frequently made more difficult as the nature of the person's psychosocial problems means that they tend to lack motivation, hope, interest, drive, to say nothing of having limited coping skills. On top of this, the person may well feel anxious about their illness and situation, and even have fears of dealing with 'a therapist'. The therapist, in turn, has to gain the person's trust and inspire confidence in the treatment, often in the face of a certain degree of hopelessness. The therapist, as part of ensuring that the therapeutic experience is meaningful, needs to *engage* the individual in their treatment.

The following four case examples offer a glimpse of the complex relationship dynamics involved when we engage someone in treatment. Although you are only being presented with snippets of dialogue, you'll hopefully be able to set these in broader contexts.

---

### Case example 6.2 Rosie

Rosie, a 76-year-old women being assessed for dementia, belligerently tells her occupational therapist that she does not want to cook scones and that she does not want to do occupational therapy. The therapist nods an acknowledgement and with a gentle smile says, 'Shall we just sit then and chat while we have a cup of tea?'

Rosie agrees. After a while she begins to share how she has spent many years baking for her husband, children and grandchildren. Being diabetic, she has never eaten what she baked. 'I guess you've made enough scones to last a lifetime', the therapist responds. 'Perhaps it is time for you to do some cooking purely for yourself?'

Rosie's eyes fill with tears. 'Its difficult to do things for yourself when you never have. And now I'm so hopeless and forgetful it's too late.'

'I don't agree, Rosie. Why not start today? Is there anything you can think of that you'd like to learn to cook and then would enjoy eating?' the therapist asks. After a rummage through the kitchen cabinets and some negotiation, Rosie happily settles down to make a salmon mousse.

---

### Case example 6.3 Cara

Cara is a profoundly and multiply handicapped child who spends most of her day rocking and gazing blankly into space. The occupational therapist works to find a point of contact. On their first meeting the therapist notices that Cara's attention is momentarily caught by the jingling noise the therapist's shiny silver and glass bangles are making. The therapist deliberately jingles her bangles again, which elicits a small smile from Cara. She reaches out to touch them. For the next five minutes, the therapist and Cara play with these bangles. The therapist encourages her to touch them, play with them, put them on. Everyday thereafter, the therapist begins Cara's treatment session by making a connection through the bangles.

---

---

**Case example 6.4   Sanjeev**

Sanjeev has been admitted to hospital with a diagnosis of schizophrenia. He is severely withdrawn and appears locked in his own world. The therapist comes to sit with him for a few minutes each day. She speaks gently to him and does not push for a reply. For instance, one morning she says, 'Hello Sanjeev. Did you know that today is Diwali? I went to a Diwali party last year. I really loved all those beautiful fireworks and the wonderful hospitality shown. You've probably been to many great parties around Diwali. When you feel ready to, maybe you can tell me about them.' After a pause she adds, 'I understand that you just want to sit quietly today.'

After several days of trying to make contact verbally (and getting no response) the therapist brings along a small sketch pad and pastel crayons, doodling as she talks. She puts some paper and crayons in front of Sanjeev. On the third day, he tentatively reaches for a crayon and begins to create a picture. This moment begins a long-term therapeutic process whereby Sanjeev uses art to explore some of the disturbing images and thoughts he experiences.

---

**Case example 6.5   Niall**

Niall has just started to attend a woodwork class in an occupational therapy outpatient unit as part of an early 'work hardening' programme. He has been off sick, out of work, for seven months. Now, as part of his therapy, he is trying to push himself to sustain concentration and his activity level for four hours a day. He starts by making a picture frame, which he is currently sanding and polishing. As the therapist observes Niall's work, he points out an area that has been missed. 'Come on Niall', he cajoles. 'This is a bit shoddy here. I'm sure you want to do a good job or you're not going to feel proud of what you've made. Just ten more minutes, let's see you give it an extra push.' After 10 minutes of 'extra effort', Niall is pleased with the result and gives the therapist a rueful nod of acknowledgement and respect.

---

In Case example 6.2 we see the way in which the therapist tries actively to understand Rosie's experience and needs. It is important for the cooking activity to be meaningful to Rosie if she is going to be motivated to engage in the activity. The therapist's skill lies in being alert to that motivation and finding a way of adapting the activity to suit.

Mattingly (1998, p. 76) notes, 'Therapists make an extraordinary effort to talk with patients, to find some way of making contact.' This can be seen most clearly in Case examples 6.3 and 6.4.

In Case example 6.3, we witness something of the challenge of working with people who have profound handicaps. While the connection made through the bangles is serendipitous, the therapist is open to the slightest possibility of contact. She is alert to Cara's non-verbal cues, which suggested some interest.

She does not push Cara to relate directly to her, instead letting Cara set the pace. Similar lessons can be drawn from the example of Sanjeev in Case example 6.4. Here, the therapist is careful to not push for a response. Instead, she waits until Sanjeev is ready. At the same time, she offers him different opportunities to communicate, both verbal and non-verbal. The use of drawing as an activity is an effective vehicle for both building the relationship and giving Sanjeev a way to express himself.

The example in Case example 6.5 provides direct contrast. The therapist is more directive and critical as he pushes Niall to perform to a higher standard. The therapist communicates the fact that he has higher expectations of Niall, something to which Niall responds positively. That Niall also recognises that he is being challenged as part of a work rehabilitation programme is important.

## Negotiating and collaborating

All therapeutic interventions are characterised by the dynamic interaction that takes place between therapist and client. They are engaged in a process of constant, mutual negotiation and collaboration. The therapist strives to engage and understand the client and collaborate in their project and life decisions; clients participate and share themselves, and collaborate in treatment decisions. As the therapist pushes, the client may choose to resist or to rise to the challenge. Together, they manoeuvre to find a way forward. This is the basis of **interactive clinical reasoning** (Schwartzberg, 2002).

Because our brand of therapy usually requires active co-operation and collaboration from service users, therapists need service users to have a stake in their therapy and to incorporate the process into their own lives. As Mattingly (1998) explains, 'Therapists work to create significant experiences for their patients because if therapy is to be effective, therapists must find a way to make the therapeutic process matter to the patient, to make it meaningful' (Mattingly, 1998, p. 82).

Mattingly is referring here to the need for both patient and therapist to be committed to the therapeutic process, sharing a view about why engaging in particular activities makes sense and also about different possible futures. We respect service users' right to own their treatment and choose what future path to take. The process of coming to share the same therapeutic story involves complex negotiation and collaboration that occurs over time. The narratives in Case examples 6.6 and 6.7 illustrates something of this.

---

**Case example 6.6   Joining the world again – Jani's story**

I was feeling overwhelmed with my life. The turning point was when I started to see the therapist. I was depressed and anxious and felt I couldn't cope. I had stopped going out unless I absolutely had to, like to collect my benefits. It was really weird. It was like I became scared of just meeting people. It was easier to stay at home and to just watch TV all day. I had just 'shut down', my therapist said. She came to see

---

me once a week for counselling. She was very gentle and patient with me. I was such a wimp! She encouraged me to slowly start going outside. First, she'd walk with me to the local park. We'd just sit and talk for a bit and then go home. At other times she went shopping with me. Once we went to [a big supermarket] on the outskirts of town. I really enjoyed that. I had been using the Net for all my shopping and I'd forgotten how much I enjoy going around that superstore. Of course it was a lot harder when she made me go out by myself. Well, she didn't 'make' me exactly. We talked about it and I could see the point. It was like I was in a bad habit of isolating myself and I needed to teach myself to join the world again. The therapy was, sort of, all about leading me to the water, but I had to do the drinking.

In Jani's story, we can see that the therapist had an important role, being both a supporter and encourager. It was important that Jani understood the point and nature of her graded desensitisation programme. It seems that one significant step was to go to the big supermarket. This intervention worked as the therapist cued into Jani's previous interests. Together they had negotiated a meaningful treatment.

Such an intervention would be consistent with all the occupational therapy models described in Chapter 3. In fact, this therapist had employed the model of human occupation. The therapist focused on Jani's **volition** by taking care to understand Jani's values and what she would find satisfying and enjoyable. The concepts of **habituation** led the therapist to encourage Jani to restructure her daily habits by getting Jani out into different **environments**.

In the model of human occupation, the therapeutic relationship is seen to *support* the client's occupational engagement and change rather than being the primary dynamic of change. This view contrasts with the psychodynamic perspective, which would argue for *the primacy of the relationship*. Case example 6.7 offers a narrative more along these lines.

---

**Case example 6.7   The evolving relationship with my therapist – Susie's story**

My memories of my therapy early on are quite blurry. I just remember my therapist being there. She was like a rock. Sometimes we wouldn't even speak but she'd be sitting beside me and somehow I knew it would be all right. She'd keep me safe. I remember sometimes wishing she had been my mother – she was so warm and loving. She would hug me sometimes. Although I'd pull away, I really wanted to have the hug go on, to let my inhibitions go.

She would often come to sit next to me as I was learning to do my macramé and other crafts. She would gently show me and laugh at my fumbling when I made mistakes. And I didn't mind. As long as she stayed there with me, I was okay. Sometimes she had to go see to other patients and she left me alone. It was like the world went dark. Once I even had a panic attack. She talked to me then about the importance of being able to cope when she wasn't there. She got me to visualise

---

her safe presence and to hear the kinds of comments she always made. Then she said, 'No one can take that away. Part of me is always with you.'

Then I remember she was there in the group – a little further away but still my rock. I would watch for the little encouraging smiles she'd give me. Slowly I found myself being with others as we did different activities. It was as if I didn't need her so much, others were there. That was when I began to talk and laugh again.

I remember later when I was heaps better that I'd only be able to see her once every week or so for a 'catch-up' session. I'd save up stories through the week to tell her. I'd ask her opinion about things. She would often just smile that smile and ask me what I thought or how well I felt I had handled something. At first, I felt quite angry with her not giving me what I wanted. I eventually got the message: what she thought was not important. What was important was me. It was my life and I had to live it.

It seems strange that I haven't seen her for two years. I still feel sometimes that she is right here.

Here, Susie describes a long-standing and evolving relationship with her therapist. Underneath the references to working collaboratively on activities, we gain a sense of how they negotiated their relationship over time, with the therapist slowly guiding Susie through stages of dependence, attachment and autonomy. In psychodynamic terms, it seems that Susie may well have experienced some transference feelings, particularly wanting the therapist to be her 'mother'. Together, they had to work through Susie becoming too needy, investing too heavily in the therapeutic relationship. These themes are followed through in the final stage of the relationship: letting go.

## Letting go

Susie's story reminds us that the process of ending relationships can be as critical and as complex as beginnings. Therapists need to take care of how they withdraw from the therapeutic relationship and how they enable clients to disengage from therapy.

Ending therapy means stopping, separating and leaving. If the therapy has become important – if the individual has a substantial investment in the experience – then they will feel the loss acutely. Some people may try to resist ending (by asking for more time or producing 'new' problems); others may try to rush or avoid the ending altogether (e.g. by not turning up to sessions). Feelings of hurt, anger or rejection associated with losing the therapist may arise and may resonate with earlier separations. A special opportunity is then offered to recapture and work through these emotions. The therapist may have to 'hold' the feelings, allowing grief, anger and fears to be expressed, and accept them as part of a process. The individual needs the time and opportunity to talk through what this and other endings mean. The therapist, too, perhaps in supervision, needs to acknowledge losses. As part of exploring how to move on, both client and therapist need to anticipate ways in which they will feel distressed and relieved, acknowledging things they'll miss the most and the least.

Exactly how the process of letting go is negotiated varies considerably. Primarily, it depends on the type of the relationship and the depth of involvement in the first place. Many of our interactions with patients and clients will be time-limited and fairly focused; the process of letting go occurs almost from the beginning and is less of an issue. Sometimes all that is needed is to offer a 'safety net', for instance offering a follow-up appointment a month after discharge or letting the person know they can get back into contact should they feel the need in the future.

In longer-term relationships, the process needs to be more carefully considered, even orchestrated. When a long-standing group is wound up, many of the group's activities are likely to centre on 'endings' and 'leavings' or doing various 'recap and review' activities. For instance, group members might be asked to think back to when they first started in the group and to reminisce. Group members might give each other either real or imaginary 'leaving presents' or they might choose to have a group 'goodbye lunch'. Activities such as these can help by offering some rituals to mark and celebrate a 'passage' while also acknowledging the inevitable pain of loss.

Mattingly (1998, p. 82) reminds us:

> *Therapists are with patients only a short time, often a few weeks or less. They might teach a few skills ... but generally their effectiveness depended on using therapy as a catalyst to help patients begin to see how they might 'do for himself' even when the therapist was no longer there.*

## 6.2   RELATIONSHIP SKILLS

Every relationship has its unique qualities and the therapeutic relationship is no exception. Individual therapists and clients will negotiate their relationship to suit their needs and the demands of the situation. That does not mean, however, that therapists are without guidelines for developing relationship skills. Both the literature and reported experiences from therapy practice suggest that certain behaviours, attitudes, skills and qualities of the therapist can be helpful in enhancing positive relationships that enable another's growth.

This section discusses 10 overlapping dimensions (Theory into practice 6.1) of these 'relationship skills'. Rather than being prescriptive, I offer this list to suggest a direction toward which we might strive. How, and to what extent, we each enact these skills will vary according to our personal styles and the broader situation involved.

---

**Theory into practice 6.1**———————————————————

**Ten dimensions of relationship skills**

- Listening actively
- Communicating empathy

---

- Being caring
- Holding and communicating safety
- Showing respect
- Conveying warmth
- Enabling and empowering
- Clarifying meaning
- Inspiring hope and confidence
- Being reflexive and self-aware.

## Listening actively

The skill of listening actively involves tuning into – trying to hear and absorb – what the person is saying. It requires us to have a genuine interest in the other as we seek to understand something of their experience. Its also about giving the person time to try and find a way to express what they want or need to say. In listening actively, we are called to attend to the nature of experiences the individual has, such as their experience of disability. At the same time we are striving to understand the story the individual is living in which they are making sense of life. Active listening involves first observing and interpreting the client's non-verbal behaviour and then listening to and interpreting the verbal messages (Egan, 1982).

The value of listening is summed up by the anonymous poem entitled 'Listen' (cited in Bauer and Hall, 1986).

*When I ask you to listen to me*
*and you start giving advice*
*you have not done what I asked.*

*When I ask you to listen to me*
*and you begin to tell me why I shouldn't feel that way*
*you are trampling on my feelings.*

*When I ask you to listen to me*
*and you feel you have to do something to solve my problem*
*you have failed me, strange as that may seem.*

*When you do something for me that I can and need to do*
*for myself, you contribute to my fear and weakness.*

*So please listen and just hear me*
*and if you want to talk, wait a minute for your turn; and I'll listen to you.*

## Communicating empathy

Empathy involves achieving an understanding of another person's world from their perspective (Peloquin, 1995). It is a *felt* experience. For instance, when working with someone who flinches in sudden extreme pain, we might find ourselves unconsciously flinching as well. The skill involved is in signalling this understanding through our body language and what we say and do. Empathy is not the same as sympathy – the person may not even want our sympathy. They may, for example, want to be handled in a business-like, unemotional manner. Being empathetic, we would respect this and work from there. Sometimes it can be difficult to grasp another's world when it is different from our own or when the person is paranoid, chaotic or filled with delusion. At such times, we might need to work harder to let go of our assumptions and to keep focused on the other's perspective.

## Being caring

Care is generally agreed to include both 'caring for' and 'caring about'. In other words, the skill involves both the *doing* of caring and the *feeling* of caring. 'To care means to be affected just as surely as it means to affect' (Yerxa, 1967, p. 8). Care is demonstrated when we seek to respond to an individual's particular needs, preferences and circumstances. Case example 6.8 contains an illustration taken from a chapter by Brechin (2000). The staff in this unit set up 'to care' may have been caring in the way they continued to try to give care in the face of Hanif's abuse. They had, however, forgotten to care in terms of respecting his individuality.

---

### Case example 6.8   Thoughtless practice – forgetting to care

Hanif, a 14-year old Asian boy with learning disabilities, was diagnosed as being 'autistic' with 'challenging behaviours' and was placed in a 'special' unit for young people with challenging behaviours. He became increasingly disturbed. He began to throw his food away and would also make attempts to get into the kitchen and throw things about in there as well. All the white staff had assumed he was 'too disabled' to have any concept of his race, culture, religion or diet and no provision for these issues was made in his care at the unit, although his parents were devout Hindus and had always encouraged Hanif to participate in prayers and attend festivals. An Asian visitor immediately attracted the boy's attention and, when he was offered an Indian snack, he accepted it without a fuss.

Brechin, 2000, p. 146

---

## Showing respect

To respect another means to genuinely value that person – their identity, dignity, privacy and feelings in general. We show our respect by acknowledging the person's uniqueness and perspective, by believing in their capacity to choose and by accepting their choices. Sometimes the simplest of actions, such as using the person's preferred name, can communicate this. Conveying respect also involves accepting and valuing the person's particular cultural and religious beliefs, no matter how much at odds to our own they may be. Case example 6.8 shows how care and respect go hand in hand.

Respect is also shown in the way that we handle confidences and are mindful of our privileged position. Respecting confidentiality is a specific value enshrined in our professional codes of practice (e.g. in *Standards of Conduct, Performance and Ethics*, Health Professions Council, 2003).

## Conveying warmth

The value of warmth came home to me one day when a client turned round to say, 'I feel so cold, hopeless and dead inside. Coming to therapy is like being warmed by a fire.'

The warmth we display within relationships needs to be genuine. It is conveyed through our smile, eyes, tone of voice, a touch of a hand, a hug, and so on. We show our warmth by responding spontaneously, and perhaps playfully, with humour and charm. 'There is nothing worse than a therapist who lacks a sense of humour!' (Mosey, 1986, p. 202).

## 'Holding' and communicating safety

'Holding' refers to the way that therapists aim to communicate to service users that they are emotionally (and perhaps physically) safe. For instance, if the therapist can stay calm and solid in the face of an individual's turmoil and fear, then that person is likely to feel safer too. The therapist's skill is in being able to communicate strength, acceptance and quiet confidence.

Kitwood (1997, p. 91) describes the concept of 'holding' beautifully:

> To hold, in a psychological sense, means to provide a safe psychological space, a 'container'; here hidden trauma and conflict can be brought out; areas of extreme vulnerability exposed. When the holding is secure a person can know, in experience, that devastating emotions such as abject terror or overwhelming grief will pass, and not cause the psyche to disintegrate. Even violent anger or destructive rage, directed for a while at the person who is doing the holding, will not drive that person away. As in the case of childcare, psychological holding in any context may involve physical holding too.

## Enabling and empowering

We enable and empower by collaborating with service users and through believing in, and respecting, their resources to heal themselves. Enabling their growth and independence, we may help them to feel empowered. The reverse also applies – being pessimistic or having low expectations can be disempowering (Research example 6.1). The skill of enabling and empowering another involves validating what they say, i.e. accepting the power and subjective truth of the other's experience. At the same time, we have a role to not *over*-support and to encourage others to do more or, perhaps, to do it better. Here, we enable and empower by constructively giving feedback, probing, offering suggestions and advice, and confronting denial and challenging games. Kielhofner and Forsyth

(2002), for instance, outline nine therapeutic strategies to enable clients' occupational engagement. These enabling strategies include advising, coaching and encouraging towards both enhancing skill and influencing volition.

---

### Research example 6.1

#### Depersonalising tendencies

In his research on caring for people with dementia, the geriatrician Kitwood (1997, pp. 46–49) identifies the danger of carers' profound pessimism and helplessness. He describes how, at its worst, individuals being cared for can become invisible. He offers a list of 'depersonalising tendencies' (i.e. behaviours that strip away an individual's persona) for carers to guard against. These include:

- **Disempowerment** – not letting a person use abilities they have; failing to help them do so
- **Disparagement** – Giving messages that are damaging to self-esteem
- **Mockery** – Making fun of, teasing, making jokes at their expense
- **Stigmatisation** – Treating a person like an alien or outcast
- **Treachery** – Using deception to achieve compliance
- **Withholding**– Refusing attention or refusing to meet needs.

---

## Clarifying meaning

The skill of clarifying meaning involves being able to reflect back accurately what has been said and being able to check out whether you have understood what the person meant to say. Paraphrasing, i.e. being able to capture the essence of what someone has said using different words, demonstrates that you have been listening. At the same time it enables the other person to clarify their own thoughts and feelings. Its about creating space to allow the person to come to their own understandings. 'Meaning arises at the intersections of the two worlds', say Cara and MacRae (1998, p. 13). Here, they are reminding us about the *intersubjective* nature of our relationships. Meanings are created through interactions, by both the people involved, as they continually influence, and react to, each other.

## Inspiring hope and confidence

It is a real skill to be able to offer someone hope and to enable them to feel more positive and confident about themselves and their future. Often it means encouraging a person to see things and themselves in a different way. In particular, we have a special role to play in offering a different vision of the future.

Offering this kind of hope can be a powerful motivator. Research has shown that, if staff have limited hope, so too will service users. It is hard to hang on to dreams in the face of pessimism and negativity (Repper *et al.*, 1998).

Helping someone feel more positive about themselves is achieved through accepting and validating what they say. At the same time it also means having expectations that they might be able to do or be more. It is not about bolstering people uncritically and always being unconditionally positive. Such responses are invariably perceived as ungenuine, if not downright condescending. If our aim is to help someone be *realistic* about their abilities, we need to incorporate such realistic assessment into our own approach.

Hope can also come from other service users. It can be very powerful to see a person who has had problems similar to your own find a way of coping effectively. Yalom (1975) suggests that group therapists should exploit this process by having group members at different stages of the 'coping–collapse continuum' and by calling attention to improvements individuals have made.

## Being reflexive and self-aware

Perhaps the most important skill of all is being able to be reflexive (i.e. to self-reflect and be self-aware). Being reflexive is about being sufficiently aware of one's strengths, weaknesses, limits and capacities. If we are to draw on ourselves as 'therapeutic tools', we need to understand our goals, needs and potential blockages. We need to be able to analyse, for instance, the impact of our emotions and any unconscious transferences or counter-transferences we might experience in our relating. We need to be aware of the impact of our behaviour on others and be sensitive to the way relationships are mutually negotiated. As part of all this, we have an ethical responsibility to be alert to the potential use (and abuse) of our professional power. Here, we can demonstrate reflexivity by challenging and resisting disempowering social practices and by engaging in strategies that empower others. We can only do this if we remain open and are prepared to be self-critical (Finlay and Gough, 2003).

To summarise, the 10 interlinked dimensions described above offer us some guidelines about the directions in which we might develop our relationship skills. In practice, these relationship skills are applied holistically and fluidly rather than mechanically. In practice, the 10 dimensions usually overlap, as Theory into practice 6.2 demonstrates. In this example a therapist aims to engage the individual in some kind of 'doing' – something therapists do routinely. The therapist here seeks to engage the reluctant Suli by first showing that he empathises with, and understand something of, her experience. He then talks through her options, drawing on various metaphors/images to which she can relate. Through this process he demonstrates some respect, warmth and caring. The therapist shows his confidence in Suli's progress and this inspires her to hope that she might soon begin to feel different. Suli clearly gains enough in that week to motivate her to continue treatment, or at least to feel safe enough to try.

---

*Theory into practice 6.2*_____

**The use of relationship skills: engaging an individual in treatment**

Suli is depressed and reluctant to do anything. The therapist explains his view that Suli is in a vicious cycle of inactivity which is making her feel worse. If she could begin to do 'a little something' each day, he advises, she would find that a change would come about.

Suli disagrees. 'Nothing is going to make a difference. You don't understand!'

'You're right, I can't understand exactly how you feel but I think I can understand a bit of what you may be experiencing. I wonder if it's like you're at the bottom of a deep black hole and you're so far down you can't see any light'. Suli nods slowly, somewhat surprised that the therapist could describe it so well. 'There's only one direction to climb, Suli and that's up.' He continues. 'You've got to move and see if you can find the light again.'

After a pause, the therapist suggests, 'How about giving my way a chance? After all, it might work. Just try it for a week.' The therapist goes on to suggest a few different options.

'What do you want me to do?' she capitulates.

'You need to try to do one concrete thing a day where you force yourself to go out and mix with people.'

Suli and the therapist then plan some activities for Suli to do. The therapist visits Suli daily to help her reflect on her experiences. Together they begin to build a picture of the sorts of thing Suli finds helpful. At the end of the week Suli asks to continue seeing the therapist.

---

## 6.3 CONSCIOUS USE OF SELF

### Adapting our approach

Conscious use of self refers to the deliberate use of mind and body. It refers to the decisions we take about how to present ourselves and approach our patients and clients. It refers to the way we communicate and engage individuals in therapy.

'Conscious use of self', states Mosey (1986, p. 199), 'is the use of oneself in such a way that one becomes an effective tool' used in therapeutic interventions. It is a skill to be employed alongside other personal qualities. The two case studies in Case example 6.9 demonstrate this skill. In both, the therapist is strategic and makes a conscious decision about how best to approach, and respond to, the individual. Jennifer's therapist is concerned to validate and be non-judgemental while not colluding with Jennifer's excessively negative self-image. Rowena's therapist settles on a more practical, directive, problem-solving approach. Importantly, although they take different approaches, both therapists aim to respond with empathy and sensitivity to the individuals concerned. The therapists use their responses to make an intervention – they are, in effect, using *themselves* as therapeutic tools.

---

**Case example 6.9   Approaching different individuals**

Jennifer says she feels fat, ugly and horrible. She is in fact attractive and has much to offer. Her therapist thinks through how she should handle this:

*I don't think Jennifer wants reassurance here. She may find it useful to hear me state the reality as I see it. Yet I suspect she isn't going to be able to take any compliments on board. Anyway, if I entered into evaluation (however positive) I would give off messages that I am judging her. Her perception is what is important. So my approach will be to acknowledge her poor self-image and focus on trying to change her negative thinking.*

Rowena says she feels dowdy and horrible after two weeks in hospital. Her therapist decides that a practical response is needed. She confirms that it is the hospital stay that is bringing Rowena down. They then discuss what might counteract the effects. Rowena settles on spending an afternoon at the hairdresser's when she goes home at the weekend. In the meantime, she takes up the therapist's suggestion of putting on some make-up.

---

Theory into practice 6.3 suggests some general strategies for how to approach people who present in different ways. At the same time, our approach is guided by the individual. Does the individual respond best when we are gentle? Forceful? Humorous? Directive? Demanding? Consoling? What role should we play? Are we a teacher/advice giver?, a supporter/facilitator?, a psychotherapist?, an equipment supplier?, a model? ... the list goes on.

---

**Theory into practice 6.3**

**Approaching different people**

**An anxious person**

Genuine reassurance given in a quiet, calm manner should be the main strategy used. Also valuable is our use of any 'relaxing', absorbing (thus diverting) activity, if the person can be persuaded to join in. The key decision to make is whether he or she will benefit most from an undemanding or structured environment. The person may appreciate being free to settle when ready or they may need the security of an external structure where the onus for any decision-making is removed.

---

### A suspicious/deluded person

Two basic rules of thumb apply here:

- Try to keep the conversation or activity on a concrete, straightforward plane
- Avoid getting locked into circular discussions in an attempt to reason the person out of his or her beliefs.

An initial clear explanation about the situation is important (e.g. 'The way I see it is … '), but it is unlikely to help to keep repeating your view. Diversionary tactics may work, such as: 'Before we talk more about that, can you try to concentrate on this activity for a few minutes?' Another possible strategy is to empathise with what is 'real', e.g. not responding to the person's fear of 'outer space electricity' but responding to their fear. With some individuals, it might be best to simply accept the delusion or hallucination and just move on.

### A potentially suicidal person

The highly emotive issue of potential suicide can only be handled if we take threats seriously and try to minimise our own value judgements (and advice as to why he or she should live). When faced with a person expressing a wish to die, our best role is to listen and allow them to express the tensions that have led to this point. Any suicidal person should be carefully monitored by the team, using general precautions (e.g. not leaving the person alone, removing scissors) as necessary. An actively suicidal person shouldn't be in a group unless there are adequate staff resources to give one-to-one attention if necessary.

### A confused, disorientated person

Reassurance, routine, repetition and structure are the important elements here. The person's daily programme and environment should be well organised and consistent. Devices such as written timetables and clear signposts are helpful, especially when combined with the human touch, where the therapist gently and clearly repeats basic information. At times it may be appropriate to focus on the here-and-now, for example enjoying moments of interaction rather than always seeking to 'correct and orientate' the person. As with any management strategy, this approach is most successful when applied consistently by the team.

### An aggressive person

Possibly the most difficult aspect of coping with verbal or physical aggression is controlling our own reactions to violence. In most circumstances the therapist needs to set and maintain clear, consistent limits on what is acceptable, and enforce them when necessary (telling the person to leave the group). If there is no physical danger to anyone at stake (e.g. if the aggression is confined to verbal abuse), the situation should be handled in a calm, matter-of-fact way designed to diffuse rather than provoke. The three A's might be useful here: **Acknowledge** the anger; **Agree** where possible; **Apologise** if appropriate. If physical violence occurs, it needs to be dealt with immediately, so be clear about your unit's policy/procedures. While we must try to ensure the safety of all patients/clients, we also have a right to keep ourselves free from physical harm. The team is an important support when any of us suffer from the understandable stress responses that tend to follow violent incidents.

Our conscious use of self involves more than just finding the 'right' approach, however. Crucially, the key is how we modify and *adapt* our role as treatment progresses. In rehabilitation, for example, we often *grade* our expectations by increasing service users' autonomy and opportunities for independence. At the same time we try to reduce the amount of support and direction we offer as we hand over responsibility to the service user.

In psychotherapy (to give another example), much thought and care is given to managing dependency. For many in therapy it is the fears that surround what it means to become attached that need addressing. In the initial stages the client may well be encouraged to allow themselves to feel dependent on the therapist as part of highlighting and working through such issues. Gradually, the client will then be encouraged to separate – their sense of autonomy evolving in the context of a meaningful, sustained psychotherapy relationship.

## Deciding what approach

Our approach to patients and clients is influenced by a number of factors. Firstly, the **situation and activity** is a key determinant of our approach. We are likely to be more directive if we are working with a large group of people, as opposed to being in a one-to-one situation. Different activities also require different role-taking, such as being a 'teacher' when introducing a new task. The respective personalities involved also need to be considered. For example, a manner that works for one therapist could fail with another simply because it comes across as artificial (a lesson here from counselling, where 'genuineness' is seen as a core quality).

Next, the **team approach** will often guide our methods – for example when the team decides a patient needs consistent handling or assigns a key worker to respond in a certain way (e.g. to be confrontative). Our approach also has to mesh with colleagues with whom we may be working. For example, a co-therapist may take a directive role, controlling a group, while the therapist is supportive of individuals. (At times when staff shortages pre-empt such careful structuring, extra efforts should be made to guide nurses, students and helpers when they join in therapy sessions regarding how they may best contribute in an unfamiliar situation).

Thirdly, the **theoretical framework** within which we are working is a major influence. At a broad level our professional philosophy suggests that we should be person-centred and foster an egalitarian relationship that invites participation. More specifically, our treatment approach can guide our responses. For instance, in the humanistic tradition we would incline towards being non-directive and accepting, to encourage self-expression. As behaviourists we might be more directive in the way we reinforce behaviour and offer a structure for the patient. Case example 6.1, for instance, shows the therapist being guided by a person-centred approach while in Case example 6.6 we saw the way the model of human occupation was used.

Lastly, and most important of all, our approach to patients and clients is determined by **their needs**. We take our cue from the individual and manage the mood of the session based on our perceptions of the person's mental state, interests, abilities, and so forth. One person might enjoy being jollied along while another needs a quieter, gentler approach. Often the most able therapists are skilled because, seemingly intuitively, they have the ability to 'strike the right note' and respond in a way that respects others' needs. That so-called intuitive response is usually a learned skill and comes from being reflexively self-aware.

Mattingly and Fleming (1994) emphasise how such interaction is both very subtle and very complex, both automatic and contrived. Describing their observations of therapists' clinical reasoning, they note:

> *Often the therapist's facial expression and posture 'mirrored' that of the patient and reflected an immediate involvement in their concerns. At other times, therapists took a slightly different tone or stance, as if trying to give some of their own energy to the patient or to invest some of their enthusiasm in the project they were doing together . . . . She would begin with a look of concern and a quiet, deep tone of voice. Gradually . . . she skilfully guided the conversation to a brighter . . . side of the problem.*
>
> Mattingly and Fleming, 1994, p. 128

Therapists constantly adjust to patients' moods, wants or needs. At the same time there is an attempt to gently guide the person through a process. This is not an easy skill to learn – there are no cookbook recipes for managing interactions. The therapist needs to be natural and, at the same time, to think strategically. It helps to be as aware of one's own responses as one tries to be with the responses of patients and clients.

## 6.4   CARE, POWER, COLLABORATION

We have seen how the therapeutic relationship contributes to positive treatment outcomes and sets the scene for positive (and, by implication, negative) therapy experiences. It is an essential element in engaging clients in treatment. It is a source of meaning and renewal for both client and therapist. The process of helping others is 'satisfying, therapeutic and curative' (Devereaux, 1984, p. 796). What this relationship involves, however, is hard to describe. This section aims to capture some of the complexities of relationships by examining three inter-linking aspects that have been highlighted in the literature: care, power and colla-boration.

## Care

Caring has been identified as a crucial element of the therapeutic relationship. For occupational therapists, to be caring means to 'know and understand the emotions of illness ... and to acknowledge this in empathic, yet therapeutic, responses' (Devereaux 1984, p. 792).

Schwartzberg (2002) identified 'engaging/connecting and creating a holding environment' as one key theme of good interactive practice. In her study, thera-pists' caring was revealed in the way they listened actively to validate the client and in the way they aimed to establish trust, empathy and mutual regard.

Different types of care have been found to influence clinical reasoning. Peloquin (1990), for instance, described how three images of occupational thera-pists dominated patients' stories of their relationships with therapists: those of technician, parent or collaborator/friend. Technical therapists were seen to equate expertise with care, while parental therapists sought to make decisions in the patient's best interests and collaborative therapists aimed for more equal and mutual interactions. When occupational therapists acted as technicians or parents, they seemed to value competence rather than the more caring aspects of relationships favoured by the collaborative therapist. Peloquin suggested that therapists who act as technicians and authoritarian parents reflect society's preference for rational problem fixing but that this can compromise more personal caring. She also discussed how the routinisation and rationalisation of health care institutions may, while promoting efficiency, curtail the element of care.

Well over a decade ago, Burke and Cassidy (1991) echoed these arguments, pointing to the changing nature of the therapist-patient relationships in the context of practice in the USA. They suggested that growing numbers of occupa-tional therapists were being obliged to use technical protocol-driven approaches to treatment, in the process moving away from care that emphasises an individua-lised, humanistic treatment approach. Similar pressures are now being experi-enced in the UK (Finlay, 2001).

While many health professionals strive to 'care', others aim to establish a professional distance within day-to-day interactions as it is impossible to care with great intensity for every patient and some distance is necessary for self-preservation (Research example 6.2). Rosa and Hasselkus (1996) argued that therapists' personal and professional identity is tied up in their relationships. For instance, some therapists described their relationships with patients in terms of being a 'friend' or 'parent'. Such personal involvement has been shown to make work rewarding and contribute to personal growth although it can also be a source of stress and burn-out.

---

**Research example 6.2**

**Striving for control**

Lyons's (1997) qualitative study of student–patient relationships in Australia suggested that occupational therapy students experienced difficulties in reconciling their inclination towards intimacy with conflicting expectations for emotional and social distance. On the one hand, students attempted to be supportive, to develop rapport and even to give friendship. On the other, 'friendship' was seen as an inappropriate professional role. Students therefore struggled to put aside personal feelings in case these contaminated their professional judgement and responses. Lyons also found that they needed to assume authority and maintain control in their interactions with patients/clients. He suggested that the game plan for an inexperienced, unconfident student is to maintain control (particularly over patients' or clients' unruly, undesirable behaviour) in order to survive.

---

## Power

A number of studies point to such tensions between 'care' and 'control', highlighting the power dimension embedded in all therapeutic relationships (Finlay, 2004a). 'Social power is an integral aspect of the daily working lives of professionals' (Hugman, 1991, p. 1). Hugman argues that power in the remedial professions is seen not only within formal hierarchies (e.g. within the team) but also in the way those hierarchies intersect with relationships with service users and structures of gender domination and racism. Power is enacted at both an interactional level and at an institutional level.

Control over the therapy process typically resides with the professional who has the expertise and authority to define the problems of patients/clients – and this applies even when therapists aim to be client-centred. Professionals then control the solutions to these problems by their capacity to prescribe and control access to treatment. Professionals maintain control, for instance, by not respecting service users' opinions. Alternatively, the therapy process can become a 'battle' when the patient/client acts aggressively, complains and refuses to comply or take responsibility for treatment (Rosa and Hasselkus, 1996).

Many commentators have demonstrated how power is exercised through the use of language – in the labels and social evaluations that health professionals apply (Research example 6.3). Numerous studies over the last thirty years have highlighted how health professionals tend to categorise and represent service users in terms of moral and social evaluations. In particular, people can be seen as 'good'/'bad' patients (see Finlay, 1997a). Good patients are co-operative, appreciative of their treatment, cheerful and uncomplaining despite being seriously ill. They allow staff to practise their skills or specialities and usually get better. Bad patients are demanding, uncooperative and ungrateful. They make staff feel ineffective and tend to be condemned by staff. Professionals would claim that they are forced to judge the social worth of people in order to balance competing claims on time and resources.

---

### Research example 6.3

### Disempowering discourses

Much current research arising from a social constructionist perspective calls for health professionals to become more aware of and reflexive about the problems of differential power between clients and professionals. As Opie explains, 'Working reflexively includes acknowledging the inevitability of differential power relations between clients and health professionals and the development, and on-going critique, of modes of interaction which seek explicitly to minimise that difference' (Opie, 1997, p. 273). Her research examined the ways in which professionals in teams discussed their clients and formulated care plans. She found that the teams' discourses were dominated by medical/physiological concerns despite the fact that they defined themselves as being holistic and client-centred. Of greater concern was how issues of power and control surfaced in competing representations. While team members sought to consult with and empower clients, their practice was disempowering.

One team Opie analysed talked about a patient who was admitted into hospital to stabilise a bowel condition. Medical, social and psychological complexities (e.g. the fact that the patient had not accepted that his condition was degenerative) made for further challenges. Words and phrases used to describe this patient in team meetings included: 'unrealistic'; 'difficult'; 'threatening to discharge himself'; 'Often he'll come up with an excuse'; 'He has to co-operate with us more'. One of the staff was to 'get heavy' with him.

Opie (1997) suggests that these representations defined the patient as 'deviant, uncooperative, ungracious'. They produce a 'binary of "proper" patients as grateful, docile, and above all, rational, able to make choices which complemented the team's understanding' (p. 272). Opie goes on to point out the presence of competing representations of the concept of 'adult'. The team, she argues, drew on discourses where adulthood was equated with rational, logical behaviour, including the acceptance of dependency. The patient, on the other hand, referred to discourses that emphasised independence and choice. The task for the team in this instance was to become aware of such processes with a view to actively deciding whether or not to maintain them.

## Collaboration

Much occupational therapy literature argues for professional–patient relationships to be based on a more equitable distribution of power – one based on mutual collaboration, participation and partnership. As Crepeau (1991) and others note, empowering relationships depend on the willingness of professionals to drop their expert position and become an ally. In practice this means creating learning opportunities and enabling patients/clients to participate actively in treatment (Schwartzberg, 2002).

In tune with this approach, occupational therapists' client-centred values emphasise the need for a collaborative rather than prescriptive relationship with patients/clients. Yerxa (1980) refers to a mutual co-operation model where power, ownership and responsibility for treatment are shared. Sumsion (1999a) describes a model of client-centred practice based on her research into the approach taken by British therapists.

'A special dynamic takes place when the occupational therapist and the client are in sync.', notes Schwartzberg (2002, p. 92). She goes on to offer numerous case examples and narratives of **interactive clinical reasoning** where collaboration lies at its core. Rosa and Hasselkus (1996) explore how therapists seek to 'connect with' patients through both helping and working together. Therapists were found to rejoice in their patients' successes and despair at their failures. This process of helping was seen as a collaboration between therapist and patient: therapists would not perceive themselves as able to help if they could not work together with a patient. 'The essence of the concept of working together', they explained, is 'a sense of joining together in mutually supportive partnerships characterised by compatibility, reciprocity and rapport' (Rosa and Hasselkus, 1996, p. 261).

Such studies, which exhort therapists to be collaborative and client-centred, have a tendency to proffer easy prescriptions of the 'ideal relationship'. In practice, our approach can fall short (see, for instance, research by Corring and Cook, 1999, which demonstrates how clients sometimes do not feel valued as human beings). Different situations demand different levels of collaboration and each relationship needs to be negotiated on its own individual terms. Crabtree and Lyons (1997) go some way to recognising this process of negotiation, noting that, while the relationship can never be completely 'equal', a balance can be struck whereby the professional relinquishes some power to gain patients' co-operation. They observe how a therapist, armed with her own idiosyncratic humour, turned away from offering a directive challenge and instead engaged in interactive reasoning, which avoided alienating her patient.

The literature reviewed in this section suggests that, in practice, therapists often struggle with, and have ambivalent feelings about, their professional relationships. As we seek to enable, support and connect with others, we are personally and professionally challenged. We experience both satisfaction and struggle as we give of ourselves in caring, empowering and often intensely personal ways. In return, we get close to, and identify with our patients and clients, gaining much pleasure, warm feelings and a sense of being valued. At the same time, these relationships can be experienced as a battle for control and a source of stress (Finlay, 1998).

## 6.5 CONCLUSION AND REFLECTIONS

This chapter has approached the complex topic of the therapeutic relationship from four different angles. We've explored the kinds of skills, qualities and approaches therapists can draw upon as they seek to use themselves consciously as tools in their interventions. The multi-faceted nature of the relationship, such as how elements of care, power and collaboration interact, has been emphasised. I hope the chapter has revealed something of the profound impact that relationships have on therapeutic interventions.

Building relationships with service users takes time. Sometimes the constraints of the system mean that we cannot spend as much time as we would like to develop these relationships. Sometimes we can find it difficult to establish a rapport with users and relationships do not always unfold in positive ways. Sometimes the process involves two steps forward and one step back. However, when we do engage and connect with individuals, the satisfaction that it brings affirms the struggle.

Occupational therapy literature emphasises the need to care, collaborate and be person-centred in our therapeutic relationships. Findings from my own research (Finlay, 1998) suggest that this is easier said than done, particularly when we are faced with patients and clients who are passive, or resistant to change, or who refuse to take (or are unable to take) responsibility for themselves. Our good intentions can be quickly undermined when we are confronted by abusive and aggressive individuals. That we sometimes fail to meet the ideal and are less than caring is no surprise – particularly given the pressures and constraints arising from the wider health-care context. Yet we often feel guilty when we perceive, or react to, our patients and clients in less than positive terms. The darker side of therapeutic relationships often stays unexpressed, unexplored and un-worked-through and this is something we need to address.

I would say that our therapeutic relationships are what makes our work worthwhile. As in all relationships, we need to take the rough with the smooth. As I look back and reflect on numerous therapeutic relationships, I feel honoured and privileged to have worked with those individuals.

# 7 ASSESSMENT

*It is time to open our eyes and see what is there, without making too many value judgements ... . It is time to lend our ears to our clients' preoccupations ... [with] recognition and resonance.*

Emmy van Deurzen-Smith

Assessment involves gathering information as part of trying to understand the needs of individuals, their problems and their situations. Rather than seeing assessment as a mechanical first stage of the occupational therapy process, we need to view it as part of our ongoing therapy interventions and team approach. Assessment goes hand in hand with clinical reasoning (discussed in Chapter 8) as the therapist moves back and forth between analysing the implications of assessment findings and deciding what intervention can and should be made. Therapists, in collaboration with the individuals concerned, strive to visualise the person's situation, both now and in the future. In these ways, therapists are engaged in a complex scientific, moral and interactive reasoning process (Mattingly and Fleming, 1994).

It perhaps goes without saying that the assessment stage is of vital importance, not least because the effectiveness of an intervention depends on accurately identifying service users' needs. After all, how can we know what to treat, and to what level, if we have not specifically identified the area of need? How can we treat people as individuals if we have not discovered what is special about them? How are we to evaluate progress if we don't have a baseline for treatment?

Yet the process of carrying out assessment is not straightforward. We have many choices to make. Are formal assessments better than casual or unstructured ones? What methods should we use – interview, observation, self-rating? Which standardised or published tools might be suitable? How much assessment should we do? Is there a risk that we spend too much time assessing and not enough on treatment?

This chapter sets out to discuss these questions. In the first section we examine the assessment **process**. The section starts by addressing the questions of What? When? How? and then explores the experience of doing assessments (from the viewpoint of both therapist and service user). Four sections then deal with the different **methods and types of assessment** available for our use:*

---

* Dividing assessment up into these four categories is somewhat artificial, as our assessments often involve a combination – for instance, when we interview someone we are also observing them. Also, standardised tests are not really a separate 'method' in themselves – they are usually based around observation and interview. I discuss them as a separate category to explore some specific issues about their application in practice.

- Standardised tests
- Interviews
- Structured observation
- Self-rating methods.

Each of these is explored by examining their *aims* and the type of information they can elicit; and the issues surrounding their *application* in practice. Some specific, well researched *published tools* are also described. Published tools are usually backed by substantiating research. For this reason some people refer to them as 'standardised assessments'. To be strictly accurate, a standardised assessment should offer both detailed administration instruction and test norms, and their validity/reliability should have been established through research. Many published assessments (e.g. many of the tools arising from the MOHO) do not have or refer to test norms. For this reason, I prefer to distinguish between 'published' and 'standardised' tools.

## 7.1 THE PROCESS AND EXPERIENCE OF ASSESSMENT

### What do we assess?

As problem-solvers, occupational therapists needs to be clear about 'the problem' and its parameters. Consider the individual who 'lacks concentration' and is referred to the occupational therapist. In order to plan treatment, the therapist needs to find out what exactly is meant by this:

- What happens (e.g. are there lapses into non-productive behaviour)? When does this occur (e.g. during tasks)? How does this affect the individual's functioning (e.g. is the person unable to return to the task)? Asking these questions will help define the specific problem.
- How many minutes can the individual concentrate when carrying out daily tasks? This becomes the baseline against which to measure any improvement.
- What situations increase/decrease concentration? This is important both to help the individual develop strategies to cope better with the problem, and to enable a graded treatment to be planned.
- What level of concentration does the person require for daily living? For example, a university student about to take exams and a long-stay patient likely to remain in hospital require qualitatively different levels of concentration. This information is needed to establish the goals of treatment.

In general terms, assessment involves gathering of information, from any relevant source, about the person and his or her circumstances. Our assessments will normally focus on how individuals cope with their daily life **occupations** in work, leisure and self care (see Law *et al.*, 2001 for a comprehensive account of measuring occupational performance). Here, occupational balance and occupational engagement are key dimensions to be alert to. The assessment should pinpoint a person's specific **functional skills and problems** related to emotional, cognitive, social and physical areas. The assessment also needs to probe aspects of **the individual**: his or her needs, interests, motivations, strengths and potential for or resistance to change. These are the positive areas upon which interventions are built. The assessment also needs to take into account the person's **situation**, including expected environment (including physical factors and the amount of social support available) and cultural practices or meanings, as these will determine long term treatment aims (Figure 7.1).

Our general focus on occupations and occupational performance needs to be seen within the context of any assessments made by other **team** members. This becomes particular pertinent in units where the Single Assessment Process (Department of Health, 1999) is being implemented. Here, agencies in each locality have been advised to adopt a common approach to assessment, specifying appropriate tools or approaches that they are going to use. The ethos of the initiative is that service users (and their carers) are expected to be centrally involved in assessments and decision making, and that agencies need to develop joint-working arrangements. While assessment documentation has been indicated (to include basic personal information, needs and health, and a summary of the

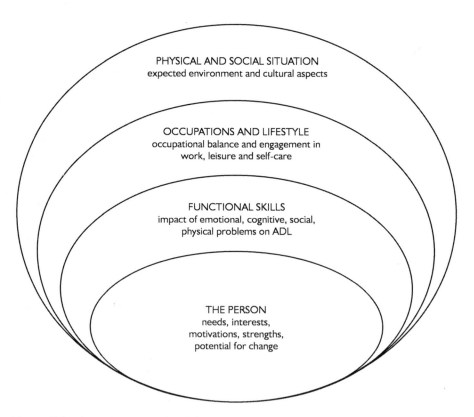

**Figure 7.1** Areas for occupational therapy assessment

care plan) no one tool has been prescribed for national use. Instead the Department of Health has developed criteria against which localities can evaluate their assessment systems. At the time of writing, guidance documents are still emerging.

Over and above having a co-ordinated team approach it is likely that different team member will have a slightly different focus according to their role and concerns: If everybody simply duplicated their assessments it would be a waste of time and effort (Theory into practice 7.1). Ideally the team should have an overall strategy for assessment: either one person takes on the job of doing a generic assessment (e.g. of general mental health) or a division of labour is negotiated where different areas of the individual's life are covered by different team members. In hospitals, for example, doctors and nurses usually take primary responsibility for assessing patients' mental state during the acute stages of their treatment, while social workers and occupational therapists become involved at the later stages, assessing the person's needs and functioning as related to discharge. In this way the assessments carried out by individual team members are partial but the overall assessment strategy is more holistic.

---

*Theory into practice 7.1* _____

**Making the assessment count: avoiding duplication in the team**

One of the most thoughtless institutional practices is repetitive serial inter-viewing, where different professionals all ask a service user similar questions. We see this most commonly in hospitals where, in the first week of a patient's admission, they may well be separately interviewed by several doctors, nurses and therapists, all asking about their mental state! There is no justification for this. Unless occupational therapists are undertaking more generic assessments on behalf of the team, their assessment should be distinctive and focused on occupation/function. The process of negotiating such an assessment can itself help educate patients about occupational therapy, as the following excerpt indicates:

**Therapist**: Rob, I'd like to arrange to see you tomorrow to chat about what occupational therapy might offer.

**Rob**: More talk! I'm getting sick of the sound of my own voice. I just go round and round in circles. I've told the doctors, I've told the nurses, I've told them: life feels very grey. I surprised myself when I took those tablets. It was just a way of taking the pain away. I've told this story so many times.

**Therapist**: It must be very tedious to keep saying the same things over and over again – particularly when it's such a difficult story. Can we take a different angle? Instead of talking about your depression, I'd like to try to understand how its been affecting your life in terms of the things you do each day – your work and how you've been managing to care for yourself. I'm thinking you're going to face all those same pressures again when you get back home this weekend and it might be worth thinking through some new ways of coping better.

**Rob**: Yeah, they said they'd probably only keep me in till the end of the week and I don't know how I'm going to cope.

**Therapist**: So can we meet up tomorrow to talk this through some more?

## When do we assess?

Assessment occurs continuously throughout our interventions (Figure 7.2). In the **initial** stages the occupational therapist (in concert with the team) will be involved in formally collecting data – observing, interviewing and testing the patient or client (and possibly the family/carers) using whatever methods seem appropriate. The information collected is then analysed, preferably in negotiation with the individual, to identify the priority problems and central issues to be dealt with during treatment. The therapist may then carry out other specific assessments at **set points** during treatment (e.g. doing a home visit prior to discharge home).

Over and above these formal assessment periods, therapists try **constantly** to monitor any changes in the patient's/client's functioning and seek to be alert to their responses and new information as it presents itself. For example, if a patient mentions that he is due to see his child that weekend the therapist, alert to this new information that he is a part-time parent, might take the opportunity to discuss the way he copes with being a parent.

The time we have available for assessment and treatment will guide and constrain how much and when we assess, as well as the type of assessments we use. A common complaint in practice is: 'We do not have the time or staffing available to do extensive one-to-one assessments'. This is an important issue and one that needs to be probed further. Is it not about choice of priorities? If we choose to offer more treatment by doing less assessment we run the risk of applying vague or inappropriate treatment. If we assess each person individually we are more likely to ensure interventions are going to be appropriate, meaningful and relevant. The skill comes in selecting the appropriate type and level of assessment. We want to select only those individuals who are going to benefit from occupational therapy intervention. For instance, if we know we are not going to be able to intervene constructively (e.g. the patient is due to be discharged that day), then assessment/treatment is probably not justified. If we know our time is short (e.g. the patient is due to be discharged this week) we then select and tailor our assessments methods accordingly, choosing relatively time efficient assessment methods.

Rather than avoiding assessment because it gets in the way of treatment, we should view assessment as part of therapy. When we listen carefully and sensitively to what a person is saying in an interview, for instance, we're already making a therapeutic intervention – in this case giving the message that what the person has to say is valued and that saying it is important. The process of

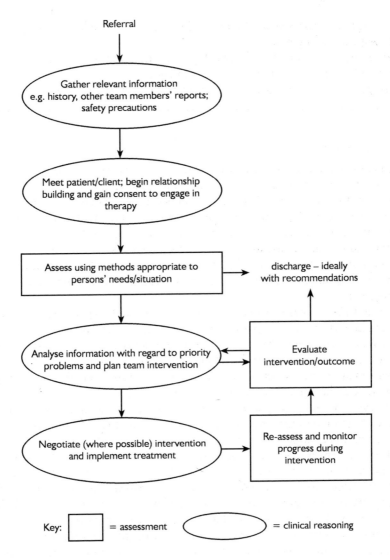

Referral

Gather relevant information
e.g. history, other team members' reports;
safety precautions

Meet patient/client; begin relationship
building and gain consent to engage in
therapy

Assess using methods appropriate to
persons' needs/situation

discharge – ideally
with recommendations

Analyse information with regard to priority
problems and plan team intervention

Evaluate
intervention/outcome

Negotiate (where possible) intervention
and implement treatment

Re-assess and monitor
progress during
intervention

Key: □ = assessment ⬭ = clinical reasoning

**Figure 7.2** The assessment process

assessment and the feedback afterwards can help give patients/clients insight into their own problems areas. Just this step may be enough for them to follow through their own problem-solving and not to need further intervention.

### How do we assess?

We assess in different ways, at different levels, using different tools, at different times. Deciding what assessment/s to use requires professional judgement and occurs as part of our clinical reasoning. We might assess a person's needs using a relatively unstructured, casual approach such as having a 'chat' over a cup of tea. Assessment also occur more formally, for instance when we set up a structured interview or observe someone do a specific task. (In Sections 7.2–7.5, I distinguish between four formal methods: standardised tests, interviews, structured observation and self-rating tools.) In practice, we will often use a combination of informal and formal methods (see Theory into practice 7.3).

The initial stages of the assessment process set the scene for subsequent interventions. This is when the therapist begins to **establish a rapport** with the person, and this in turn helps them decide what method of assessment is going to be useful. Sensitively applied initial assessment can mean the difference between success and failure of treatment. For one thing, the assessment period is the stage where service users give their consent and engage themselves in treatment. Further, encouraging individuals to be actively involved in working out their needs sends a message that they can have control over, and responsibility for, their treatment. This is likely to increase their motivation.

When doing an assessment, therapists should try to adopt **methods and tools** that are appropriate to people's needs and situation. For example, a person who is very withdrawn may well respond better to a non-verbal task than to an interview, while someone suffering from performance anxiety and high emotion might prefer to talk initially. With some individuals it may be appropriate to use formal standardised tests, while others might benefit from more informal strategies. As with any intervention, it is important for the therapist to be **flexible**, adapting the assessment activity when necessary. For example, if a person is becoming overly anxious while doing a standardised test, the therapist might decide either to suspend the test or to offer some additional assistance/ support (accepting that this would, in effect, nullify the test). Likewise, we should respond sensitively and with respect when individuals say they are 'not up to talking today' or 'don't fancy doing OT'. This is a necessary consequence of being person-centred.

After carrying out an assessment we have to **analyse the results** and share the findings with both the person concerned and the treatment team. Future interventions can then be planned and **negotiated**. Assessment doesn't end there, of course. We continue to assess and evaluate throughout the person's treatment (Figure 7.2). Or if it is decided that no intervention is to be offered, this should be justified and any specific **recommendations** made.

The assessment process is neither a linear nor a completely systematic procedure. Sometimes the therapist seems to function at an instinctive level and may even be unaware of picking up on subtle verbal and non-verbal behaviour. The therapist may also make imaginative assessment judgements that seem to be based on 'gut feeling' rather than tangible evidence. In other words, the therapist's clinical reasoning is multilayered (Theory into practice 7.2). The most important point for therapists to remember is that the assessments are *tools* to be used judiciously and selectively. Some individuals respond well to having 'an informal chat' while others find this patronising and would not perceive it as a professional approach. Some individuals respond well to structured tasks (such as the Rivermead battery or AMPS) while others prefer more fluid interactions (as with OPHI-II). Experienced therapists get a 'feel' for what assessment to apply as well as how and when to apply them (Theory into practice 7.3).

---

**Theory into practice 7.2**

**Assessment involves multiple layers of clinical reasoning**

| | | |
|---|---|---|
| On receiving a referral the therapist is likely to formulate provisional and tentative ideas | For instance, on being given a diagnosis, the therapist could estimate information about length of treatment, prognosis, individual's likely level of insight and cognitive function | Scientific reasoning |
| Then the therapist sets out on an initial interview geared to building a relationship with the individual concerned. Together they construct a picture of the individual's particular needs and situation | For example, a woman discloses she is being abused her husband but fears being alone in the future and having to cope as a single mother | Narrative reasoning |
| Throughout the assessment, and as the relationship evolves, the therapist adapts his or her approach in response to the patients'/clients' cues | For instance, a therapist sees that a patient is lacking in motivation during an activity so he suggests that they take a break in order to work out what is going wrong | Interactive reasoning |
| As they work together to plan treatment, the therapist considers wider social factors and practical constraints | For instance, knowing the patient is likely to be discharged shortly, they concentrate on daily life occupations in the community rather than arranging treatment in the hospital itself | Pragmatic reasoning |

---

**Theory into practice 7.3**

**Selecting and combining assessments**

Often several methods of assessments are used in combination – some formal, some informal; some standardised, some developed and practised locally. The following case examples indicate one therapist's provisional choice of assessments for different individuals (see Sections 7.2–7.5 for details about the published assessments).

**Masha**, aged 56, is depressed, labile and says she is a failure. Assessment methods selected: a) counselling interview b) Occupational Questionnaire

**Thomas**, aged 76, has a possible diagnosis of dementia and some mobility problems. Assessment methods selected: a) 'chat' over a cup of tea b) AMPS c) home visit specifically observing safety, mobility and the environment.

Leroy, aged 45, suffers from chronic schizophrenia. He lacks drive/ motivation and has poor social skills. Assessment methods selected: a) Volitional Questionnaire (using cooking, painting and printing activities) b) Social Functioning Scale

Jamie, a boy of 8 with an apparently deprived childhood, has been referred because of destructive behaviour. Assessment methods selected: a) observation during one-to-one free play session b) observation while in small-group cookery activity.

Carrie, aged 30, is recovering from a manic-depressive episode and has been referred to therapy to prepare for discharge. Assessment methods selected: a) OPHI-II b) home visit c) general 'chat' while travelling to and from the home.

Pat, aged 45, has multiple functional problems resulting from the neurological damage sustained in a head injury. Assessment methods selected: a) COPM b) AMPS c) COTNAB.

## Doing assessment – making judgements

The process of doing an assessment is not easy. Therapists commonly experience some tensions when making evaluations of patient's/client's performance. Often evaluations are crucial and involve major quality of life decisions. For instance, a person's discharge may depend on our judgement based on carrying out a safety-risk assessment. We also routinely make moral judgements. Making such judgements carries heavy responsibility.

Such 'power' can sit uncomfortably on our shoulders. Do we have the right to make judgements about others – particularly on the basis of one or two relatively brief formal assessments? While acknowledging this problem, we still have to make judgements – they are part of our role and cannot be avoided. The point is to learn to make judgements responsibly and professionally, avoiding decisions jaundiced by our personal moral standards, religious beliefs or political views. While we are entitled to have and advocate these, we should not subject others to them.

How do we make these professional judgements? Here are some pointers:

- **Be as objective as possible**, so as to limit the possibility of being blinded by unduly subjective or stereotyped perceptions. This is particularly pertinent when we read notes, or hear other team members' reports, prior to meeting a patient/client. Here we especially need to guard against being swayed by labels or diagnoses that could act as self-fulfilling prophesies. For example, when working with institutionalised people, we should resist the tendency to reduce the goals we set for them simply because they are institutionalised.
- **Acknowledge any gaps or limitations in the specific judgements made** to avoid possible misinterpretation. An example here is: 'Mary is safe using our department cooker. Further assessment is required to confirm her safety at home.'

- **Devote more energy to collecting data rather than making inferences.** For example, consider the situation of seeing a person cry. We could fall into making all sorts of interpretations, for instance that he or she is inadequate or being manipulative (Figure 7.3). Therapists need to avoid over-inferring or over-interpreting. We should be wary of making instant judgements on the basis of limited evidence.
- Constantly **monitor judgements** to confirm, deny or adjust to changes in the individual or their circumstances. Here team members can help each other by sharing their findings and impressions of the person in different contexts and at different points in the day.
- **Acknowledge assumptions** about what is 'normal' or 'desired behaviour' that may underlie our judgements. This is particularly important over time as views and fashions change. If an individual is behaving promiscuously, do we assess this to be his/her habitual pattern or a sign of a hyperactive mental state? Also, we each have our own cultural standards, which may be prejudicial – a point that should be taken into account. An illustration of this is a person who eats with their fingers being assessed as disinhibited and confused when eating thus is in fact his or her normal cultural practice.
- Always try to **offer feedback** on evaluations to the person, remembering to present it carefully and sensitively. The challenge is not simply to point out problems and failures but to work with the person to identify their difficulties and strengths. A useful tip is to get into the habit after an assessment of asking individuals how they felt they performed and if the assessment showed them anything. Then the therapist can give his or her view, owning the fact that it is just one view.

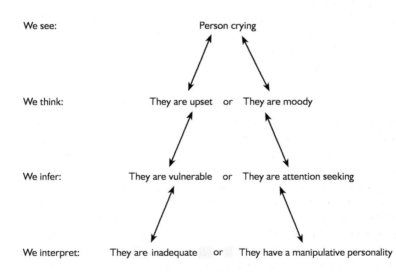

**Figure 7.3** Two different over-interpretations of data

## Being assessed – feeling judged

Sometimes as therapists we can become blasé about the assessment process. It is such a routine part of our work that we forget how difficult – even traumatic – the experience is for some people. Understandably, people feel nervous about their performance and test results – all the more so if they recognise the possible implications (e.g. that discharge might be postponed). Other people may find the assessment process itself threatening. We are so accustomed to receiving personal details from others that we may forget how difficult and painful self-disclosure can be. As therapists we need to be sensitive to these different reactions, to try to have empathy and to offer appropriate explanations. We should feel honoured and humble when someone shares something of themselves and not resent it when they are defensive and non-communicative. When we feed back results we need to remember that sometimes the results themselves can be alarming to the person (e.g. when they learn that they have something 'wrong' with their brain).

Sometimes our concerns about assessments generating tensions lead us to wonder if we should observe unobtrusively rather than assess more formally. While much depends on the individual concerned and the team approach, covert assessment is problematic. We need to remember that we have a professional–legal responsibility that requires that 'consumers' have access to reports and are informed about their treatment. The professional–moral argument emphasises the need to collaborate with our patients/clients in treatment planning. Maintaining a 'professional silence', or finding non-transparent, covert ways to uncover problems, works against encouraging mutual trust and goes against the spirit of our person-centred philosophy.

If an individual feels overly threatened or anxious on being observed or assessed, we should explore the situation further, as a number of factors may be involved. Firstly, the person may feel upset that he or she is being judged (which they are) and judged negatively (which they may be). Here the problem seems to lie with how the therapist is presenting assessment in the first place. Alternatively, the person may feel a certain amount of natural performance tension on being given set tasks. We must take this into account, of course, and consider his or her performance in several contexts over time. Lastly, we may be inadvertently appearing too distant or threatening, for example by our non-verbal behaviour. The writing of notes during assessments is an example of this: while it may be perfectly acceptable, even desirable, it has a negative side if human contact is broken.

A person-centred approach gives service users a degree of control over what information is gleaned from assessment, and how. This is what we aim to offer. Service users should be encouraged to alert us to what is important to them and what they wish us to know (see Law *et al.*, 2001, for details of measuring occupational performance while being client-centred). A good place to start in our thinking is to consider how we would like to be treated if we were in a similar situation.

## 7.2 STANDARDISED TESTS

### Aims

In the current climate of evidence-based practice and increasing demands for us to demonstrate efficacy and effectiveness of our interventions, standardised assessments are being used increasingly. A standardised test is a formal procedure that has been carefully researched and developed to establish its objective and 'scientific' status (de Clive-Lowe, 1996). Three main elements are usually addressed when a test has been standardised:

- Consistent, clear **administrative and scoring procedures** are detailed. All the people who are given the test use the same materials and experience the same instructions, and assessors score the results in the same way.
- The **test norm** is defined – i.e. details of the accepted standard given a particular population are provided as a yardstick for interpreting results. Tables of norms show the distribution of scores and statistical analysis provides information about the spread of scores normally obtained.
- The instrument's **validity and reliability** has been researched and established (i.e. the test measures what it is supposed to measure in a consistent way across assessors and across time). Usually this process evolves over a sequence of trials where appropriate adjustments are made to successive versions (as seen with the progression from OPHI to OPHI-II).

### Application

There are many good reasons to use standardised assessments. First, we can have **confidence** in their results. Second, they are likely to improve **communication** in the team, ensuring a better understanding of, and respect for, our contribution. As our credibility improves so will the appropriateness of our referrals and confidence. Third, they provide a concrete **framework for practice** – a clear focus for both service user and therapist. (For this reason, we tend to prefer function- and occupation-based assessments.) Finally, they provide a solid baseline measure of performance and a means to **measure outcomes**. To give an example, Cook (2001) used the Social Functioning Scale, among other assessments, to act as a baseline against which to measure improvement – in this case, improvement in social functioning. The results of her study showed statistically significant improvements in people's social functioning, demonstrating the value of their primary care and occupational therapy service.

In practice, some therapists remain reluctant to use these assessments – often because they lack the knowledge of what is available or would be appropriate. Sometimes therapists feel that certain standardised assessments go against our philosophy of being person-centred and focused on occupations (Research example 7.1). Standardised assessments need to be used judiciously – they need to be selected to suit our occupational therapy values and practice aims (for a discussion on this see Payne, 2002).

---

**Research example 7.1**

**The use of standardised assessments in practice**

- Managh and Cook (1993) studied the use of the Bay Area Functional Performance Evaluation (BaFPE) by American occupational therapists. The reasons the therapists gave for using the test included: departmental habit, time efficiency, for screening/selection purposes, to have a task-based assessment of functioning and team preference. The authors found that, although specific guidelines for administering the assessment are provided, therapists often deviated from these (e.g. excluding the social interaction scale). Mostly, the therapists adapted the test in response to perceptions of clients' needs. Most of the therapists indicated mixed feelings about the use of standardised assessment. The authors concluded that the values of client-centred practice outweighed the values of a scientific approach. Therapists are thus challenged to develop assessments more consistent with our philosophy.
- Craik *et al.* (1998b) surveyed 200 British mental health occupational therapists about their practice. Less than half of the participants reported using standardised assessments. Preferred assessments that were in use were the Canadian Occupational Performance Measure (18% of participants) and the AMPS (7%). The authors reported that the participants were eager to learn more about outcome measures and evidence-based practice.
- Haig (1997) surveyed occupational therapists working in head injury rehabilitation units in the UK. Of the 97 therapists surveyed, 96% stated that they used both standardised and non-standardised methods (only 4% said they never used standardised measures). Of the measurement scales most commonly used, 44% used Barthel, 39% used the Functional Assessment Measure (FAM), 33% used the Functional Independence Measure (FIM) and 13% used AMPS. Of the assessments that examined component skills, 73% used both the Rivermead and Rivermead Behavioural Memory test while 68% used COTNAB. The therapists emphasised the need to assess patients in both hospital and everyday environments. Team objectives and realistic goal-setting were described as being easier when standardised assessments were employed because a common language was in use.

---

With all standardised tests, four points need to be stressed to avoid their misuse/abuse.

- First, **it is important that assessors are properly trained** to administer and score the test according to standard methods in order to maximise the test's reliability and validity. The AMPS test, for example, requires users to attend a five-day course.

- Second, testing is not just a matter of following procedure – **testing also requires interpretation of results**. Here the occupational therapist must have a good understanding of the rationale behind the test and/or the comparisons with available norms. Without this, tests remains an observational tool only.
- Third, **each test has limitations and weaknesses**. Tests are usually designed for specific populations, types of problem and/or situations and are only applicable to such areas. Some tests are weak in certain areas, such as being vague in their instructions. Also, some tests stir up considerable performance tensions in people, which could unduly affect the result (to say nothing of the patient's/client's response to occupational therapy as a whole).
- Finally, **care must be taken when reporting results and making recommendations**. If a test is not administered precisely (e.g. if tasks are modified or the client is prompted) it may invalidate the assessment. It is legitimate (and may even be desirable) to adapt an assessment, as long as we do not report results as having been produced by a standardised procedure. We need to use tests responsibly.

Overall, standardised assessments offer an objective, systematic and scientific way of assessing service users' needs providing baseline and outcome measures. While they are invaluable for comparing results and communicating findings to other professionals, they remain a tool to be used selectively and judiciously alongside other (perhaps non-standardised) tools.

## Published tools

The available pool of standardised tests (and their respective norm tables) is increasing every year as demand grows for valid assessments and reliable outcome measures. The following are some psychosocial assessments commonly used in the UK.

### Assessment of Motor and Process Skills

The Assessment of Motor and Process Skills (AMPS; Fisher, 1999) simultaneously assesses **functional performance** in activities of daily living tasks (ADL), such as meal preparation, and underlying **motor/cognitive skills**. The person carries out a specifically defined ADL task of choice while the assessor (who has been specifically trained and 'calibrated') carefully observes. A total of 16 motor and 20 process skill items are scored using a four-point rating scale (4 = competent, 1 = deficit). The scores are then analysed by computer using a many faceted Rasch analysis to provide measures that are adjusted to account for the challenge of the task, the severity of the rater, the ability of the subject and the difficulty of the skill items.

The strength of this specially developed occupational therapy assessment is its highly scientific, well-researched approach. Findings from numerous studies support its **validity and reliability**. For example, research by Robinson and Fisher (1996) supports the validity of the AMPS as an evaluation of the interactions between cognitive impairments and disability in complex activities of ADL.

McNulty and Fisher (2001) demonstrate the validity of using AMPS in the clinic in assessing home safety levels in persons with psychiatric conditions. Doble *et al.* (1999) demonstrate the test-retest reliability of using AMPS with elderly people. The clinical **research base** for AMPS is now extensive (see, for example, Baron, 1994). Early problems with **cross-cultural applications** have been addressed to a reasonable degree and research/training in AMPS around the world continues to grow, providing a bigger pool of data. The computer scoring of the precise level of motor and process skills allows therapists to **predict** how well a client can be expected to perform on many other ADL tasks.

On the negative side, some therapists feel uncomfortable using this tool as the requirements to ensure reliability can be restrictive. Tasks need to be done a certain way or be scored down and this may not suit the therapist's own methods. Some therapists are challenged by the time it takes to become trained while others feel inexperienced when it comes to installing and using computer software.

Assessors need to attend a five-day training and calibration workshop (held regularly in the UK and around the world) to develop the skills for scoring and interpreting results. Therapists wishing to attend should contact: AMPS Project, Occupational Therapy Building, Colorado State University, Fort Collins, CO 80523, USA.

**The Rivermead Perceptual Assessment Battery**

The Rivermead Perceptual Assessment Battery (RPAB; Whiting *et al.*, 1985) is one of the more widely used standardised perceptual tests available to occupational therapists in the UK. It consists of a battery of 16 timed tests that take approximately an hour to administer. Tasks range from matching simple pictures to copying a complex three-dimensional model. The assessment is designed to measure deficits in visual perception and so is most relevant for assessing people with schizophrenia or with neurological disorders.

One of the strengths of this assessment is that it has been well produced and researched. Donnelly *et al.* (1998), for instance, assessed 35 people who had had strokes using RPAB and three functional activities (packing a lunch box, putting on a cardigan and setting a table). A statistically significant relationship was found between these, suggesting that assumptions can be made about a person's functional performance simply on the basis of RPAB results. A drawback of this test as far as occupational therapists are concerned is that it does not specifically analyse occupational/functional performance.

The RPAB is relatively easy to apply, although care needs to be taken to follow the instructions precisely. Some service users find the formality and timed elements stressful, while others appreciate its professional packaging and presentation. Arguably, its focus on visual perception limits its value and broader cognitive-perceptual tests, such as the COTNAB, may be more useful.

The attached manual includes information on interpretation of scores and illustrative therapy case studies. This battery can also be obtained from Fern Nelson Publishing, Unit 28, Bramble Road, Techno Trading Centre, Swindon SN2 8EZ, UK.

## The Social Functioning Scale

The Social Functioning Scale (SFS; Birchwood *et al.*, 1990) has been created for people with severe mental health problems. It offers a comprehensive assessment of seven different aspects of social functioning:

- Social engagement/withdrawal (hours spent alone)
- Interpersonal behaviour (number of friends; quality of communication)
- Pro-social activities (e.g. sport)
- Recreation (e.g. hobbies)
- Independence-competence (ability to perform independent living skills re: loss of skills)
- Independence-performance (ability to perform independent living skills re: use of skills)
- Employment/occupation (productive activity).

The self-report SFS questionnaire can be used as part of an interview or can be answered by carers. Options are offered to answer questions (e.g.: 'How many hours of the day do you spend alone? 0–3 hours = very little time, 3–6 = some of the time, 6–9 = quite a lot of the time, 9–12 = a great deal of time, 12+ = practically all the time). Each answer is scored and the means of the seven area scores are totalled to give an overall score. The value of these are then scaled using a pre-set table. Scaled values give a normative average of 100 for 'unemployed people with schizophrenia'. Scores of 115 or less indicate a cause for concern. Scores of 116 or more indicate that the person does not need clinical intervention for their social function.

The advantages of this assessment are that it is reasonably easy to apply as the questions are concrete and relatively straightforward. If service users find the questionnaire too difficult, their carers can be consulted. Results are often valued by the team as the scale has been well researched and normatively standardised. The scale offers a useful indicator of social function, even if occupational therapists are likely to supplement findings with more specific assessments of occupational functioning. Research indicates that the SFS is both valid (it distinguishes between people with and without schizophrenia) and reliable (it has high inter-rater reliability).

For further information about the use of this assessment, contact Dr Max Birchwood, Department of Clinical Psychology, All Saints Hospital, Lodge Road, Birmingham B18 55D, UK.

## Life Experiences Checklist

The Life Experience Checklist (Ager, 1990) is used primarily with people with learning disabilities. It identifies whether deficits in clients' cognitive learning are the result of limitations in cognitive skills or lack of opportunities to learn. The interview questions asked touch on areas to do with home, leisure, relationships, freedom and opportunity. The questions (which require simple yes/no answers and can be answered by the client or by the therapist on the client's behalf) are appropriately straightforward: 'My home has more rooms than people'; 'My home is carpeted and has comfortable furniture'; 'I visit friends and relatives for a meal once a month'. Scoring with norms is standardised against the general population (recognising urban, suburban and rural differences).

The checklist is quickly administered and can be used flexibly as an individual assessment tool or for group treatment. Although very simple, it offers insight into the person's quality of life and pinpoints possible environmental problems.

The assessment can be obtained from the British Institute of Learning Disabilities (available online at www.bild.org.uk/publications).

**The Chessington Occupational Therapy Neurological Assessment Battery**
The Chessington Occupational Therapy Neurological Assessment Battery (COTNAB) is one of several assessments occupational therapists can use to assess neurological functioning (e.g. in the case of people who have suffered a head injury or stroke). There are 12 sub-tests, which assess:

- Visual perception (overlapping figures, hidden figures and sequencing)
- Constructional ability (two-dimensional, three-dimensional and spatial ability)
- Sensory-motor ability (stereognosis, dexterity and hand–eye co-ordination)
- Ability to follow instructions (written, visual and spoken).

The person's scores on each test are compared with norms for that age group in terms of ability, time and overall performance.

This professionally packaged (but expensive) assessment is one of the best known tools as it was specifically designed for occupational therapists' use. It has a good research base (see, for example, Laver and Hutchinson, 1994). COTNAB is often favoured by therapists over the Rivermead as it tests wider cognitive function as opposed to just visual perception. In common with the Rivermead, the limitations of this test are the performance tensions it can generate and the fact that it does not specifically measure occupational/functional performance. On the other hand, many people enjoy carrying out the interesting and challenging puzzles and tasks.

COTNAB is available from Nottingham Rehab Ltd, Ludlow Hill Road, West Bridgeford, Nottingham NG2 6HD, UK.

## 7.3   INTERVIEWS

### Aims

Interviews are the use of structured conversation to gain insight into a person's world. They are our most widely used tool, both for initial assessment and to monitor progress. Often they are the only relatively formal procedure the occupational therapist applies alongside the impressions we gain through general observations and interactions with the patient or client. As Mosey comments, 'Interviewing is probably the most powerful, sensitive and versatile evaluative instrument available to the occupational therapist' (Mosey, 1986 p. 314). Where other tools are being used, e.g. specifically focused functional assessments, interviews can be useful to keep the 'whole' person in mind.

Different interviews do different jobs. The interview that takes place as the first contact between therapist and patient or client is primarily a relationship-building exercise, with the occupational therapist sharing as much information about her role as the patient or client shares about his or her situation. Subsequent treatment-planning and evaluation interviews will have greater focus on the person's attitudes, interests, and view of problems he or she is prepared to work on.

The main aim of the interview is to gain information – both from what is said and how it is said. At a **verbal** level we seek relevant factual information about situation and interests, feelings, attitudes, the person's own view of his or her problems, verbal skills and intellectual capacities. At a **non-verbal** level the person's appearance and behaviour may communicate much about their mood, mental state and attitudes. The specific information obtained depends not only on the person's specific problems but also on their motivation, abilities and situation.

## Application

Every interview should be planned, or at least thought through, carefully. Decisions need to be made about the specific aims and structure of the interview, taking into account the context and the individual's previous experiences (e.g. of occupational therapy). Prior to the interview, the therapist should be clear about what he or she hopes to achieve and why. If the primary aim of the interview is to build a **relationship**, then the therapist might choose to start with a quick, relatively informal 'chat'. If the aim is **fact-finding**, then the therapist can usefully go into the situation armed with a few already-formulated, pertinent questions. This pre-empts vague interviews and can help in those moments when we 'go blank' and do not know what to ask next.

The structure of the interview itself is, of course, determined by its aims. The one important guideline that applies to any interview is to remain throughout an **active listener**, putting effort into listening instead of formulating your next question. We should strive to really hear what another person is saying (or, perhaps, not saying). While this is not always easy to do, we need to remember that service users' stories are important and should be valued (Theory into practice 7.4).

---

*Theory into practice 7.4*

**Tips for good interviewing**

- Ensure that the environment is as 'safe' as possible to encourage the individual to feel comfortable and to open up.
- Establish boundaries at the beginning of the interview – by, for example, negotiating how much time the interview might take. This will help the

---

- individual to gauge what depth/detail to go into and will give them some control over the process.
- Interviews offer an opportunity to develop the therapeutic relationship. Being warm and responsive is more important than remembering to ask a set number of questions.
- Ask open-ended questions, such as 'How are you settling in?' (as opposed to 'Do you like this ward?') or 'What does your typical day look like?' (as opposed to 'Do you have a job?'). This way of asking questions allows a person more opportunities to expand his or her comments and open up, rather than responding with a 'yes' or a 'no' answer. Further, it implicitly respects the individual's capacity to take responsibility and share what is important for them. Possible exceptions to this, however, are when we are working with people who are cognitively impaired or who are acutely ill. They may well need the structure of being asked simple, direct questions.
- Respect what it must feel like to be the person being interviewed. We are privileged to receive any information, let alone the deep confidences often offered.
- Remember that assessment is part of treatment. The patient/client needs to understand the purpose of the interview to be motivated to answer. It helps to explain why you need to know the answers to the questions you are asking.

As a general rule the interview **environment** should enable individuals to feel comfortable and safe, in order to encourage them to open up. If the interview is to take place in the person's home, they themselves should decide where they would feel most comfortable. When the interview is to take place in a unit, a quiet room off the main ward or a quiet area with which the individual is familiar is a good start. The key to ensuring 'safety' is to try to respond to what works for each individual. While some people react positively to a relaxed, informal approach, others may experience this as unprofessional and would prefer a more structured, formal interaction. Safety and trust are also promoted by listening sensitively, giving enough time and being free from interruptions.

## Published tools

### Occupational Performance History Interview – Version 2.1

The Occupational Performance History Interview – Version 2.0 (OPHI–II; Kielhofner *et al.*, 1998) is a semi-structured interview that was devised as a generic interview tool and is suitable for most occupational therapy contexts. Although developed as part of the model of human occupation (MOHO), it is readily applicable by raters subscribing to other theoretical frameworks. Questions are designed to elicit information about a person's occupational roles, daily routines, occupational behaviour settings, activity/occupational choices and critical life events. Three rating scales (Occupational Identity, Competency and Behaviour Settings) used for scoring the interview offer a way of quantifying information (Theory into practice 7.5), while space is available for a 'life history narrative' to capture qualitative information. The OPHI-II works best if the therapist can develop a conversational style.

---

**Theory into practice 7.5**_____

**Summary of OPHI-II categories for rating**

Occupational Identity Scale

- Has personal goals and projects
- Identifies a desired occupational lifestyle
- Expects success
- Accepts responsibility
- Appraises abilities and limitations
- Has commitments and values
- Recognises identity and obligations
- Has interests
- Felt effective (past)
- Found meaning and satisfaction in lifestyle (past)
- Made occupational choices (past)

Occupational Competence Scale

- Maintains satisfying lifestyle
- Fulfils role expectations
- Works towards goals
- Meets personal performance standards
- Organises time for responsibilities
- Participates in interests
- Fulfilled roles (past)
- Maintained habits (past)
- Achieved satisfaction (past)

Occupational Behaviour Settings Scale

- Home-life occupational forms
- Major productive role occupational forms
- Leisure occupational forms
- Home-life social group
- Major productive social group
- Leisure social group
- Home-life physical spaces, objects and resources
- Major productive role physical spaces, objects and resources
- Leisure physical spaces, objects and resources.

(reprinted with the kind permission of Gary Kielhofner)

---

The strength of this assessment is an approach that is consistent with occupational therapists' interactive clinical reasoning. In practice, therapists using the interview also focus on how to engage the individuals in the therapy itself. As the person's problems are seen in the context of a their previous functioning, it is particularly useful for assessing people who have been changed (e.g. a person who used to be an alcoholic and now has stopped drinking; or someone who functioned well before suffering a breakdown or sustained a traumatic injury). The five areas of questioning offer a useful and comprehensive structure without overly constraining the therapist's style of questioning. Less experienced interviewers sometimes prefer a more structured tool, although raters can use this test without formal training.

The original version of the OPHI assessment was well researched and this helped establish both its validity and its relevance to occupational therapy. A good practice base has developed around the world (see, for instance, Fossey, 1996, for an evaluation of its use). The emphasis on qualitative information and the limited question structure are both its strength and its weakness (as rich information is obtained while inter-rater and test–re-test reliability are reduced). Version 2.1 has been studied by Kielhofner *et al.* (2001), who demonstrate that the three scales used for rating the interview are valid across age, diagnosis, culture and language.

The OPHI manual (consisting of instructions, research base information, question lists and scoring forms) can be purchased from the Model of Human Occupation Clearinghouse, University of Illinois at Chicago, 1919 West Taylor Street, Chicago, IL 60612–7250, USA (website http://www.uic.edu/ahp/OT/MOHOC/assessments.html).

**Occupational Case Analysis Interview and Rating Scale**
The Occupational Case Analysis Interview and Rating Scale (OCAIRS; Kaplan and Kielhofner, 1989) is a semi-structured interview, arising from the model of human occupation, that was originally designed for use in the field of acute mental health. Questions are carefully worded to cover all areas of occupational performance: interest, roles, habits, skills, personal causation, values/goals and other areas related to how the individual functions within the environment. The answers are then scored to aid treatment and discharge planning.

The strength of this interview is its clear and comprehensive structure. Therapists new to interviewing often find the supplied set questions helpful. Most of the questions are written in a user-friendly manner, such as 'How do you like to spend your time'; 'Overall, how satisfied are you with how you spend your time?'; and 'What do you see yourself doing one year from now?'. More experienced therapists may find the structure too constraining and rigid. The specific and detailed rating scale is both a strength and a weakness: inter-rater reliability is increased but it can be hard to rate individuals who do not fit neatly under the headings offered. The instrument has been well researched and has been shown to be a reasonably consistent tool.

The assessment consists of a manual, instructional audio tape and question/ rating forms. This package can be purchased from Slack Inc., 6900 Grove Road, Thorofare, NJ 08086, USA. Further information on the new edition can be obtained from the MOHO Clearinghouse (website: http://www.uic.edu/ahp/OT/ MOHOC/assessments.html).

At the time a writing, a new version of the OCAIRS (now called Occupational Circumstances Analysis Interview and Rating Scale) is about to come out that has been researched with people with both psychiatric and physical disability.


**Worker Role Interview**
The Worker Role Interview (WRI; Velozo *et al.*, 1992) is a semi-structured interview and observation tool based on the model of human occupation. It aims to identify the psychosocial and environmental variables that may influence the ability of the 'injured' worker to return to work. It is designed to enable the client to discuss various aspects of his or her life and job setting that are relevant to past work experience. The recommended questions cover:

- The effects of injury (e.g. 'What parts of your job do you feel you are unable to do because of your injury?')
- Life outside of work (e.g. 'What do you do in the evenings')
- Present job (e.g. 'What are you most proud of in terms of your work?')
- Past jobs (e.g. 'What other jobs have you had over the last five years?')
- Return to work (e.g. 'Do you think you will return to work?').

The therapist then rates (both interview and work assessment observations) in terms of content areas based on the model of human occupation (i.e. personal causation, values, interests, roles, habits and environment). Each content area is subdivided into specific work-related issues. For instance, the subcontent area of 'expectation of job success' is rated on a four-point scale indicating how strongly this item supports the client returning to work. The User's Guide offers detailed instructions for rating individuals' responses. Scores obtained on an initial assessment and discharge reassessment may then be compared.

Arguably this assessment has limited value in the psychosocial field given the realities of the employment market. However, it could prove to be a useful tool for any work rehabilitation programme. The strength of this interview is its clear and comprehensive structure. The fact that the interview goes beyond work questions can be seen as both a strength and a limitation (as its extends the interview time). Questions are reasonably user-friendly. The detailed guidelines offered for the scoring system ensures reliability and validity has been established through extensive literature on factors influencing return to work.

The manual can be obtained from: Model of Human Occupation Clearing-house, Department of Occupational Therapy M/C 811, University of Illinois at Chicago, 1919 West Taylor Street, Chicago, IL 60612–7250, USA (website: http://www.uic.edu/ahp/OT/MOHOC/assessments.html).

## 7.4   STRUCTURED OBSERVATION

### Aims

Observation is a method of assessment we use all the time – often without thinking. We continuously monitor (and then respond to) how service users are presenting, behaving and performing, and how they are responding to their treatment. We observe the way they interact with others and their environment (Case example 7.1). *Structured* observation is a more formal and systematic procedure where we focus on specific aspects – for instance, observing the way a task is being performed or taking note of environmental hazards on a home visit.

Therapists who are particularly skilled at observing learn to focus on specific and relevant cues. General observations like 'John is looking better today' are transformed into 'John's posture is more upright today, making him look more confident'. It is this level of specific observation that we need to encourage in ourselves. Primarily, this is because when we are more specific about a patient's/ client's areas of skills or behaviour we have a more specific yardstick to monitor the effectiveness of interventions. A second, not unimportant, factor concerns our professional presentation and our communication with both service users and other staff. Vague verbal reports are unhelpful and could even prove counterproductive.

---

### Case example 7.1   Observing on a home visit

Marli was referred to a community mental health team to be assessed for depression. The occupational therapist was chosen do the assessment on behalf of the team. She arranged a home visit, which proved invaluable for understanding Marli's situation and pressures.

| **Description of the home visit** | **What the therapist observed** |
|---|---|
| Marli greets the therapist at the door. | The therapist observes Marli's unkempt appearance and that she looks pale, thin and exhausted. |
| She shows the therapist into the living room. | The therapist notices the strong dank smell of stale tobacco, alcohol and urine. The room, like Marli, is uncared for and messy with several toys and clothes strewn around the floor. The room feels damp and mould covers the window frames and walls. Wet laundry hangs all around the room. The small gas heater in the corner is on but is unable to cope with heating the cold, damp room. |

---

A 4-year-old boy (Kenny) comes rushing in noisily, causing Marli to reprimand and remind him not to wake up Jason (the 2-year-old). Jason then toddles in sleepily.

The therapists observes that both children are wearing nappies and are drinking what looks like watered-down milk from the same nursing bottle. They both have runny noses and Jason is wheezing slightly. She notices that Marli seems to have little control over Kenny's behaviour but that she cuddles both children warmly.

Marli asks the therapist if she would like a cup of tea. The therapist nods her thanks. They both go into the kitchen and Marli invites the therapist to take a seat. After making the tea Marli joins the therapist at the table. Jason climbs up on to Marli's lap and goes to sleep.

The therapist observes Marli make the tea efficiently while also doing some clearing up. Dirty dishes are stacked in the sink but the rest of the kitchen seems clean and cosy.

As they talk, the therapist begins to understand the many pressures on Marli. Her children are the biggest worry, with Kenny being overactive and Jason being severely asthmatic. Marli struggles daily with a large amount of laundry as both children regularly wet the bed. Together they plan ways for Marli to get some social support – for instance, joining a mother and toddler group each morning at a local day centre. The therapist also suggests that social services may be able to help with rehousing or arranging for central heating to be put in as the damp is clearly exacerbating Jason's asthma.

The therapist observed that, although Marli is clearly tired, she is responsive, friendly, grateful, interested in the therapist's suggestions and interacts openly with her.

The therapist reports back to the team: in her view Marli is not actually clinically depressed – just ground down by poverty and the challenges of being a single parent to two young 'problem children'. She suggests that the most helpful intervention would be to activate a range of social support networks and to formally follow-up Marli in 6 weeks time.

## Application

To observe effectively it is helpful to utilise one or two of the infinite number of observation checklists available. For instance, **activities of daily living** checklists can be a useful prompt to highlight points such as:

| Making a cup of tea | Comment |
| --- | --- |
| Aware of use of equipment | |
| Organises task in sequence | |
| Aware of safety factors | |
| Fills kettle appropriately | |
| Turns on gas/electricity switches | |
| Puts tea in pot/cup appropriately | |
| Pours boiled water in appropriately | |
| Uses sugar/milk appropriately … | |

We can also take any developmental scale and translate it into behavioural observations, as the following example detailing **cognitive function** at the level of a 2–3-year-old child demonstrates. Having such a structure for observations helps us be clear and precise.

| | Date achieved | Comment |
| --- | --- | --- |
| … Draws vertical lines | | |
| Copies circle | | |
| Matches three colours | | |
| Points to big/little in imitation | | |
| Places objects 'in' on request … | | |

Specific observations like these can be applied to many situations and tasks. They offer an objective measure of performance (even if this cannot be called standardised) whereby a person's actual functioning can be observed rather than inferred.

## Published tools

### The Assessment of Communication and Interaction Skills
The Assessment of Communication and Interaction Skills (ACIS; Forsyth *et al.*, 1998) is an observational assessment that aims to gather data on the communication and interaction skills displayed during occupational/social situations (e.g. a cookery group). Three domains are assessed, consisting of 20 action verbs that indicate skills that can be observed, for example:

- **Physicality** (e.g. contacts – makes physical contact with others; gazes – uses eyes to communicate and interact with others)

- **Information exchange** (e.g. articulates – produces clear, understandable speech)
- **Relations** (e.g. collaborates – co-ordinates one's own action with others toward a common end goal).

The manual provides details of the standard scoring system used for each action verb. For example, a score of 2 for information exchange implies:

*ineffective ability asserting which impacts on social action; seems to procrastinate, be stubborn, get in others' way; has difficulty making effort for self; speaks with some confidence but also with some doubt; uses indirect approach with others which causes delay in social action; and makes requests without being specific which causes delay in social situation.*

This assessment was initially developed by Simon (1989), revised by Forsyth (helped by 52 Scottish occupational therapists). Research suggests a high level of validity and reliability, aided by the detailed action verb measures (e.g. Forsyth *et al.*, 1999). The assessment manual emphasises the need to observe patients/clients in **meaningful situations** and how therapists should assess the behaviour in terms of the social and cultural context. While it takes time to get used to the jargon and use of terms, the meanings are well spelled out and growing familiarity with the tool makes it easier to use.

The manual, containing research to date, rating guidelines and score sheet, can be purchased from the Model of Human Occupation Clearinghouse, University of Illinois at Chicago, 1919 West Taylor Street, Chicago, IL 60612–7250, USA (website: http://www.uic.edu/ahp/OT/MOHOC/assessments.html).

### The Volitional Questionnaire

This questionnaire (de las Heras *et al.*, 2002) arises from the MOHO and was developed to assess volition in people with chronic mental health problems or with learning disabilities (i.e. people who have limitations in cognitive or verbal abilities). The assessment involves observing the person in different activity sessions in terms of 14 volitional indicators related to:

- Intrinsic motivation
- Personal causation
- Values/interests.

The patient/client is rated along a four-point scale (passive, hesitant, involved, spontaneous) for each indicator. Examples of rated item are: 'Spontaneously demonstrates interest/curiosity in the environment' and 'Is hesitant about trying new things'.

The strength of this assessment is that it offers a reasonably simple, systematic way of observing many aspects of volition and motivation as part of therapy sessions – a significant problem for this client group. The assessment has been used in research in the USA and has been positively received in practice around the world. Given some therapists' idiosyncratic scoring patterns, reliability may

|                                              | 0 | 1 | 2 | 3 | 4 |
|----------------------------------------------|---|---|---|---|---|
| *1. General behaviour*                       |   |   |   |   |   |
|   A. Appearance                    |   |   |   |   |   |
|   B. Non-productive behaviour      |   |   |   |   |   |
|   C. Activity level (hypoactive or hyperactive) |   |   |   |   |   |
|   D. Expression                    |   |   |   |   |   |
|   E. Responsibility                |   |   |   |   |   |
|   F. Punctuality                   |   |   |   |   |   |
|   G. Reality orientation           |   |   |   |   |   |

    Subtotal

*2. Interpersonal behaviour*
  A. Independence
  B. Co-operation
  C. Self-assertion (compliant or dominant}
  D. Sociability
  E. Attention-getting behaviour
  F. Negative response from others

    Subtotal

*3. Task behaviour*
  A. Engagement
  B. Concentration
  C. Co-ordination
  D. Follow directions
  E. Activity neatness or attention to detail
  F. Problem-solving
  G. Complexity and organisation of task
  H. Initial learning
  I. Interest in activity
  J. Interest in accomplishment
  K. Decision-making
  L. Frustration tolerance

    Subtotal

Scale: 0 = normal, 1 = minimal, 2 = mild, 3 = moderate, 4 = severe.

**Comments**

Therapist's signature

**Figure 7.4**    COTE scale

be improved with special training. A further limitation is that there is a ceiling effect for clients with higher volition (Chern *et* al, 1996).

The Volitional Questionnaire and User's Manual (which includes two useful case simulations) can be obtained from the Model of Human Occupation Clearinghouse, University of Illinois at Chicago, 1919 West Taylor Street, Chicago, IL 60612–7250, USA (website: http://www.uic.edu/ahp/OT/MOHOC/assessments.html).

## Comprehensive Occupational Therapy Evaluation

The Comprehensive Occupational Therapy Evaluation (COTE; Brayman *et al.*, 1976) is a useful, structured observation scale (if now somewhat dated) used primarily for initial assessment (Figure 7.4). In addition to the basic scale, official definitions detail the problems at a specific level to maximise reliability as the following example shows.

> *1. A. Appearance – the following six factors are involved: clean skin, clean hair, hair combed, clean clothes, clothes ironed and clothes suitable for the occasion.*
>
> *Rating:* 0 = no problems in any area; 1 = problems in one area; 2 = problems in two areas; 3 = problems in three or four areas; 4 = problems in five or six areas.

The form has been designed for flexible usage: it is an observation checklist; a record of performance over time; and a proforma report that can be included into the medical notes.


## 7.5 SELF-RATING TOOLS

### Aims

Self-rating assessments tend to suit our **person-centred** philosophy because they elicit the person's own views as they formally complete a rating scale or question-naire. Self-rating tools are used in a variety of ways: They can measure people's own perceptions of themselves, their attitudes, feelings and interests and also their perceptions of their world. Often used in conjunction with counselling interviews, they can act as a tool to promote insight and self-awareness. Self-rating assessments can help with individuals' motivation for treatment as they ensure that the person is actively involved in identifying their needs/problem areas. Also, some people enjoy filling out questionnaires (perhaps because they remind them of the fun self-scoring quizzes that crop up in popular magazines).

Recording something in black and white can be more powerful than simply saying it. To illustrate this, consider the person who ticks a box saying that she would like to have a work role in the future. She is admitting that it is a possi-bility and she may have taken the first step towards committing herself to such an action. As it is recorded in black and white, she cannot deny having said it. Simply saying 'I might like to have a job in the future' can be offered as a throw-away line and reneged on later.


### Application

Self-rating methods can be used on their own or (more commonly) as part of a wider interview/discussion process. Some forms cover largely factual material and can be easily and quickly filled out by people (e.g. forms that relate to address, type of dwelling, home circumstances; or forms that act as a checklist of interests). Other forms are more complex and may be best discussed in tandem with the patient/client. For instance, when using the Role Checklist, some people may be unclear about the term 'role' or feel unable to determine what category their roles come under. They may want to explore their feelings/attitudes before committing themselves to putting something down in writing.

The following excerpts from four different assessments – focusing on hobbies, work, social anxiety and self concept – illustrate the range of self-rating assessments available.

**Hobby interest checklist**
This type of form (see example below) is often best used in the early stages of treatment when a lot of information can be recorded, stored and possibly used towards planning treatment. It can easily be filled out by the individual to cover 'factual' information quickly. Do not, however, fall into the trap of dehumanising the process by reducing the person's view of themselves to a few ticks. Discussion after the person has completed the form will increase its value.

*Hobby interest checklist*
Please tick the activities that interest you most:

| Activity | Interest |
|----------|----------|
| Pottery | ☐ |
| Dressmaking | ☐ |
| Woodwork | ☐ |
| Watching TV | ☐ |
| Play-reading | ☐ |
| Gardening | ☐ |
| Sport | ☐ |
| Cooking | ☐ |
| Typing ... | ☐ |

**Work assessment form**
On the basis of performance over the week, apply rating criteria of 0 = no

serious problems; 1 = some problems; 2 = definite problems needing further help:

| Skill area | Client rating | Staff rating | Comments |
|---|---|---|---|
| ... Accuracy | | | |
| Speed | | | |
| Neatness | | | |
| Organisation | | | |
| Coping with pressure ... | | | |

The above illustration is an example of an ongoing week-by-week evaluation form where the individual is actively monitoring his or her own performance in co-operation with the therapist. The aim of this method is to increase the individual's awareness of their functioning and their involvement in assessment, thereby improving motivation. If a significant discrepancy between the client's and therapist's score arises, that can be interesting in itself, or it may highlight the need for further observations. This type of form is perhaps best used on a regular basis (e.g. during weekly interviews), with the same therapist able to measure any improvements over the week.

**Social anxiety rating scale**
Select the choice of difficulty that most closely fits how you feel about the following social situations: 0 = no difficulty; 1 = slight difficulty; 2 = moderate difficulty; 3 = great difficulty; 4 = avoid area.

| Situation | Rating 1 | Date | Rating 2 | Date |
|---|---|---|---|---|
| ... Going to parties | | | | |
| Going into restaurants | | | | |
| Meeting strangers | | | | |
| Initiating a conversation | | | | |
| Maintaining a conversation ... | | | | |

The illustration above is an example of a behavioural rating scale that could be used both prior to and after communication or social skills training. Its value lies in how it specifically pinpoints the person's problem areas. As the material is potentially emotive, care needs to be taken on presenting this to service users. It is perhaps best used within a counselling-type interview, where answers can be expanded on and discussed. If the questionnaire can be filled out honestly (in the context of a safe therapeutic relationship), then it can act as a valuable baseline to which the individual concerned can subsequently refer.

**Self-concept questionnaire**
Please tick yes or no

| I would like to learn: | Yes | No |
| --- | --- | --- |
| . . . That I am a person of worth and value | ☐ | ☐ |
| To be less self-destructive | ☐ | ☐ |
| To feel better about my appearance | ☐ | ☐ |
| To feel I am competent | ☐ | ☐ |
| To be more assertive . . . | ☐ | ☐ |

A range of self-rating tools like the one above has been designed in an attempt to grapple with individuals' views of themselves and their emotional responses. They are particularly valuable for promoting insight, and can be useful when comparing the person's own view with that of others. Given their nature they are potentially threatening, and are certainly not easy to complete. At the very least, people may have difficulty with the jargon or in giving yes/no responses to complex concepts. Moreover, individuals may not be ready to apply such concepts to themselves. Given these potential pitfalls, care must be taken both in choosing people who would find this technique useful and in presenting it to them in a caring, sensitive way. Often the tests are best used within ongoing counselling sessions or as part of a personal 'diary' in which the person monitors his or her own feelings more privately.

**Summary**
To summarise, a range of self-rating questionnaires/forms exist that are adaptable in how they can be used by both therapist and patient. They can act as:

- A motivator, where the person can be active in his or her own treatment
- A casual checklist to touch on verbally or in writing
- A vehicle for further discussion/counselling
- Written evidence to refer back to as treatment progresses
- A tool to promote insight and awareness
- An opportunity to explore the individual's own view of the world compared with that of others.

Whatever type of self-rating method is used, care must be taken not to reduce our clients' view of their world to a few ticks. As with any method involving personal reflection, some people may feel threatened or become distressed in the process. A self-rating assessment can be a powerful tool but needs to be presented in a caring, sensitive way.

## Published tools

### The Canadian Occupational Performance Measure

The Canadian Occupational Performance Measure (COPM; Law *et al.*, 1991), arising out of the Canadian Model of Occupational Performance, combines a semi-structured interview with self-rating measures. Questions are asked about self-care, productivity and leisure. When the patient/client identifies a problem area, he or she is asked to rate/weight its importance on a scale of 1–10. The person is then asked to choose the five most important problems and rate them in terms of performance and satisfaction. A numerical score is then calculated.

The main strength of this assessment is that it was developed for occupational therapists and emphasises our person-centred approach. The focus is firmly on the patient's/client's own values and view of their occupational performance. As such, it is very helpful in setting goals for therapy and offers outcome measures that may determine the degree of change in occupational performance.

Extensive research, largely stemming from Canada, has taken place to develop this tool. Several studies show that it is easy for therapists to administer and that it provides a useful client-centred framework. From service users' perspectives it can help them define their occupational problems/priorities more clearly. A number of studies have demonstrated the fairly good reliability, responsiveness and validity of this tool (for a review, see Pollock *et al.*, 1999). While the validity of the subjective response scores can be questioned, they are meaningful for comparison on reassessment.

Although limited in scope and in what it measures (e.g. it does not deal with mental health in general), COPM's concentrated focus on occupational performance has made it popular tool for occupational therapists, particularly those concerned with physical and practical problems. Many clinical research studies now use this tool to measure outcomes (e.g. Chesworth *et al.*, 2002; Bodium, 1999).

There are a number of factors to do with adopting a client-centred approach that make the COPM challenging to apply (Sumsion, 1999b). Some clients need extra time to understand and respond to questions. Some may need the process to be made more concrete (e.g. talking through a typical day's schedule) and some need extra help in rating the scales. Perhaps not appropriate for some client groups, the COPM is also difficult to apply in service contexts dominated by biomedical approaches where there is less interest in occupational performance in general.

The assessment can be obtained from: The Canadian Association of Occupational Therapists, 110 Eglinton Avenue West, 3rd floor, Toronto, Ontario M4R 1A3, Canada.

## Interest Checklist

This checklist was originally devised by Matsutsuyu (1969) and then revised by Kielhofner and Neville (1983) and others. It is a self-rating tool that requires the person to rate 68 different activities or areas of interest (e.g. gardening, sewing/needlework, playing cards, foreign languages, church activities) according to:

- Level of interest in the past 10 years/past year
- Whether or not he/she currently participates
- If he/she wishes to pursue it in the future.

This assessment is a valuable tool (particularly when combined with discussion) for identifying patterns of interest, as it offers such a comprehensive checklist. It has also been extensively used in clinical research studies. Scaffa (1991), for instance, found that clients beginning rehabilitation for alcoholism and those with extended periods of sobriety had similar numbers of strong interests. The latter group, however, had more frequent participation in pleasurable activities.

Therapists practising in the UK are likely to want to modify the tool by translating some of the American words (such as 'visiting' and 'yardwork') and adding some others (such as DIY, horse racing and cricket!). If therapists do modify the list, they need to remember this when looking at research that would only apply to the original.

The (modified) Interest Checklist can be printed out from the Model of Human Occupation Clearinghouse website at: http://www.uic.edu/ahp/OT/MOHOC/assessments.html).

## Role Checklist

This checklist (Oakley, 1981) is a self-rating form designed to obtain information about the types of roles a person engages in, comparing past, present and future roles. The checklist describes 10 roles (student, worker, volunteer, caregiver, home maintainer, friend, family member, religious participant, hobbyist/amateur, participant in organisations). The significance of these roles for the person are then rated (e.g. not at all valuable, somewhat valuable, very valuable).

The checklist is a valuable simple tool (particularly when used in conjunction with discussion – at least to explain what 'role' is!) for understanding the person's own perceptions of their life roles and can be applied in many situations. Information about mismatch of roles regarding frequency of performance versus their perceived value can be highly significant (e.g. if a person does not value the carer role yet performs it frequently, or *vice versa*). With its focus on occupational roles, it has become a popular tool for occupational therapists around the world. Research carried out when it was first developed and subsequently demonstrates reasonable validity and reliability (Oakley *et al.*, 1986). Since then, the Role Checklist has been used frequently in research to measure role performance and satisfaction (e.g. Elliot and Barris, 1987).

The Role Checklist can be obtained from Frances Oakley, National Institutes of Health, Building 10 Room 6S235 10 Center Drive MSC 1604, Bethesda, MD 20892–1604, USA (e-mail: foakley@nih.gov).

**Occupational Questionnaire**

This questionnaire (Smith *et al.*, 1986) is a self-rating tool that can also be used as a semi-structured interview. Individuals describe their typical use of time (activities carried out are listed for every half-hour). The person then rates each activity on a Likert-type scale according to:

- Whether it is work, daily living, recreation or rest
- How competently he/she does it
- How important it is
- How much it is enjoyed.

A variety of scores can be calculated to give an insight into the person's pattern of occupational activity.

The strength of this tool is its focus on occupational activities and the insights it yields about the person's own view of how he/she copes. The questionnaire can be applied in a variety of settings and it can be useful for understanding the needs of different types of service users (including individuals with physical problems). The process of filling it out can feel laborious but it offers a clear-cut account of the person's daily life activities, any changes to which are easily measured. It can also be used to discover a person's strengths and weaknesses towards setting treatment goals.

The Occupational Questionnaire can be downloaded from the Internet (http://www.uic.edu/ahp/OT/MOHOC/assessments.html). Otherwise, the guide is available from the Model of Human Occupation Clearinghouse, University of Illinois at Chicago, 1919 West Taylor Street, Chicago, IL 60612–7250, USA.

## 7.6 CONCLUSION AND REFLECTIONS

This chapter has covered much ground, looking at the range of assessment tools available and issues around applying them in practice. Four types of assessments and their applications have been analysed. Each one has been shown to have both strengths and limitations – see Table 7.1 for a summary evaluation.

Throughout the chapter I have implicitly advocated the use of fairly *formal*, specifically focused assessments, as opposed to *informal*, off-the-cuff and unstructured methods. Therapists like me who support the use of more systematic methods argue that:

- They promote a clearer understanding of particular issues/needs and facilitate more focused interventions
- They reduce the influence of our own biases, values and idiosyncrasies by providing standard routines
- Patients/clients often trust and respond better to procedures that feel 'professional'
- The stronger the research base backing the assessment, the more interprofessional credibility it has as a tool.

I have also specifically emphasised the use of *published tools* that have been well

**Table 7.1** Summary evaluation of types of assessments and their application

| Type of assessment | Main focus of assessment | Value/strengths | Limitations/weaknesses | Application implications for use |
|---|---|---|---|---|
| **Standardised tests** | Occupational performance and behaviour; cognitive/ perceptual/social/motor skills | Scientific rigour<br>Validity/reliability increased<br>Respected by colleagues and patients/clients<br>Baseline/outcome measure | Can be impersonal and anxiety provoking<br>Value lost if modified or incorrectly applied<br>May not have local relevance<br>Assessor may need special training | Strict adherence to standard practice important<br>Times before and after testing important for explanations, relationship building and feedback<br>Use norms relevant for that patient/client group |
| **Interview** | Life situation, self-perception, attitudes, interests, behaviour, mood | Individuals can communicate what they feel is important<br>Relationship-building facilitated<br>Factual and subjective aspects can be covered | Responses often depend on skill of therapist e.g. being sensitive/ listening and asking the right questions)<br>People can lie<br>People may not be skilled verbally or is too withdrawn to talk | Be clear about the aims of the interview – particularly as the patient/client may well go through several interviews<br>Develop skills of active listening |
| **Structured observation** | Skills, behaviour, task performance, group interaction | Judgements made on the basis of what is seen, not on inferences or assurances from patient/client – therefore fairly objective<br>More practical/activity based so fits our role | Validity/reliability not assured as it relies on therapist observation skills and accurate interpretation<br>Limited contexts for observation<br>Subjective experience cannot be easily observed | Consider using structured forms and tasks in preference to general observation<br>Recognise limitations and continue to develop skills<br>Draw on observations at different times and situations |
| **Self-rating** | Feelings, attitudes, interests, self concept and factual information | Taps more abstract material and subjective experience<br>Person can communicate what he or she feels is important<br>Respects person's capacity and responsibility for treatment | People can lie<br>Process can be impersonal<br>Certain forms may threaten, irritate or be too abstract | Use the forms as a vehicle for patient's/client's growth and development<br>Be flexible with how they are applied – e.g. some people may wish to fill it out privately and then discuss it |

researched. Many occupational therapists (judging by some surveys, as many as half of us) still do not use published and/or standardised tools. However, given the context of evidence-based practice, the requirement that we measure our outcomes, and imperatives coming from team colleagues who are under similar pressures, it is becoming hard to justify not using them. In my view, rather than arguing the case for using published well-researched assessments, we really should be explaining why we're not using them!

Any assessment can only be a *tool* for an occupational therapist to use – a tool that should be applied selectively, judiciously and sensitively. The best assessors are the ones who remember they are also therapists. The best assessments are the ones that occur as part of a wider therapeutic process. Once the therapist has begun to build a relationship with the client and preliminary assessment findings are established, the therapist is ready to start planning treatment – the subject we turn to in the next chapter.

# 8 CLINICAL REASONING AND TREATMENT PLANNING

*There is a certain fluidity in this practice from the ridiculous to the sublime, from the trivial to the essential, as therapists shift from playing endless games of checkers ... to engaging patients in intense discussions about why they shouldn't just give up and die.*

Cheryl Mattingly

---

**Case example 8.1    An everyday occupational therapy story ...**

Dowie is a 52-year-old unemployed, married man. He lacks motivation and drive. He doesn't want to do anything other than lie around at home in bed all day. As his extreme inactivity and passivity becomes entrenched in habit, his functioning deteriorates. His family despairs and don't know how to help. They turn to the GP, who calls in an occupational therapist to advise.

The occupational therapist, Kevin, observes how seemingly intractable Dowie's inactivity has become. He asks Dowie if this is what he wants for the rest of his life. Dowie denies this, saying he wishes he had the energy to do things but he doesn't. Kevin explains the value and importance of doing some level of activity every day to prevent Dowie from going on a downward spiral. Dowie agrees to a treatment contract. He'll give Kevin's ideas one month. If he hasn't improved significantly by then, he is free to withdraw from therapy.

Together, Dowie and Kevin plan a daily activity regime that gradually demands more activity from Dowie each day. (For example, in the first week he agrees to help cook a dinner. By the end of the month he is to plan and cook a large family meal. See the detailed plan on p. 202). Kevin visits two afternoons a week to encourage and cajole Dowie and engage him in different activities. As sport has been a particular past interest of Dowie's many years before, they decide to go to the local sports centre. On the third week, Dowie meets some friends at the sports centre whom he hasn't seen for some years. They encourage him to join their over-50s badminton team. With some trepidation, but good humour, he does. A few weeks later, Dowie is a changed person. He enjoys doing things with his family once again and he makes an effort to get out of the house at least once a day.

The occupational therapist in this story has managed to creatively engage Dowie in treatment. The activity programme was well graded (achieving the right balance of stimulation and pressure) and appropriately drew on Dowie's past interests and current motivations. This seemingly simple intervention disguises complex clinical reasoning. Clinical reasoning is the process where the professional thinks through, plans and negotiates a treatment plan or intervention. This process is simultaneously logical, creative, intuitive and interactional. It involves science, art and ethics.

---

Our clinical reasoning involves both rational problem-solving analysis and creative envisioning of a range of possible therapeutic interventions to fit service users' problems, needs, interests, environment and lifestyle. It involves the way we think, plan and negotiate interventions in relationship with the service user. While service users may take the lead in identifying their own needs and preferences, it is the therapist who focuses and facilitates the person's thinking. It is the therapist who, in the context of the team approach and decision-making, lays out the options and possibilities. Then, when it comes to designing the treatment or intervention, our challenge is to be both realistic and imaginative as we engage the patient or client in a collaborative journey. In addition to using ourselves as a therapeutic tool (see Chapter 6), we adapt the environment and activities (grading the amount of stimulation and pressure) towards therapeutic goals.

This chapter begins to explore some of these complexities by breaking down the stages of planning an intervention or treatment into component parts and then examining the clinical reasoning as a whole process. We look, in turn, at:

- Organising assessment information
- Establishing aims and goals
- Designing the programme
- Clinical reasoning.

## 8.1 ORGANISING ASSESSMENT INFORMATION

Our assessments often produce a mass of data where emotional, cognitive, physical, social and functional problems intertwine in complex ways. Confronted by numerous problems, we can find it tricky to see the wood for the trees. It is vital, however that we work to understand the underlying and dynamic nature of our service users' problems if we are to intervene effectively. Having a specific theoretical approach can help focus and guide our clinical reasoning (see Chapters 4 and 5). Even then, we still face the challenge of trying to translate our global, and sometimes ambiguous, findings into a well-defined problem and intervention strategy. The first step is to organise the information gleaned from assessment, which involves:

- Identifying the problem/s
- Identifying positive aspects
- Selecting the priority problem on which to focus initially.

### Identifying the problem/s

The first step in identifying problems is to move away from focusing on service users' clinical diagnoses and, instead, see their needs in terms of occupational performance and functional problems (Theory into practice 8.1). (This is our version of 'diagnosis'.) The process of understanding these problems, however, is made more difficult because of the subjective way individuals experience them. A large problem to one person may be irrelevant to others. For example, one person may be devastated by losing their job whereas another person might accept it phlegmatically. Three main considerations apply when we try to identify a person's problems:

- Focus on function
- Focus on individual in his/her social context
- The need to be realistic.

---

***Theory into practice 8.1***_____

**Use and limits of diagnosis**

Occupational therapists try to avoid depersonalising labels and blanket diagnoses, recognising that illness is only one aspect of the whole person. Two main dangers of employing diagnosis are:

- It takes us down the route of the medical model, focusing us unduly on the course of illness rather than on coping/health
- Stereotyping people can result in stereotypical treatment where individuals' needs are not noticed.

However, diagnosis does have a role to play in our work. First, knowing a person's diagnosis gives us clues about the likely course, prognosis and contraindications of that particular condition. Armed with this information, our clinical judgement and long-term aims will be more realistic. Second, we need to know about diagnoses in order to work with others in the treatment team who do use diagnosis as a starting point. This is particularly true in acute in-patient settings, where much discussion will take place along medical model lines. Third, some therapists may play a role in the team determining differential diagnoses. In principle, however, our focus is on functioning and occupational performance, not the person's illness.

---

**Function not illness**

When a person becomes ill or stressed, their ability to function in daily life and occupations is impaired. Occupational therapists focus on these functional aspects rather than the illness itself. For example, take two people, one with schizophrenia and the other with depression. Different diagnoses but, from our point of view, both may display similar functional problems and need similar occupational therapy. For both, their daily occupational performance is affected by their state of being withdrawn, apathetic and passive. They may have both stopped looking after themselves so self-care will be poor. They may both tend to sit around all day doing nothing, have few interests and find difficulty in relating to others. They may both have reduced cognitive and task performance skills that impair their ability to work. Their psychiatric history may make future employment problematic. They may both require long-term support in the community. These are the functional problems that we would address.

### Focus on the individual in his/her social context

Having recognised that service users may have similar problems, we still try to value the uniqueness of each individual. Each person has his or her own skills, issues, needs and motives, along with their particular wider social/cultural heritage. Each person will have different hopes and expectations about what they need to be able to do in the future. Therefore each person requires individualised interventions. Even if we use the same occupational therapy activity with two different people, the intervention planned is likely to be very different. Everything we do needs to be tailored to the needs of the specific individual – whether it is the way we approach that person or how we use occupations as part of the person's overall treatment.

Consider the different ways that cooking has been used with these three individuals:

- Annie is a 20-year-old on the point of leaving home. She has been dependent on her family and lacks both skills and confidence in her ability to cope as an adult. As part of a wider programme of skills training and developing her *sense of agency*, Annie learns to cook during her occupational therapy sessions.
- Rufus is a 40-year-old man who has been in and out of hospital for years. He is passive and lacks the drive to do anything. He enjoys cooking, however, and it provides a useful way both to activate him and to assess his *task performance*.
- Meena is 65-year-old socially anxious women. She is a confident cook so the therapist recommends that she join a local advanced cookery class with the aim of *enabling social interaction* in a relatively non-threatening way.

### Being realistic

Being realistic means that we sometimes have to make difficult choices. We may need to accept that treatment will not result in a 'cure' or full employment or whatever. Relapses, deteriorating functioning and the need for life-long medication are real probabilities for some people with enduring mental health problems. Occupational therapists need to be realistic (without being unduly pessimistic). For one thing, we may be called upon to help a person come to terms with their likely prognosis. Ignoring potential future problems is not usually helpful. It is also important to be realistic about which problems we can do something about and which are likely to be beyond our scope and/or professional skills (Case example 8.2).

---

***Case example 8.2   Winnie – Being realistic***

Winnie is 53 years old. She lives on the streets, except when it is very cold, when she goes into a homeless shelter. She survives by a combination of begging and charity, moving from place to place with her carrier bags of belongings. Her self-care is extremely poor as she has limited opportunities to wash and she lacks both the

---

awareness and the motivation to be concerned about her appearance and hygiene. Several times each year she relapses into an acute psychotic episode that involves her experiencing hallucinations/delusions, causing her to behave in a bizarre and aggressive manner. At these times she is admitted to hospital, only to be discharged as soon as possible, partly because she wants her 'freedom' and partly because the team feel unable to do anything positive with her.

Winnie's problems are long-standing and interventions are unlikely to have much impact. For a start, her social problems of poverty, homelessness, unemployment, exclusion and poor health/hygiene are probably intractable. Winnie's self-care problems are largely a result of her situation. Implementing a self-care programme would be both an imposition of our values and also a relatively pointless exercise, as she is returning to the streets. Winnie's psychotic symptoms are also beyond our scope as only medication can stabilise her mental state. It might be possible for Winnie to be referred to a Rehabilitation Unit (of which occupational therapy is a part), after which steps could be taken to try to rehouse her. Realistically speaking, this would take many months and Winnie is unlikely to be sufficiently committed to the treatment and to changing her habits. For many reasons, Winnie may not receive or follow through long-term rehabilitation. Arguably our best role is to offer her sanctuary in times of particular need and brief periods of pleasure to enhance her quality of life. We might also consider acting on her behalf as her advocate. In this role, we should work to ensure that she has adequate supportive follow-up in the community when she is discharged.

## Identifying positive aspects

Successful interventions usually build on service users' strengths, interests and motivations, as we saw in Dowie's story at the beginning of the chapter. Strengths are important, as often we use a person's skill in another area to help the problem area (e.g. a creative bent being harnessed to learn a craft in order to improve task skills). At the very least, we must always remind the individual (and ourselves) of his or her positive points to help balance our emphasis on problems. Interests should be taken into account as part of appreciating the individual's social and cultural background and needs. The process of incorporating strengths and interests usually goes some way to ensuring a person has some motivation to engage in the therapy (Case example 8.3).

---

### Case example 8.3 Bernie – Finding something positive to work with

Bernie, a large man with a history of extremely violent (often drug-related) behaviour, is a resident in a forensic unit. He has a reputation for being aggressive and abusive, particularly when asked to do anything. On first meeting the occupational therapist, Bernie threatens her, saying she will regret it if she tries to push him. The therapist replies mildly that he can make his own decisions. She offers him (with some trepidation!) an open invitation to come down to the activity room if ever he is interested to do so. When one day Bernie suddenly presents himself, the therapist acknowledges him but is careful to leave him to look around on his own. She notices that he returns several times to look at some model aeroplanes that have been painted by a patient. She asks him what has caught his eye. Bernie is disparaging and tells the therapist they are using the wrong type of paint brush. A few days later, unasked, Bernie produces a paint brush for the therapist. She asks him if he will show her the proper technique for using it. Bernie starts to come down to the occupational therapy activity room, on his own volition, regularly. Eventually, he takes the lead in starting up the 'model aeroplane group'.

### Selecting the priority problem

We are rarely able to treat all the problems identified in assessment. Firstly, occupational therapy is not, and cannot be, a panacea for all ills. Secondly, if we sought comprehensive coverage of problems, our treatment would stand in danger of being far too wide-ranging and vague. Consider, for example, the chronically institutionalised individual who has received minimal therapy in recent years. The problem list is likely to be long (possibly encompassing poor social skills, low motivation, poor concentration, difficulties in carrying out tasks, stooped posture, unkempt appearance, slowed and passive behaviour, poor reality orientation, and so forth). In the initial stages it would be impossible to work on all of these problems. It is far better to select a particular area for focus. Any success we achieve is likely to have additional payoffs in the manner of a domino effect (Figure 8.1).

Once a person starts to function better in one area, they may be able to take it from there and sort out their own situation. We are not responsible for 'fixing' all areas. Take the example of Mick, a 50-year-old deep-sea fisherman who had lost his business. As a result, he started to drink heavily and suffered marital problems. He spent his time either sitting morosely at home or in the pub. The

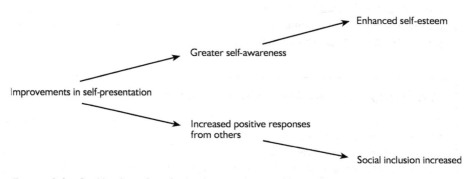

**Figure 8.1**  Positive benefits of selecting one key problem

occupational therapy intervention simply focused on trying to develop some meaningful, productive activities that would positively activate Mick. Treatment was successful. As Mick felt happier, his marital relations improved and he no longer felt the need to abuse alcohol.

Where possible, therapeutic interventions should be negotiated with service users. The individual needs to agree the problem or the focus of intervention, providing they are able to do so. Research (e.g. Jenkins *et al.*, 1995) has shown that treatments are more likely to be effective when individuals' attitudes and beliefs about disease and treatment are elicited and when they are enlisted as therapeutic allies. These researchers describe an interactional approach and demonstrate that best practice arises when the therapist invites client partici-pation. If the person is unable to participate actively, the therapist, and the team as a whole, must be extra concerned to make decisions that are both ethical and well justified.

One of the therapist's skills is to select, with the service user, one or two key problems to work on initially. This can be done on the basis of:

- **Agreeing the most basic or underlying problem** – For example, poor social skills may be at the root of the difficulties of a person who is having problems in both relationships and finding and keeping a job
- **What the individual (or carers/family) perceives to be important** – Service users might be invited to arrange their 'problem list' in a hierarchy; on this basis, their motivation to follow through any intervention is likely to be higher
- **A problem with a relatively easy solution** – An 'easy problem' could be worked on first, as part of confidence-building and developing trust in the therapist–client relationship, e.g. teaching relaxation techniques for coping with anxiety or supplying a communication aid
- **Whichever theoretical framework is being used** – For example, therapists who favour a humanistic approach are more likely to select emotional problems as being fundamental, whereas behaviourists would direct their attention towards behaviour.

This last point reminds us that we negotiate therapeutic interventions as part of **team decision-making** and strategy. This applies most clearly when we work within teams that adopt particular theoretical approaches (see Chapter 5) and it is necessary for us to co-ordinate our interventions. In practice, however, this process is not always straightforward: therapists can feel themselves pulled between competing conceptions of 'good practice'. Mattingly (1998) argues that the need to structure interventions to fit a medical model of clinical work while trying to address the individual needs of the service user generates tension. 'Even during the best of times', she suggests, 'this dual focus is likely to result in a sort of jagged dance in which both the patient and the condition are addressed and in which therapeutic plots are created, interrupted, resumed, and sometimes abandoned altogether' (Mattingly, 1998, p. 131).

*Theory into practice 8.2*_____

**Discovering the priority problem**

Therapist: During this interview, Jean, you've mentioned a number of problems ranging from what you're feeling inside to the strains of work and home life.

Jean: Yes, everywhere I turn there seems to be another problem.

Therapist [nods, acknowledging Jean's comment]: I think we'd find it difficult to work on all those problems at once. Is it possible to narrow them down a bit to see if we can come up with one or two areas to work on first?

Jean [unsure]: I guess so.

Therapist: Okay, let's see .... . Which problem do you think causes you the most stress? [The therapist could equally have asked: Which problem do you want to get rid of the most? or Which problem has the most/least effect on your life?]

Jean: Oh, I don't know ... . I can't cope with the children and their screaming ... . The biggest problems are at home, I'm so tense all the time when I'm at home and I can't seem to relax.

Therapist: You know, that might be a good place to start? One of the things we find in therapy is that sometimes, if you get one problem area sorted out, the other problems sort themselves out too. For example, if you were feeling less tense, do you think you might cope with your children's screaming better?

## 8.2 ESTABLISHING AIMS, GOALS AND OBJECTIVES

Once the problem(s) to be worked on have been identified, the aims and goals of the therapy intervention need to be devised, then regularly revisited.

### Aims and goals

**Aims** are general statements of intent and provide the basic direction of treatment. The overall long-term aim is usually established by the team, and occupational therapy aims are similarly negotiated. Long-term aims in occupational therapy usually relate to a person's life roles and occupations. Examples of **long-term aims** are:

- To discharge home, resuming an independent life
- To undertake graded rehabilitation, aiming for discharge to a sheltered environment
- To resettle into part-time employment
- To teach how to use community resources.

More **specific aims** can then follow from the general statement, e.g.:

- To *improve* a problem area or to increase a skill (e.g. develop conversation skills)
- To *maintain* skill or prevent deterioration (e.g. maintain dressing independence)
- To *minimise* the problem or help adjust to difficulties (e.g. learn an alternative way to communicate).

**Short-term goals**

Once the general direction or strategy has been agreed, we narrow down our focus to think in terms of tactics and the smaller steps and goals that need to be worked on. Here, for example, is a plan of Dowie's treatment (see Case example 8.1):

| | |
|---|---|
| Long-term aim: | To encourage productive activity |
| **Specific aims:** | To develop a range of regular daily activities and leisure interests |
| **Goals:** | |
| *Week 1* | Plan activity programme with Kevin |
| | Help cook family meal on one occasion |
| | Visit sports centre to decide preferred activity for next week |
| *Week 2* | Help cook family meal on two occasions |
| | Go with wife to shop for weekly groceries |
| | Sports centre activity with Kevin |
| | Go into town for coffee |
| *Week 3* | Help cook family meal on two occasions and help clear up afterwards |
| | Meet Kevin at the sports centre having found own way there |
| | Go with wife to shop for weekly groceries |
| | Go to see a local football match |
| | Visit pub one evening for a drink and meal with wife/family |
| *Week 4* | Cook family meal on own |
| | Go with wife to shop for weekly groceries |
| | Help to cook and clear up after at least one other meal |
| | Meet Kevin at the sports centre and go there alone at least once |
| | Visit pub at least one evening |
| | Have one other family outing, e.g. bingo, drive in the country. |

Aims and goals should, ideally, be written down and explicitly stated at the beginning of treatment sessions. Non-specific, mental goals are insufficient. It is too tempting to devise them retrospectively! Once written they can act as something tangible for the service user to work towards, and can also be more easily communicated to relevant team members.

The manner in which these goals are written will vary from unit to unit. Some units might adopt highly regularised procedures for recording problems and goals. For instance, teams might employ the SOAP system (using the headings of 'subjective, objective, assessment and planning' to record goals) or POMR ('problem-oriented medical records' where the team identifies and prioritises problems and goals). Practitioners may write goals from the service users' perspective (*learn* a skill) or from their own (*teach* a skill).

### Objectives as outcome measures

Objectives are precise statements of intended results or outcomes, and serve as realistic, measurable targets for both service user and therapist. An effective objective records *what* is to be achieved and *how* it is to be achieved. It also offers criteria for *measuring* achievement. For example, the aim 'to improve the ability to concentrate' can be transformed more precisely into the objective of: 'At the end of a month of regular practice, Mr Brown will be able to concentrate for a minimum of 20 minutes on a basic familiar task'. (This might be broken down further: say, by the end of the first week he will be able to concentrate for 10 minute periods.)

Objectives are most relevant when modifying behaviour and skills, as these can be quantified in terms of observable outcome measures. The process of learning to type, for instance, can be measured via the ratio of number of errors to the total number of words typed. It is quite a different matter to measure the extent to which someone is feeling better (although it is possible to have some measures, like the number of minutes spent engaged in productive activity).

---

### Case example 8.4   Setting objectives – Irina's programme

Irina becomes acutely anxious when she is required to interact with others. In order to work on this difficulty, she joins a photography group in occupational therapy. She has always wanted to pursue photography as a hobby and is keen to develop her skills. The therapist and Irina negotiate a hierarchy of goals where she is required 'to interact with others, without undue anxiety, over the course of 10 sessions' (graded exposure).

1. Be a nominal member of the group; work alone taking photographs; interact only with the therapist
2. Work on an individual activity alongside others doing a group activity
3. Work outside with one other person from the group, taking photographs
4. Work with the same person in the group room and dark room
5. Work with another person in the group room and dark room
6. Join the group when they are being taught a technique; no particular interaction required
7. Work with others in the group
8. Join the group on an outing to a photography museum.

---

Irina manages goals 1–4 fairly easily by the third session. Involvement with the photography tasks enables her to achieve the goals for interacting without too much anxiety. During the fourth session, however, she has a panic attack prior to going in the dark room with a male member of the group. The planned dark room activity is adapted to accommodate her difficulties. She had not anticipated her reaction to being in an enclosed space with a man and is able to explore this further in her individual psychotherapy sessions. With extra encouragement and support she achieves the rest of her goals.

For therapists working in the psychodynamic or humanistic traditions, setting specific goals or objectives is often inappropriate. For instance, the emphasis within the humanistic tradition on being non-directive and letting the client lead leaves the therapist little scope to structure future action. In cases like this, aims such as 'gain greater self-awareness' may suffice and, providing the therapist is very clear about the design of treatment (e.g. structure of activity) and evaluates the intervention carefully, vague treatment will be avoided.

## Constructing effective goals/objectives

The following points should be remembered when establishing goals/objectives:

- Goals should, if possible, be **negotiated** with the person. At the very least their agreement is needed to ensure their co-operation and motivation. If an individual does not realise he or she is meant to interact with others to practise social skills, how can we expect him or her to do it? Service users must know what is expected of them and what they can expect from themselves. Ideally, goals/objectives should be made explicit and agreed at the beginning of a treatment session. Then at the end of the session, you have criteria to evaluate what has taken place, and future goals can be modified accordingly.
- Goals must be **achievable but challenging**. While the overall aim of treatment may require a large leap in the person's functioning (e.g. from being 'ill' to being 'well') it is essential that the person feels able to manage the immediate mini-steps. Herein lies a difficulty. There is a fine balance between stimulation and too much pressure, between underestimating the person's capacity (which results in boredom) and overestimating it (which may result in failure and loss of confidence). Because of this, failure may need to be formally acknowledged as 'understandable' or 'acceptable'.
- Goals should be **flexible** and regularly revisited. Therapy rarely proceeds according to a pre-set sequence: aims are modified. Sometimes treatment starts with a therapy activity and then planning occurs subsequently. Also, service users change and progress in unpredictable ways. As Kielhofner puts it, 'Change involves periods of stability and instability, dramatic transformation and uneven progression' (Kielhofner, 1995, p. 259). Planned interventions need to remain flexible so that they can accommodate such evolution.

- Finally, we should recognise that **the process of negotiating goals may in itself be therapeutic**. A person who has grandiose or unrealistic views of their ability, for instance, may benefit from a discussion that aims to establish realistic goals. Another person may have a condition where their functioning is deteriorating in an unpredictable way (such as in dementia) and may well appreciate the opportunity to explore what they should realistically anticipate being able to do in the future.

## 8.3  DESIGNING THE PROGRAMME

Once the basic aims/goals have been formulated, the more creative side of designing the therapy intervention comes into play. This often involves manipulating and grading two key elements: the *activity* and/or the *environment*. Activity and the environment become the tools we use in our interventions.

### Using activity in treatment

Central to occupational therapy is our focus on occupation. This may include the use of activities as a key therapeutic tool. Here, we adapt and use activities purposefully to achieve therapy goals, for instance increasing the social, cognitive, perceptual or physical demands of the activity. Alternatively, service users may carry out purposeful activities at home on their own as part of the therapy (as Dowie did in Case example 8.1).

The **choice of type and level of activity** and how its used to meet therapeutic goals varies enormously. One of our core skills as occupational therapists is being able to creatively harness the inherent potential of purposeful activities towards making therapy useful, meaningful, interesting, even fun. When we design treatment, we aim to adapt and grade activities to provide levels of increasing stimulation and challenge. Activities are lengthened, shortened, made more complicated, spiced up with competition, rearranged for smaller groups, and so forth. Cara and MacRae (1998) distinguish between different characteristics of activities:

- **Structured versus unstructured** – Structured activities (e.g. certain crafts and games with rules) can be helpful for people who lack motivation/drive, have limited functional abilities, or who need the security of having something clearcut on which to focus. Unstructured activities, such as creative arts, can be useful for generating energy and self-expression.
- **Passive versus active** – Passive, non-threatening activities, such as watching TV or listening to music, will suit some people as they appeal to their interests or because they are enjoyed at a shared/symbolic social level. Active activities (from cooking to jogging) will suit those who need more motor, sensory or cognitive stimulation or who enjoy physical challenge.
- **Simple versus complex** – Simple tasks can increase individuals' self-esteem as they can be completed successfully, while complex tasks may invite a sense of

frustration or failure. However, simple tasks can be viewed as boring, childish and not providing sufficient opportunities to learn and grow.

- **Process- versus product-orientated** – Process-orientated activities where the emphasis is placed on the doing (as in projective art, when feelings are expressed on paper and then torn up), help clients to experiment. Other individuals may prefer having a concrete end-product to show for their efforts (as in a craft piece).

The use of activity will be explored more fully in the next chapter. For now, the following are the key factors that need to be taken into account when designing treatment.

### Aims of treatment

Which activity or activities can best fulfil the aims of treatment and have scope for grading, while being appropriate for the specific service user? For example, the structured activities of woodwork or printing are arguably more suitable for improving task performance than an open-ended 'paint what you like' session.

### Patient's/client's choice

Which activity is going to be most *meaningful* to the person at both a personal and cultural level? Motivation to do an activity is increased if it has some meaning for the person and only the individual can decide this. While the therapist may set some of the parameters, he or she should offer choices to patients/clients respecting their capacity to make their own decisions (Case example 8.5). As Yerxa points out, 'The meaning of the activity, its choice, and satisfaction in it are determined by the individual patient's needs, interests, and motivations. They should not be determined by the occupational therapist's view of meaning' (1979, p. 29).

---

#### Case example 8.5   Planning the use of music in a leisure group

A twice-weekly leisure group was created for 10 elderly clients in a day unit. In the first session, with the therapist's help, the group members decided what kinds of activity they would like to do together. Working with music in different ways came out as the number one choice. At the day unit, music was often used already – for instance in regular sing-alongs and dance sessions. The therapist was charged with the responsibility to come back the following week with different ideas for what they might do using music. The therapist suggested the following activities.

**Ideas for different activities**

- Discuss the life and times of a composer/band leader/music group and the culture/history of the time
- Each member brings in or suggests a special piece of music to be played – group members would then share reminiscences about that piece

---

- Listen to a new piece of music and share personal reactions with other group members

**Aims of treatment**

- Reactivate an interest in music and encourage its use as a hobby
- Stimulate interest in studying topics in their historical context
- Encourage group interaction and relationship building
- Enable personal reminiscences and expression of feelings

**Grading**

The therapist explains that it might be a good idea to start gently with some prepared talks and discussions. As the group get to know each other better they can move on to activities that involve more personal disclosure and interpersonal sharing.

### Therapist's choice

Sometimes the person is not able to choose which activity he or she would like to do (e.g. when a person is acutely ill or severely disabled and unable to communicate). Occupational therapists must choose on behalf of their client, applying their professional judgement. In such situations, therapists should adopt an ethical stance, trying to resist imposing our own values (Case example 8.6).

---

**Case example 8.6   Resisting imposing one's own values**

Therapists need to guard against imposing their own values/assumptions/stereotypes when selecting activities. Take, for example, the cases of Hilda, Karen and Bill:

- **Hilda** is 72 years old. She is invited to come to the unit's kitchen to cook a meal as part of her domestic assessment prior to discharge. In fact Hilda has always hated cooking. At home she never cooks, tending to buy in frozen TV meals or get a take-away. The activity that Hilda really wants to do in occupational therapy is to give the computer a go but she feels too shy to ask.
- **Karen**, aged 16, is encouraged to help a group of adolescents put up Christmas decorations. At first she is reluctant but after much persuasion she makes some streamers. Later the occupational therapist finds out that Karen has got into trouble with her parents for taking part in this activity. Her parents are Jehovah's Witnesses and do not support celebrating Christmas in this way.
- **Bill**, aged 65, watches television all day. The therapist feels that Bill should be engaged in something 'more productive and active' and suggests a range of community activities. Bill is not interested and disengages from treatment.

## Practical constraints

What activities are currently in operation? Taking these into account may help make the best use of existing resources. For instance, if treatment is to take place in a client's home our intervention might be limited to talking or to paper-and-pencil exercises. Limited funds may constrain opportunities to buy expensive equipment such as computers and kilns, while insurance and safety considerations may prohibit the use of heavy machinery. Limited staff resources may prevent certain activities, for example those that need two therapists to run a group. Limited resources can also be a source of inspiration, though – for example 'rubbish collages' are both fun to make and potentially attractive!

## Balance of total activity programme

It is important to consider the shape of a person's day/week and how interventions may impact on the person generally. For instance, if treatment is to take place in a unit, then the balance of the person's overall programme needs to be taken into account. Is the service user going to experience an appropriate balance of activities that are new and challenging or reassuring and safe; active or passive; diversional or emotionally charged; restful or stimulating; structured or free-ranging; staff-directed or patient-directed; abstract or concrete? It is a thoughtless institutional practice to apply treatment without considering how the patient/client will experience it in the context of their day. I once witnessed the absurd situation of a patient who was required to do cooking all morning with a helper, then had a kitchen assessment with the occupational therapist at teatime, and in the evening was pushed into cooking a meal on the ward!

## Environment

In addition to being concerned about service users' environments in terms of identifying the skills they need to cope in these, occupational therapists exploit and adapt environments as part of their therapeutic interventions. Specifically, we manipulate the physical, emotional and social dimensions of the environment to achieve a range of goals. The process of grading the environment (adding more or less stimulation, pressure, stress) is the foundation of most of our therapeutic interventions (Case example 8.7):

- **Physical environment** – The physical environment (in terms of type of room, seating arrangements, positioning of equipment, noise, stimulation, light) can have a dramatic impact, prompting certain expectations and behaviours. For instance, we could simulate an office environment to encourage work-like behaviour; use floor cushions and darken a room to induce relaxation; and put chairs in a circle to encourage interaction. Where we have several occupational therapy rooms to work with we would creatively and carefully balance noisy areas with quiet spaces, messy ones with neat ones, and structured activity areas with unstructured, relaxed zones. People have different preferences, needs and thresholds in relation to noise, stimulation and mess. Some people need to have a quiet space before they can engage in activities, while others like to have music and lots of things happening around them.

- **Emotional environment** – Although less tangible, the emotional environment is important for making people feel safe and supported. When we work in units, it is worth considering the impact of the atmosphere around us. What 'feel' does the unit have? Caring? Busy? Accepting? Do patients/clients feel encouraged? If the answers are in the negative, is there anything that can be done to change the 'feel' in more positive directions?

- **Social environment** – The influence of the therapist's role has already been discussed in Chapter 6. Beyond this, the influence of other people can be crucial. If a client is being treated at home, what are relationships with family members like? In groupwork, what supporting roles can other group members play? Here, choice of group size is particularly relevant. Generally, six to eight members is the preferred size, but a smaller group may be indicated if members are disturbed or functioning at a developmental level that reduces their ability to interact.

---

### Case example 8.1   Grading and adapting the environment

Two examples of grading the physical, emotional and/or social environments are offered below:

Neeta, aged 25, is admitted to hospital suffering from acute anxiety. Her anxiety is so extreme that she becomes paralysed whenever she is in the same room as other people. Yet, on a one-to-one level, Neeta is able to function well and is bright and articulate. As part of the wider team treatment strategy, the therapist and Neeta negotiate a systematic desensitisation programme, to be carried out for an hour a day, in which she is exposed to increasing levels of social contact while doing activities.

**Goal 1** = Work one-to-one with therapist in a large workroom but away from others behind a screen

**Goal 2** = Screen partially removed so Neeta catches glimpses of others

**Goal 3** = Screen removed but therapist stays beside Neeta and acts as a protective screen

**Goal 4** = Neeta and therapist work in the open (other people are around doing their own activities but keep away)

**Goal 5** = One other person (of Neeta's choice) joins the activity session

**Goal 6** = Size of group increased.

Neeta progressed through her goals relatively swiftly, achieving them all within three weeks.

Stella, aged 50, suffers from recurring bouts of depression that eventually respond positively to medication. She is referred to a community mental health occupational therapist to assess the degree to which environmental pressures play a part in her

---

condition. At the first interview, they discuss Stella's work environment. She tells of being in her job for five years and how she has mostly managed to cope with the stressful working environment, which offers little by way of positive benefits. In particular, Stella perceives her boss as over-critical and exploitative. The therapist and Stella seek new ways to make the work experience more palatable. For instance, Stella is encouraged to renegotiate her work tasks with her boss to include more fulfilling and satisfying aspects. This proves unsuccessful but, with the therapist's support, Stella makes the positive move of changing jobs, which has a major impact on her quality of life and reduces her vulnerability to depressive episodes.

## 8.4  CLINICAL REASONING

So far, I have focused on the component parts and the decisions involved in planning interventions. This runs the risk of failing to capture the artistry and the complexities of the way therapists actually think and act in practice. In practice, our reasoning can often be tacit (unstated); our planning intuitive, rather than systematically logical. We think 'on our feet', pulling together our knowledge, skills and experience of different problems and strategies. Also, the planning process does not simply occur in the therapist's head as a series of clear-cut decisions. Instead, planning occurs continuously, negotiated in the context of an evolving therapeutic relationship. The wider, ever growing, literature on clinical reasoning better reflects and demonstrates the rich, flexible and multidimensional way we think, plan and act in practice (see Table 8.1 for a summary of different types of clinical reasoning; examples of clinical reasoning in a range of practice contexts are offered in the *British Journal of Occupational Therapy* 58(5), 1996).

Mattingly and Fleming (1994) famously describe occupational therapists as having a 'three-track mind', simultaneously engaging in what they call procedural, interactive and conditional reasoning. On the basis of their extensive study of therapists' practice, they found that: 'Therapists could process or analyse different aspects of the problem, almost simultaneously, using different thinking styles; and they did not "lose track of" their thoughts about aspects of a problems as those components were temporarily shifted to be in the background while another aspect was brought into the foreground' (Mattingly and Fleming, 1994, pp. 120–121).

**Procedural reasoning** is the term Mattingly and Fleming give to the problem-solving process. Here, therapists focus on the disease or disability, identifying the functional problems and selecting interventions to reduce the impact of these problems. **Interactive reasoning** cues into the co-operative nature of practice, which requires occupational therapists to tap into the meanings, commitments, values and motives of patients/clients as part of engaging them collaboratively in treatment. With interactive reasoning we continually use our own feelings as a reference point and interpret patients'/clients' meanings either to modify treatment or to persuade them to see their disability in another light. **Conditional reasoning** focuses on the particular kind of enquiry therapists use when they

**Table 8.1** Different types of clinical reasoning

| Type | Description | Example |
|------|-------------|---------|
| Conditional reasoning (e.g. Mattingly and Fleming, 1994) | Striving to understand 'the whole person in their life world context' | Devising purposeful activity a person might do when discharged home, in order to keep them active |
| Interactive reasoning (e.g. Mattingly and Fleming, 1994; Borg and Bruce, 1997) | Reasoning arises out of the interaction between therapist and client. The therapists acts on subtle cues in order to motivate and engage the individual in treatment | Therapists modifies approach during treatment sessions to relieve some of the client's tension, e.g. by lightening the interaction with some humour and small talk |
| Narrative reasoning (e.g. Mattingly, 1998; Schell, 1998) | Phenomenological process where stories are used to understand an individual's meanings. Thinking involves empathy, improvisation and attention to values/beliefs | Therapist and client share their pictures of how the individual experiences his or her disability. They explore occupational meanings in terms of past, present and future scenarios |
| Pragmatic reasoning (e.g. Schell and Cervero, 1993) | The sociocultural context, setting and practical/environmental constraints, plus therapist's own life experiences, all influence decision making | Therapist plans a client's discharge programme that takes into account limited home support and day-care provision |
| Predictive reasoning (Hagedorn, 1997) | Therapist imagines different scenarios for the future, weighing up possibilities and probabilities while trying to predict the effects of different interventions | Therapist considers how the use of a piece of new equipment might transform the individual's ability to communicate with others |
| Procedural reasoning (e.g. Mattingly and Fleming, 1994) | Therapist identifies problems and problem-solving goals through hypothetico-deductive reasoning | Therapist identifies that a person is not performing a task correctly because of an underlying cognitive-perceptual problem rather than an emotional block. Steps to remediate this problem are then taken |
| Scientific reasoning (e.g. Rogers, 1983; Schell, 1998) | The focus is on the nature of the condition and likely consequences for activities. Systematic thinking process based on hypothesis testing and scientific model making plus use of research and evidence-based practice | Therapist formulates problems based on knowledge of client's condition, prognosis and the results from a standardised assessment |

strive to understand 'the whole person in their life world context' and to create meaningful experiences. Here, therapists seek to understand what is meaningful to the person. They have to imagine the individual as they were before their illness and in the future. As Mattingly and Fleming put it, conditional reasoning 'requires an ability to understand and "see" people as they see themselves, and the ability and energy to project a picture for a person's future, one vivid enough that the person will be willing to participate in the image making' (Mattingly and Fleming, 1994, p. 197).

Other researchers have studied how clinical reasoning varies between practitioners – for instance, between 'novices' and 'experts'. Strong *et al.*, (1995) found that experts considered a wider range of factors when making clinical decisions than did students. Both experts and novices employed narrative reasoning, but experts were found to utilise scientific reasoning to a greater extent than did novices, who tended to rely more on pragmatic reasoning. Research (e.g. Ryan, 1995) has also established that experienced therapists are able to form a clear procedural and interactional image before they meet a client, even if this image is subsequently revised. In contrast, novice therapists need to be with the client before they can form images and start reasoning. McKay and Ryan (1995) found that expert practitioners were able to formulate a more total picture of the client and were more rapid and accurate in their assessments. Novices needed to break the situation down into component parts, were more rule-bound and tended to focus on the immediate situation rather than the larger picture.

## Clinical reasoning in practice: Thomas's experience

While different types of clinical reasoning tend to operate simultaneously, it is possible to highlight moments when one type of reasoning seems to take precedence or is more relevant. The story of Thomas's occupational therapy experience given in Case example 8.8 is a case in point:

---

### Case example 8.8   Thomas's experience

Thomas, aged 35, had a long-standing history of unstable epilepsy and a tendency to be passive and dependent in his behaviour. He was admitted to a hospital to stabilise his medication **[scientific reasoning].** On initial assessment the occupational therapist learned that he lived in a flat with his parents and spent most of his time watching television. When he was feeling better, he helped around the house **[narrative reasoning]**.

Thomas was likely to be discharged within a couple of weeks and the team recognised that there was a limit to how much treatment could be accomplished. However, they were concerned about what was likely to happen on his discharge **[predictive reasoning]**. Based on his previous pattern of being erratic about taking his medication, it seemed likely that he would be readmitted within a few months **[pragmatic reasoning]**. It was agreed that the occupational therapist would try to follow him up after his discharge home. The team decided that the most useful intervention would be to help Thomas develop some new productive activity that he would be able to continue once discharged. The therapist reasoned that having a new role or interest would not just give Thomas more drive/motivation, it would also offer a way of structuring his day, thus helping him to maintain his mental health **[conditional reasoning]**.

The first step to treatment was to search for a meaningful occupation. Thomas was unresponsive when the occupational therapist tried to interview him **[interactive reasoning]**. She returned to the occupational therapy records from his previous admissions and discovered that Thomas had always loved plants and

---

nature: he was often to be found wandering around the local parks and gardens. Also, he had functioned well in previous occupational therapy gardening groups, though this had not been taken further **[narrative reasoning]**. The therapist returned to Thomas and asked if he would like to come to the occupational therapy department to do some gardening. For the first time since his admission, he showed a spark of interest **[interactive reasoning]**. They agreed the short-term objective that he would come down to occupational therapy daily to re-learn and practise his gardening skills, potting plants, taking cuttings and so on. For the long term the therapist hoped he would become sufficiently engaged to take on the responsibility of creating a patio garden at home **[conditional reasoning]**.

Thomas spent two weeks tending the department's plants. Towards the end of his admission, he went with the therapist to a garden centre to design and plant a new tub of flowers that was to be placed in the entrance of the hospital. On his discharge, the therapist arranged to visit him at three-weekly intervals, with the aim of continuing to encourage the new hobby **[narrative reasoning]** and to monitor his use of medication **[scientific reasoning]**. Together (and with the support of Thomas' parents), they planned a new patio garden for Thomas to create and work on at home **[interactive reasoning]**.

## 8.5 Conclusion and reflections

This chapter has explored the components and stages of the treatment planning process, examining how therapists reason and the criteria they bring to bear when making clinical decisions. In the process, therapists necessarily draw upon science, art and ethics. 'Science' comes to the fore when we analyse problems and apply our knowledge of conditions and appropriate theoretical frameworks. The 'art' emerges in the way we engage service users in treatment and we intuitively and creatively design interventions therapeutically blending elements of our approach, activities and the environment. The ethical dimension is evidenced in our attempt to be person-centred and to work with what is meaningful and purposeful for the individual concerned. Our clinical reasoning is therefore multi-layered.

The stages of planning an intervention are summarised in Figure 8.2. However, clinical reasoning in practice is considerably more fluid and complex. Much of our reasoning and planning emerges out of a continually evolving negotiation between the team, service users and ourselves. At the same time, we still need to try to be systematic and clear when planning interventions. This is the only way to ensure that our interventions are both coherent and effective. Tacit clinical reasoning is not enough. If therapists cannot be clear about their clinical reasoning and interventions, what chance do service users have of understanding what they are supposed to be doing? Therapists must articulate the value of particular interventions if other team members are to understand and make use of our potential contribution.

*Organise information* using scientific, procedural, interactive and narrative reasoning:
- Identify problems in functional terms
- Identify strengths to build on
- Select priority problem/s.

↓

*Establish aims and goals* using interactive, pragmatic and predictive reasoning:
- Establish overall aim
- Identify short- and long-term aims/goals
- Set specific goals and objectives where relevant.

↓

*Design the programme*, using narrative, conditional and interactive reasoning:
- **Activity**   The choice of which activity and how demanding to make it depends on treatment aims, patient's/client's preference, therapist's selection, practical constraints and overall programme balance. Where possible, we should try to be client-centred and only use activities that the individual finds meaningful. Consider how to grade the activity in order to achieve treatment aims; e.g. increase complexity of task to facilitate higher learning of problem-solving skill
- **Environment**   Consider how to adapt the physical, emotional and social environment in order to achieve therapy aims, e.g. we might reduce amount of tools available for use in a group activity to encourage sharing between people

**Figure 8.2**   Summary of stages of planning an intervention

# 9
## OCCUPATIONAL THERAPY INTERVENTION

*A common sense practice in an uncommon world.*

Maureen Fleming

Ten contrasting case studies are outlined in this chapter, which aims to integrate the different aspects of the occupational therapy process discussed in previous chapters. While the case studies are not a representative sample, they show something of the breadth and scope of our work. Each case study offers, in broad brush strokes, an indication of the variety of individuals we treat and the different kinds of intervention we make. I have tried to demonstrate our eclectic theoretical base, short- and long-term aspects of treatment, and some of the issues that can arise from our interventions. Although these case studies are not verbatim accounts of actual records, the material for them is drawn largely from clinical experience and so reflects the kinds of problems and treatments encountered in occupational therapy.

Space does not permit a more in-depth exploration of the complexities of the individuals' problems or treatment and the different satisfactions, frustrations, disappointments and uncertainties we experience in practice. Despite this, I hope the case studies will encourage deeper reflection. To this end I offer a couple of points of discussion at the end of each case study to stimulate debate and highlight particularly important practice issues.

To assist ease of reading and the drawing of comparisons, I have organised all the case studies under the following headings:

- Problem issues
- Summary of history
- Team strategy
- Occupational therapy assessment
- Treatment plan
- Progress
- Points of discussion.

As you go through each case study you might find it useful to reflect on the following questions:

- What is the key occupational therapy role identifiable in each study?
- What theoretical framework underpins each intervention? Select an alternative theoretical framework or approach. How would this change the intervention applied?
- In your view, how should the problems identified in each study be prioritised and handled?

- How could the occupational therapist grade each suggested activity to meet the associated aims and goals effectively?
- Would any of the individuals be assessed or treated differently in your own, familiar clinical context? What would be your team's approach?

## 9.1   CASE STUDIES

## CASE STUDY 9.1    CATHERINE

- **Problem issues** – Alcohol misuse; retirement and lack of productive occupations

### Summary of history

Catherine, a 68-year-old woman, lives alone in an attractive house with her two cats. She retired eight years ago from her job as a librarian at the local university (a job she had held for 20 years). Since that time she has become isolated and inactive. She has few friends and no family nearby. Catherine has a long-standing history of being a heavy drinker but she kept her drinking largely under control when she was working. She now tends to drink alcohol throughout the day – as she says, 'It helps me feel good'. Catherine's alcohol misuse came to light after a fall where she fractured her femur. Having admitted her problem to herself, she went to her GP for help in tackling it. Her GP referred her to the Substance Misuse Team (part of the community mental health service).

### Team strategy

The team agreed that the likely focus of treatment should be on helping Catherine develop some alternative, meaningful occupations and so she was allocated to the occupational therapist. The therapist decided to adopt a cognitive–behavioural approach. She also hoped to refer Catherine to a psychotherapy group run on psychodynamic lines.

### Occupational therapy assessment

Two preliminary interviews at Catherine's home were undertaken. The therapist explored Catherine's view of the alcohol problem and her motivation to manage it. The OPHI-II was used to structure the interview, in which Catherine compared her life eight years ago to her life now. Several self-rating tools were employed alongside to explore her roles, pattern of daily activities, interests and values.

Assessment revealed that, while Catherine wanted to manage her drinking, she did not want to give it up entirely. She realised, however, that she would need some extra support to control her intake. She agreed with the therapist that her main need was to find and develop some meaningful occupations – ones that would productively fill the void that had opened up on her retirement. She expressed interest in swimming on a regular basis to help get her back into shape physically. She also agreed to return to doing some creative writing as this was a hobby she had always loved and enjoyed prior to retirement.

**Treatment plan**

| Aims/objectives | Treatment methods |
| --- | --- |
| 1. Implement a controlled drinking regime with support | a) Use of contract and a review of daily drinking habits, recording intake and associated feelings/ events in a diary |
| | b) Group work – weekly supportive psychotherapy group for 'ex' and 'controlled' drinkers |
| | c) Individual therapy sessions with the occupational therapist once a fortnight to review progress |
| 2. Set goals towards implementing a new activity programme. | a) Swimming three times a week |
| | b) Spend at least five hours a week doing some creative writing |
| | c) Join a new club or class |

**Progress**

Catherine responded well to her new activity programme and professional support. She found the diary writing difficult to maintain but, with encouragement from the therapist, she persisted and found that the process gave her insights into her situation. Initially, she had been shocked to realise how much she did drink – an insight that provided an extra spur to engage in treatment. Through writing her diary she learned about her stress points and drinking 'triggers', and this enabled her to take more control over her behaviour.

However, she found the group work threatening and stressful. After the first session she was reluctant to return. The occupational therapist acknowledged how difficult it was to be in a group and discuss such painful issues. She negotiated with her to give it a try for a month (four sessions). Catherine was also encouraged to discuss her anxieties with the group leader. She did this and soon found the group both supportive and instructive. She eventually became a long-standing attender.

In terms of her activities, Catherine joined an over-50s swimming club, which she enjoyed for both the activity and the social element. She also signed up for a creative writing evening class, which became the highlight of her week. On her discharge interview, Catherine reported that, in collaboration with her writing group, she was working to produce a volume of short stories and poetry, which they hoped to get published.

While the treatment proved extremely successful in terms of enabling new meaningful occupations, it was not without problems. Catherine lapsed and broke her controlled drinking regime on two occasions and as a result she withdrew from her 'new life' for several weeks. The important lesson for her was that she understood that she would be able to get back on track if, or when, she had similar lapses in the future.

**Points of discussion**

Two particular issues are raised by this case study:

- The therapist needed Catherine to be actively engaged in goal-setting and planning her new occupational life. For Catherine's treatment to have any chance of success, **she needed to be motivated** to carry out the controlled drinking programme and to engage in activities. Had she not wanted to change – at least at some level – treatment would probably have been pointless. Often the biggest battle is the first one, where individuals acknowledge that they have a problem with which they want to grapple.

- The case study also raises questions about **the therapist's theoretical approach**. While adopting a cognitive–behavioural approach (featuring, among other things, diary writing to identify behavioural triggers), the therapist also offered Catherine an opportunity to work through emotional issues psychodynamically. At the same time, the therapist was operating within a broader framework of using a person-centred occupationally focused model. It is quite common to see therapists draw in this way on several theoretical approaches simultaneously. While eclectic practice like this is possible, even common, there are some tensions that need to be resolved. In particular, despite generally aiming to be person-centred, the therapist was also fairly directive, for instance, when encouraging Catherine to persist with the diary and the group therapy. These two approaches could be seen as being potentially contradictory.

The key to resolving this dilemma is to focus on the *partnership* angle. There is a difference between being coercively directive and negotiating. In negotiation, the therapist acknowledges the person's understandable anxieties and explains the potential gains of a treatment. With a person-centred approach, the final decision of whether or not to carry out a certain treatment must always rest with the individual.

---

## CASE STUDY 9.2   REG

- **Problem issues** – Severe and enduring mental health problems; rehabilitation

### Summary of history

Reg, a 40-year-old Afro-Caribbean man, had his first schizophrenic breakdown when he was in his teens. Since then he has spent a significant proportion of his life going in and out of hospital. When he is ill, he is paranoid and suffers from florid delusions and hallucinations, including hearing threatening voices. Some of his delusions relate to spiritualism and voodoo – ideas that seem to relate to events he witnessed as a child while visiting his grandmother in the Caribbean. He has been sectioned a number of times as his behaviour when ill is violent and unpredictable. Although Reg's long-term medication contains most of his psychotic symptoms, he still has some residual difficulties. He sometimes says strange things or behaves in a slightly bizarre manner. His behaviour and skills also show evidence of deterioration and institutionalisation. He lives with his sister and her family, and they require some support and a break from Reg during the day. In an attempt to prevent inpatient admission and to maintain Reg's life in the community, he periodically attends a day hospital. In addition, a community psychiatric nurse seeks to provide long-term support to both Reg and his family by making regular home visits.

## Team strategy

Overall, the strategy of the day hospital team is to provide Reg with some productive roles during the day and to develop his skills. The doctors and nurses monitor Reg's medication in an attempt to find the most effective long-term dose, which the community psychiatric nurse will follow up. The psychologist at the day hospital designs a social skills training programme to be carried out with the nurses. The occupational therapist aims to work with Reg's occupational performance and skills in conjunction with the art teacher (technical instructor).

## Occupational therapy assessment

The priority problems identified from observing Reg in activities and carrying out assessment using the standardised REHAB and the Social Functioning Scales include:

- **Task performance** – Reg's skills are fairly poor: he has poor concentration (less than 10 minutes on routine work task), process skills with limited problem-solving ability and difficulty in following verbal instructions. He is only partially independent in daily living tasks and needs prompting and assistance.
- **General behaviour** – Reg tends to be compliant, dependent and passive. Some slightly odd behaviours are in evidence, such as making inconsequential remarks and staring blankly ahead. Social skills are also reduced, given his slightly suspicious demeanour and his limited ability to initiate conversation and maintain eye contact.
- **Social functioning** – Reg scores quite poorly on measures related to withdrawal, interaction and recreation. He engages in few leisure activities other than watching television. He tends to be isolated except in the evenings when he is in the company of his family.
- In terms of his **strengths**, Reg enjoys music and he shows considerable skill in drawing and painting. His self-care and presentation are relatively good, in part because of his sister's care and influence.

## Treatment plan

The day hospital staff create the following rehabilitation programme with Reg:

| Aims/objectives | Treatment methods |
| --- | --- |
| 1. To practise productive work/ leisure role behaviour towards increasing esteem/status and improving task performance skills | Daily attendance at the art workshop to develop a portfolio of art work and learn different art techniques |
| 2. To develop a greater sense of self, initiative, autonomy and responsibility | (a) Day hospital environment and consistent team approach<br>(b) Successful experience in his art work |

| | |
|---|---|
| | (c) Investigations into his home/domestic work role aiming to increase expectations of him in the long term |
| 3. To develop social skills, improve functioning, reduce problematic behaviours and widen leisure opportunities | (a) Once-weekly social skills group |
| | (b) Twice-weekly general social activities group within day hospital |
| | (c) Encouragement to take up evening activities and holidays with family |
| | (d) Consistent staff approach to challenge any bizarre speech or behaviour |
| 4. To develop domestic independence skills and encourage Reg to make a positive contribution in his domestic role | Twice weekly lunch cooking group |

## Progress of treatment

Reg regularly attended the day hospital over a period of two years. He was gradually resettled to a local day centre, which he attended three times a week. The community psychiatric nurse maintained contact over the period of discharge and continued to provide long-term support at home.

The regular art sessions proved significant in helping Reg to develop his task performance skills. By the end of his treatment he was able to work reasonably well for two-hour stretches. He enjoyed learning different art techniques and he developed a creditable portfolio of work. Several of his pieces had been framed and displayed on the day hospital walls. Reg seemed quietly pleased that his work was valued in this way.

The formal social skills training sessions proved less effective, as Reg preferred to be by himself. As he said, 'No point in talking-talking'. Through his group cookery sessions, however, he learned to handle working in parallel with others and feel reasonably comfortable. It became apparent that Reg's bizarre behaviours were reduced when he felt more relaxed, safe and not pressurised to interact with others. The day hospital staff discussed the implications of this with his family.

The latter part of Reg's rehabilitation focused on increasing his role at home in terms of his level of contribution and the amount of responsibility he took. To this end he learned how to cook four set meals for his family – a development much appreciated by his sister. He was also encouraged to make a contribution in terms of washing up and household cleaning. While he rarely initiated such cleaning activities, he was amenable when asked to help.

## Points of discussion

- While we are now much more aware of health inequalities than we were 20 years ago when Reg first required treatment, we still have an important role to play in challenging inequalities, discrimination and oppression when we see it. In Reg's case, it is likely that **institutional racism** contributed to his levels of stress, his illness and the type of treatment he received.. Statistical evidence on the incidence of mental illness in the UK shows that significant health inequalities persist. For instance, people of African descent and others from ethnic minorities are more likely than white people to be detained under Section of the Mental Health Act. Moreover, studies show that these groups of people are also less likely to be offered alternatives to drug treatment (Department of Health, 2003).

- Reg's rehabilitation also raises an important point about our responses to mental illness and **the social construction of disability** in conditions such as schizophrenia (see, for instance, Williams and Collins, 2002). It is all too easy to have low expectations of people with severe and enduring mental health problems. While the prognosis for Reg is relatively poor in that he is always likely to struggle with his illness and remain on a trajectory of deteriorating function, we still need to remain positive and enable Reg to have some hope for the future. It is likely that Reg's recovery was enabled, at least in part, because of the positive expectations of the staff and their confidence that Reg could be productive and make a positive contribution.

## CASE STUDY 9.3    IFIGENIA

- **Problem issues** – 'Mid-life crisis' issues; loss of valued occupational roles

### Summary of history

Ifigenia is a 50-year-old Greek woman who came to this country 30 years ago after marrying an Englishman. She first became depressed after the birth of her daughter and has since had a couple of other major episodes that necessitated her being hospitalised.

Recently, Ifigenia has been so depressed that she has felt unable to get out of bed in the morning. It seems that the depression has occurred as a result of a combination of factors. She has remained somewhat isolated at home and has missed her family back in Greece. She has 'lost' both her husband and daughter in the last year – the husband left her for a younger woman, while her daughter recently changed jobs and moved 200 miles away. Alone on her 50th birthday, Ifigenia took an overdose of sleeping tablets. She was discovered, just in time, by a friend. As a result of this incident she was admitted to an acute psychiatric unit.

### Team strategy

The team's overall strategy was to provide Ifigenia with a temporary safe haven and manage her depression with medication. Aware of the multiple losses in Ifigenia's current life the team are concerned to give her support and to provide some follow-up care after she is discharged. The team agree that the occupational therapist is well placed to offer this follow-up support and to help Ifigenia develop some new roles and interests. The occupational therapist decides to use the model of human occupation as her theoretical framework.

## Occupational therapy assessment

Initially, the occupational therapist attempted to engage Ifigenia in treatment by building a relationship. The therapist went on to the ward each day to talk quietly with Ifigenia and try to establish some kind of contact. Ifigenia was not interested. She was not motivated to do anything and said she just wanted to be left alone to die. She felt that committing suicide was the only way to stop the dark pain she was suffering. The therapist was gentle and empathetic in her approach. She told Ifigenia to 'hang on in there' as the darkness would lift in a few days as the medication kicks in. She also acknowledged what a difficult time Ifigenia had had during the last year, missing her daughter and coping with the loss of, and rejection by, her husband. That all this occurred around the stress of Ifigenia's 50th birthday was just more salt in the wound. Slowly Ifigenia turned to the therapist for support and shared more of her story.

Ten days into her admission, Ifigenia's mood had lifted slightly. The occupational therapist talked with her about the importance of starting to 'get out and about' and do things, while she coped hour by hour. She suggested that Ifigenia try to do something active or productive – however small – every day and gradually to increase the amount she did. With this encouragement, Ifigenia managed to wash her hair, get dressed and put on some makeup. By the end of the week, Ifigenia felt able to come down to the Occupational Therapy Department to do a little cooking. The therapist observed that Ifigenia was slow and shaky in her movements and that her concentration was poor. However, Ifigenia found that the effort of engaging in a small cooking task was helpful, making her feel more 'normal' and grounded, combating her feelings of depersonalisation. She agreed to the idea of coming down to occupational therapy every day until her discharge home.

Prior to Ifigenia's discharge, the occupational therapist used the OCAIRS interview to determine her immediate and longer-term occupational needs. The most striking finding was that Ifigenia's sense of personal causation was extremely low. She felt her life to be highly out of control and her poor self-esteem was evident in her view of herself as a failure both as a woman and as a wife. She could not identify any skills of which she was proud and felt that anything she did was worthless. While Ifigenia was able to pinpoint dressmaking, fashion and cooking as interests, she did not currently participate in these in any meaningful ways. Her roles were also problematic: having lost her roles as wife and mother role she said she had nothing left in her life.

## Treatment plan

### Short-term aims in hospital
Alongside stabilising Ifigenia's depression with medication, try to engage her in activity and increase her productive activity. Encourage her to engage in cooking and other activities of her choice in the occupational therapy department.

**Long-term aims related to home**
- Monitor and develop occupational performance in terms of volition and habituation
- Continue to offer longer-term support to help improve self-esteem and sense of personal causation
- Engage in meaningful and satisfying occupations related to her dressmaking, fashion and cooking interests

**Progress**

While Ifigenia's depression was effectively and quite quickly managed by her medication, she remained at risk when she returned home. As she said, her life had been 'so empty, what is the point?' She continued to feel unworthy and she lacked a sense of agency, believing herself unable to effect any change in her life. She could not see beyond her roles as wife and mother – roles she felt she has lost. Part of her wanted to return to Greece to be with her family. But she also felt too much of a failure to be seen by them now.

The occupational therapist arranged to visit Ifigenia on a weekly basis until she was back on her feet. She encouraged Ifigenia to focus on herself and on getting better. Bigger questions related to where she was going to live and what she was going to do with her life could wait. The therapist stressed the importance of Ifigenia doing something productive and potentially enjoyable every day. Realising how helpful the cooking and other activities in the hospital had been in terms of 'grounding' her, Ifigenia agreed. They negotiated a programme that involved her in designing and making herself a new outfit.

On her first week home, Ifigenia started by going shopping to collect ideas and to buy the necessary fabrics and dressmaking patterns. Enthusiasm for the project grew. She took the step to join a weekly dressmaking class as part of building herself a new social life. Somewhat to her surprise, she so enjoyed the class and the social contact that she decided to enrol in a cordon bleu cookery class as well.

After three months the therapist gradually withdrew her input. Ifigenia was feeling much stronger and better about herself. She had enjoyed the dressmaking and cooking activities, gaining both pleasure and a sense of achievement. She had also made some new friends at the classes. With the therapist's encouragement, Ifigenia planned a small dinner party. When her new friends saw Ifigenia's dressmaking work they were full of praise. One woman asked if Ifigenia would make her bridal gown. This request began a new phase in Ifigenia's life. She began to run a part-time dressmaking business.

**Discussion**

- Ifigenia's story reminds us that **our interventions and responsibilities may be quite small** in the context of a person's life. Here, the therapist's main role was to help Ifigenia re-engage with previous leisure interests. The therapist hoped that the satisfaction and feelings of achievement that Ifigenia would gain from these hobbies could be the start of rebuilding her life. At the same time, the therapist recognised her limits. Medication played a key role in lifting Ifigenia's depression while the work involved in coming to terms with her losses and building a new life was entirely down to Ifigenia's efforts. The therapist did not assume responsibility for sorting out Ifigenia's work, social or domestic long term plans – she was there to enable and support knowing that a focus on one area often brings benefits in others.

- This case study offers a good example of the application of the **model of human occupation (MOHO)**. The therapist used the OCAIRS, which focused on Ifigenia's volition and habituation and the dynamic interaction between these. We can see how Ifigenia's occupational engagement in her dressmaking drove change. Of particular importance is the way that the therapist interacted with Ifigenia to support this occupational engagement – what Kielhofner and Forsyth (2002) call 'therapeutic strategies'. We sense the therapist *structuring* Ifigenia's activities in hospital and *encouraging*, *advising* and *validating* her efforts at home.

---

## CASE STUDY 9.4   ED

- **Problem issues** – Work rehabilitation; problematic manic behaviour

### Summary of history

Ed, a 45-year-old man, is admitted to hospital with a diagnosis of schizo-affective disorder and a history of manic episodes. On admission Ed is 'high', with pressure of speech and a volatile temper. He has not slept or eaten for five days but is still 'buzzing'. During this current manic episode, he has spent £15,000 on computer equipment for his 'new' (i.e. not formed except in his head) business as a creative marketing expert. He is convinced he is fast becoming a world-wide success. He is brought into hospital under Section to be stabilised on medication. He does not mind this, particularly as the hospital and staff are familiar to him and he currently views them as friends with whom he can share his many ideas.

Ed's continuing mental illness has been destructive to his marriage (his wife left him six years ago) and has seriously impaired his work and social relationships. Ed has worked as a fifth-form science teacher at a local school for the last 15 years. He has a reputation as a popular, charismatic teacher. His recent record is more problematic, however, as he has had two breakdowns in three years. The school children and his colleagues have had to cope with some very odd behaviour and the fact that he has had extended periods off sick. While his head of department has been supportive and understanding, his colleagues are reluctant to have him back.

### Team strategy

The ward staff found Ed extremely difficult to contain as he reacted aggressively when any attempt was made to curb his behaviour. He was slightly calmer in the more 'normal' and quieter atmosphere of the Occupational Therapy Department. This was partly because he had 'fallen in love' with the head occupational therapist and was content to sit and watch her work, occasionally making sexual advances. She was also one of the few people (along with the consultant and the charge nurse) from whom he would accept direction. He felt only the senior staff were 'his equals'.

The team's short-term aims were to get Ed re-stabilised on medication and to try to contain his manic and aggressive behaviour. As far as possible, only the charge nurse, consultant and head occupational therapist had direct dealings with Ed in order to minimise the threat of violence. The occupational therapist reluctantly agreed to accept Ed in the Occupational Therapy Department each morning. His attendance helped to calm him down and offered an opportunity to monitor any improvements.

## Occupational therapy assessment

Ed was encouraged to engage in concrete activities in an effort to contain his behaviour and offer him a daily structure. When he was interested in the activity, Ed was able to concentrate for up to 20 minutes. He needed prompting to stay engaged and a contract was established that involved withdrawing his 'privilege' of attending occupational therapy if he did not 'hold his enthusiasm in check'. No other formal assessment was attempted at this stage as his behaviour was likely to change significantly once he was stabilised on medication.

## Treatment plan

| Aims/objectives | Treatment methods |
|---|---|
| **Short term** | |
| Engage in concrete task-orientated behaviour to develop concentration and reduce activity level | Any activity that Ed can do by himself (quietly) with the occupational therapist monitoring him at a distance. Ed frequently chooses an art activity. The therapist encourages him to do some printing – an activity she thinks would be more containing |
| **Middle term** | |
| Once stabilised on medication, begin to return home (with support from the occupational therapy staff) and begin to sort out his financial problems | Home visits with support of a therapist initially. Later he stays at his house through the afternoon by himself |
| **Long term** | |
| Prepare and carry out simulated lessons as part of a work preparation programme Work assessment to establish whether it is realistic and appropriate for Ed to return to his job as a teacher | a) Simulated teaching sessions (using other staff and patients as pupils) b) High-level printing activities to assess concentration and task performance c) Discussion with the occupational therapist and consultant about managing the difficult return to work |

## Progress

Initially, Ed's behaviour proved to be too disruptive and volatile for the Occupational Therapy Department and he was confined to the ward. After a couple of weeks he calmed down sufficiently to join in some of the art and printing sessions in occupational therapy. These sessions were helpful for developing his concentration and ability to follow through concrete tasks.

After seven weeks of admission, Ed's mental state became more stable and he was ready to begin to sort out problems at home. The occupational therapist and a nurse did a home visit with Ed. They found an appalling mess, including computer equipment still new in boxes all over the place. Ed's task for the next few weeks was to clean and tidy his home; to try to get refunds on the equipment; and to sort out his correspondence, finances and numerous unpaid bills. All of this was quite difficult for Ed to handle – not least because he was confronted by how 'mad' he had been and his inability to recognise this. He went home from the hospital every afternoon. Sometimes staff went with him to give some moral support. After a couple of weeks, the strain of the process began to tell. Ed became depressed and his home treatment had to be suspended temporarily. When he was ready, he restarted his home activities and spent increasing amounts of time there. He began to take up the reins of normal life again, going home for the weekend.

Once Ed was back home full-time, attention turned to what to do about his teaching career. He wanted to return to his job, not least because he needed the money to cover some of his debts. As his head of department was prepared to have him back for a trial period, a work rehabilitation programme was implemented with Ed attending the hospital as a day patient. First, he practised his teaching skills in a series of role-play teaching sessions, with volunteers acting as his pupils. The goals for one of his sessions were to:

- Devise an accurate lesson plan
- Describe clearly the concept of oxygen debt
- Speak clearly and confidently
- Have eye contact with everyone in the room
- Answer questions appropriately.

His teaching ability proved excellent but that only resolved one part of the problem. Ed still had to return to the school, face his colleagues and, most importantly, cope in the long term with the stress of his job. Through discussion it was decided that Ed should arrange a meeting at the school with his head teacher to consider how to handle the difficulties ahead. The Head agreed that Ed could return to the school for one day a week initially, but that he should be supervised during all the teaching sessions. Ed tried this out for a month and reviewed his progress in weekly follow-up sessions with the occupational therapist. The days themselves went fairly well, but at the end of the month Ed decided that it was unrealistic to work as a teacher again. The treatment team concurred, despite recognising that letting his job go might well also compromise Ed's future mental health.

## Points of discussion

- Ed's case highlights an **ethical dilemma** we often face when service users' interests conflict with those of the wider society. Ed's therapist was strongly committed to helping him back to work, knowing it was his only remaining productive role and that it was important to him. However, the therapist also recognised that Ed was likely to become ill again and that this would probably involve a level of damage and disturbance for his colleagues and the schoolchildren. The therapist also faced the question of whether to encourage Ed to pursue work given the severity and instability of his mental state. He was heading for another failure. Maybe it was time to cut his losses and begin to adjust to a different life? At what point should hope be replaced by *realism* where expectations need to be lowered? In this case, Ed made his own decision not to return to work, thereby resolving the team's ethical dilemma.

- That Ed **felt he had fallen in love with his therapist** and that he made sexual advances to her is a not uncommon phenomenon. It is probably not surprising that individuals respond to care, warmth and attention in this way. The issue is how the process is handled and negotiated. It can be difficult for therapists to cope with the sexual harassment and intensity of emotion coming their way, even when it is understood and rationalised as 'transference' or as a 'disinhibition' – a symptom of the illness. In this case study, the therapist faced the challenge of continuing to work with Ed and respond positively to him without giving him undue encouragement. She needed to find a balance whereby she could reject his advances without rejecting him.

## CASE STUDY 9.5     KEVIN

- **Problem issues** – Playtherapy for limited play skills; behavioural problems

### Summary of history

Kevin, aged 8, is referred to a child and family psychiatry day unit after being suspended from school for his antisocial behaviour. He has a history of behaviour problems and bullying other children. Kevin is seen to have a close relationship with his mother, who tends to overprotect and cosset him, occasionally limiting his social contact with other children. This is the result, in part, of Kevin's epilepsy, largely controlled with medication.

### Team strategy

Each team member had a specific role to play: the nurses and unit teachers worked on Kevin's social interaction/behaviour; the psychologist investigated his cognitive functioning; the social worker engaged the parents in family therapy; the doctors reviewed the medication and took an overall management role; and the occupational therapist acted as a play therapist.

### Occupational therapy assessment

The occupational therapist initially attempted to use non-directive play with Kevin, offering 'free play' and a non-judgmental approach. This proved unworkable, however, as Kevin seemed unable to play and resorted to requesting structured, competitive board games. The occupational therapist decided to use play more directively. Through puppets, painting and dressing-up activities, Kevin revealed his lack of imaginative/fantasy play (i.e. developmentally he seemed to have missed out the play stage between 3 and 7 years). Further, when uncertain about what to do next, he often became aggressive or demanded to play a competitive game saying, 'I'm going to win!' The occupational therapist hypothesised that a key problem for Kevin was his limited play skills, which in turn severely affected his peer interactions. On the positive side, he was bright and able (e.g. in relation to school work) and he wanted to make friends with others, despite his past inability to do so.

## Treatment plan

| Aims/objectives | Treatment methods |
| --- | --- |
| 1. Establish a relationship with Kevin (making it 'safe' for him to lose occasionally or feel inadequate, as well as boosting his esteem) | Twice-weekly individual sessions with the occupational therapist taking a positive and encouraging attitude, while confronting him about his difficulties |
| 2. Teach how to play – encouraging flexibility, having fun and using imagination | Grade each activity for its imagination level, acting first as a model |
| 3. Lessen intensity for winning competitive games | Discuss issues of winning and losing, trying to practise handling the latter |
| 4. Work with Kevin's mother to find a play activity he can share with other children | Session with mother and Kevin together |

## Progress

First, a contract was established whereby Kevin could choose any activity he wanted to do for the last 10 minutes of the session, providing he joined in the occupational therapist's set activities earlier. The therapist invented a structured, competitive game that eventually could act as fantasy play. On trying to work constructively with Kevin's aggression she devised a competition of 'knocking down toy soldiers in the sandpit by throwing small plastic balls'. Kevin enjoyed this and it became his 'choice game' as well. The therapist encouraged the fun element by using laughter and adding little flourishes such as 'throwing all the balls in one go, really quickly'. When the intensity of Kevin's desire to win reduced and he simply enjoyed his sessions, the occupational therapist increasingly added the element of imagination, e.g. speculating on what a soldier was thinking or feeling. The natural progression was to focus more on the sandpit, having the soldiers fight and help each other, building barriers, inventing scenarios, etc. When Kevin was thoroughly familiar with this play other children were invited in for short periods to join in 'Kevin's game' which they all found great fun.

The second strand of Kevin's treatment was for the therapist to work with his mother. The therapist explained how much of Kevin's aggressive behaviour with other children came down to not feeling comfortable playing. In addition to encouraging some imaginative play, Kevin's mother needed to find structured play activities that Kevin could engage in with other children. On discussion with the therapist, Kevin and his mother hit upon the idea of Kevin learning how to skateboard. A new skateboard park had opened near their house and Kevin expressed an interest in learning this new sport. Initially, the mother was hesitant. Reassured that Kevin would wear the necessary safety gear she agreed to let him have a go.

Kevin learned and practised the basic skills, having been taught by one of the older children who was quite skilled. He was keen to try out his new skills at the skateboard park. His mother agreed to allow him to play there for an hour after school each day.

**Points of discussion**

- Kevin's treatment lies within a *developmental* framework of teaching skills. In common with all treatments we offer, alternative methods based on **other theoretical frameworks** are possible. Kevin's problem might well have been seen as a behavioural one (as the nurse prioritised), with his aggression towards his peers being targeted as the priority area for treatment. Here, behaviour modification using star charts and modelling could have been incorporated into a group activities programme. The humanistic occupational therapist, following the Axline approach, might have diagnosed Kevin as an unhappy, lonely child who needed to explore his feelings within an accepting relationship. The decision as to which approach to take was based on negotiation within the team, which sought to balance interventions. To some extent trial and error also had a part to play (e.g. the initial unsuccessful use of free play).
- A vital ingredient in the success of this intervention was involving Kevin's mother. She was the one who was going to be with Kevin long-term and could encourage him to play in appropriate ways. Without her involvement, any gains Kevin made could well have been lost after his discharge. The lesson here is to recognise the need to look more deeply into, and take into account, the individual's social circumstances. Problems and solutions commonly lie beyond the individual **within their wider environments and relationships**.

## CASE STUDY 9.6    STEVE

- **Problem issues** – Perceptual, motor and cognitive functional performance difficulties

**Summary of history**

Steve, aged 20, sustains a head injury following a motor cycle accident. Initially, he requires intensive care as he is confused, disorientated and unable to carry out any self-care. After three weeks his functioning is greatly improved, although he is left with some residual damage. He has some physical problems involving weakness, tremor and co-ordination difficulties down his right side, plus some motor dyspraxia and cognitive deficits. He is transferred to a rehabilitation ward for intensive therapy – first as an inpatient, then as a day-patient.

Steve was in his first year of university doing a building degree. He was a popular and academically strong student. He shared a house with friends and had an active social life. His accident has required him to put university life on hold and he has returned to live with his parents for his recuperation.

## Team strategy

The physiotherapist worked on Steve's mobility/co-ordination problems while the occupational therapist focused on assessing and improving his dyspraxia and cognitive difficulties. The team envisaged that Steve would need several months of treatment and rehabilitation but they could not predict the extent to which he would be able to return to his previous level of functioning.

## Occupational therapy assessment

The occupational therapist carried out a range of assessments summarised below:

| Assessment | Findings |
| --- | --- |
| COTNAB to assess perceptual/ cognitive function | Difficulties most apparent for: hidden figures, three-dimensional construction, block printing, dexterity, co-ordination, following written instructions. Slow performance for the above as well as sequencing and two-dimensional construction |
| AMPS to assess skills related to ADL functioning. Tasks used: toast and instant coffee; making a bed with a duvet | Particular problems revealed (i.e. scores of 2) on: posture, mobility, co-ordination, strength and effort, energy, temporal organisation and adaptation. He was slow in performing the tasks and showed difficulties about accommodating/learning from experiences |
| Computer games (an activity he enjoyed) to observe general problem solving and concentration | Concentration problems exposed (he could only attend to a game for about 10 minutes at a time whereas he used to play for hours); problem-solving difficulties in relation to abstract problems also apparent |
| Occupational performance tasks (e.g. dressing, shaving) to assess his personal ADL and safety | Steve proved to be slow at these tasks but he managed them independently |

**Treatment plan**

| Aims/objectives | Treatment methods |
|---|---|

**Early stage**

1. Ensure independence in dressing/self-care
2. Develop concentration and problem-solving
3. Promote normal movement patterns for occupational tasks

a) Dressing practice and other ADL tasks
b) Computer games (for increasing lengths of time, starting with 15 minute slots and working up to one hour daily)
c) Twice weekly cooking group (including going to the shops and cooking a range of meals/snacks)

**Middle stage**

1. Develop 'normal' social interactions and movement patterns
2. Continue to improve perceptual and cognitive functioning

a) Once weekly 'social gym' session (e.g. volleyball, team badminton, swimming at the local baths)
b) Computer games and 'work' related to his university studies

**Late stage**

1. Return (if possible) to building degree course, having taken one year out
2. Arrange to discuss with course tutor preparation for course and any course work requirements

a) Computer work – revising and doing some old assignments/projects
b) Exercises in maths and technical drawing (house plans, etc.)

**Progress**

Steve worked doggedly at his rehabilitation as he was strongly motivated to return to his university course. He enjoyed all his computer games and used his computer time well to monitor his improving function. On the therapist's advice, he monitored and recorded his performance daily (e.g. he measured his increasing game scores and the length of time he concentrated). Steve's gym sessions proved effective at both a physical and a social level. The games helped with his balance/co-ordination, speeded up his reactions and encouraged him to 'lighten up' and have some fun with other group members. Steve did not enjoy the cooking sessions but he could see that they were useful for developing his functional ability.

Steve was discharged after eight months of rehabilitation. The team (including Steve) felt he would be able to return to his university course, although he gave up his honours course for an ordinary degree. His physical functioning had improved significantly though he remained a touch slow both in movement and thinking. The results from repeating the standardised assessments showed that he had retained some mild cognitive problems (e.g. his abstract thinking remained slightly impaired and he tended to be 'rule-bound'). At a social level, he appeared to have lost much of his old charm, sense of humour and ability to converse fluently. Steve recognised that he had changed but was unable to identify what was different. Steve's parents were the ones who seemed most disturbed by the personality changes and continuing impairment. In confidence, they confided to the therapist, 'We have lost our son.'

Six months after discharge, Steve returned to the unit for a follow-up review interview. The treatment team were pleased to hear that he was coping well with his course, although he had to work long hours to keep up. While he was experiencing some social isolation problems, he felt pleased about his general progress and he was hopeful for his future.

### Discussion

- Steve's case is a good illustration of **psychosocial practice in a physical context**. Depending on the rehabilitation unit, Steve could have been treated by an occupational therapist specialising in neurology or liaison psychiatry (which involves bringing a mental health practitioner into a general hospital setting as a consultant). Occupational therapists are particularly well placed (given our dual training) to offer this kind of 'holistic' treatment, encompassing a person's long-term physical, psychological and social functioning. As packages of 'seamless' care are offered across health and social care boundaries, we are likely to see more people with multiple needs. Some would even argue that we should concentrate on these complex interventions and step back from short-term work in acute settings.
- This case study also illustrates the value of standardised assessments and of having **explicit outcome measures**. That Steve specifically recorded his progress and monitored his improving function was probably crucial to keeping him occupationally engaged and motivated on a day-to-day basis. Eight months is a long time to sustain the effort needed for active therapy.

---

## CASE STUDY 9.7   SUKHJEET

- **Problem issues** – Anxiety, abuse and self-abuse; gender and race

### Summary of history

Sukhjeet, is an attractive, bright 18-year-old British Asian woman. She has been referred to a community mental health team for her anxiety. She has recently had a couple of panic attacks, which seem to have been precipitated by a traumatic incident involving racial abuse where a group of youths taunted her as being an 'evil Muslim'. They threatened to 'get' her if she didn't go back to 'her own country'.

### Team strategy

The community mental health team of two nurses, a doctor, a social worker and an occupational therapist function largely as generic therapists or care managers. They use a variety of counselling and psychotherapy approaches. At the weekly referral meeting, the team agrees that the occupational therapist should work with Sukhjeet – probably initially to teach some cognitive–behavioural strategies to handle her anxiety.

## Occupational therapy assessment

In the first counselling interview, the therapist hears how devastated Sukhjeet was by the racist attack. Until now, Sukhjeet thought that such incidents were something that just 'happened to other people'. She had positive experiences at school, where she mixed with both black and white students. Never before had she been made so aware of her ethnicity or been threatened in this way. She now feels that it will be hard to trust people again and for the first time begins to feel an outsider in her own country.

The therapist listens, letting Sukhjeet talk and express her different emotions. They both recognise that these feelings are going to take some time to work through. Sukhjeet then asks if there is anything specific that can be done about the panic attacks. The therapist explains there are techniques that she can teach Sukhjeet and they agree to spend the next session on this.

By the third session, Sukhjeet is less anxious about having panic attacks. She alludes to having 'other stresses' that she has never told anyone else about. The therapist encourages her to talk, observing that it can help to share inner feelings. Sukhjeet then admitted that she has problems with her eating. On delving further the therapist discovers that Sukhjeet has been routinely bingeing and vomiting for the last year. The therapist suggests that often such behaviours involve 'pushing down' deeper emotions and conflicts. Sukhjeet acknowledges that there are things she hasn't yet told the therapist.

## Treatment plan

Appreciating that there are deeper issues that could be usefully explored, the therapist offers Sukhjeet a couple more one-to-one counselling sessions. She also suggests that Sukhjeet might benefit from attending a women's psychotherapy group that is due to begin the following month. Sukhjeet is unsure but is persuaded to give it a try. She is reassured because her therapist will be leading the group along with another counsellor.

## Progress

In the one-to-one counselling sessions Sukhjeet discloses that she had been sexually abused the previous year by a male teacher. Although they didn't go 'all the way' Sukhjeet still feels besmirched and somehow guilty. She has kept this secret, too ashamed to tell anyone. Now she is anxious that the incident will negatively affect her in the future when she is going to be married. The therapist is a little surprised to hear that Sukhjeet is looking forward to an arranged marriage that her parents have planned for next year. The therapist wonders whether Sukhjeet feels split between her Western school experiences and friends, and her more traditional Asian home life. Sukhjeet, however, accepts these differences as 'normal' and is content to respect her parents' wishes. Only occasionally, she admits, does she have a problem with the restrictions her parents place upon her. The stress for her at this moment lies in feeling unable to share her 'guilty secrets' with her family.

In the next two sessions the therapist guides Sukhjeet to explore issues around the multiple abuse she has suffered and the possibility of a link between this and the way she is abusing herself. These issues are further explored in the women's psychotherapy group, which Sukhjeet attends on a weekly basis for several months. Here, Sukhjeet gains some relief and comfort by sharing her 'secrets' with other women in a supportive environment. Sukhjeet learns that several of the other women have had not dissimilar experiences. Somehow this knowledge is reassuring, making her feel more 'normal' and the events less threatening.

## Discussion

- One issue that emerges from this story is the therapist's **choice of approach** and intervention. The use of a cognitive–behavioural approach, followed by a psycho-dynamic one, was helpful here. Sukhjeet's story involves complex dynamics and multiple abuse experiences. Simply applying a relatively straightforward intervention related to one behaviour (namely the panic attacks) proved insufficient. It was important that the therapist could adapt her role and intervention as new problems emerged and the treatment progressed. It was also important that the therapist withdrew from the one-to-one counselling to allow Sukhjeet to use, and benefit from, a committed group experience.

- Issues relating to **culture, race and ethnicity** clearly play a profound and complex role in Sukhjeet's story. The therapist needed to be aware of, and be sensitive to, the issues at stake. First of all, she needed to appreciate some of the implications of Sukhjeet's ethnicity – for instance, how Sukhjeet gained a sense of identity from her parents and community while also feeling threatened by being racially abused. At the same time, the therapist needed to be cautious about not over-generalising and stereo-typing Sukhjeet's experience as simply being 'an Asian girl caught between two cultures'. The therapist also needed to be careful not to judge or impose her own values – for example making the assumption that Sukhjeet was being coerced into an arranged marriage and believing this to be unacceptable. Sukhjeet's cultural background and ethnicity are part of her and need to be positively valued and appreciated in those terms.

---

## CASE STUDY 9.8    PHIL

- **Problem issues** – Lack of life roles and interests; long term implications of acute psychotic episodes

### Summary of history

When Phil was 18 years old, he had a psychotic breakdown during which he became extremely disturbed and was actively hallucinating. It seems likely that the episode was triggered by drug use. In common with many of his friends, Phil smoked cannabis heavily each day and regularly took a cocktail of other drugs. On one occasion it seemed he was unable to recover from a particularly prolonged 'bad trip'. With his interest in science fantasy, many of his hallucinations and delusions concerned fears of magic, goblins, wizards and 'dark forces'. Certain objects, such as the amulet he wore around his neck, carried particular significance for him and he felt he was 'on a quest to save the world'.

Phil was admitted on Section to an acute admission unit. He had been picked up one night behaving in a particularly bizarre manner – he was found naked, shouting incoherent 'spells' in the street in a desperate bid to stop the traffic. After three weeks of assessment and medication, Phil is discharged home to continue his recovery. Three months later, Phil's care manager visits him and finds that he has become withdrawn and somewhat depressed. He has cut himself off from his friends and previous social activities and is reluctant to leave home. Phil lives in a small town and feels acutely embarrassed and humiliated by the way he behaved when he was ill. He is also acutely self-conscious, believing that everyone is talking about him and calling him 'the local loony'.

### Team strategy

The care manager tried to offer Phil support and encourage him to re-engage with life but he felt unable to face the people he had known previously. After several months, Phil made the decision to start a new life in another town. While this enabled him to escape from his sense of being in the public gaze, the move meant that he was cut off from the support of being with familiar people in familiar places. Other than a new part-time job filling shelves at a local supermarket, his life was relatively empty and he became increasingly depressed. He contacted his care manager who arranged for a new community mental health team to become involved.

The team decided that the occupational therapist, Marco, should act as Phil's key worker. Marco's brief was to assess Phil's mental state and help him develop some new life roles.

### Initial assessment

In his initial interview, Marco employed the Role Checklist to get a sense of Phil's perceptions of his participation in occupational roles and the value he placed on these. The assessment revealed that Phil had lost most of his occupational roles and that he lacked involvement in roles that he valued. His roles of student, friend and family member were particularly valued and yet significantly absent in his present role identity. While Phil valued being in employment, he did not value his particular job as he found it boring and mentally unstimulating. On the positive side, Phil still enjoyed reading (particularly science fantasy) and he felt that this helped keep his mind active. Marco felt that Phil's depression was an understandable, temporary response to his current situation.

Marco helped Phil to see that his current depression was unsurprising given the multiple losses he was experiencing. In addition, he was coming to terms with the implications of having been through a psychotic episode. They both agreed that Phil's lack of a meaningful and satisfying social life was a significant gap. Phil could see how joining some sort of social club or evening class could be useful – both to keep his mind active and to increase his social contacts. Using the Modified Interest Checklist together, they tried to identify what interests could form the basis of new social activities. Two interests were rated particularly strongly: (1) science fantasy reading and (2) playing cards (although Phil had not done this for several years).

### Treatment plan

The main thrust of therapy was to help Phil find ways to incorporate his interests into a new life and to increase his social contacts. On discussing different options, Phil showed a spark of interest in the idea of learning how to play bridge (both his parents had been good players and he had picked up a bit about the game). Marco researched the opportunities in town and found that there was a good local club, which ran beginner's classes one night a week. Phil was reluctant to take the step – the idea of going to a place full of strange new people was daunting. Marco said that he would go with him the first time, on condition that Phil tried to stick at it for at least a month. They started by going to meet the bridge teacher to discuss how the lessons worked and what preparation Phil could do.

### Progress

The bridge lessons proved to be enormously successful. Phil enjoyed the complexity and mental challenge offered by the game and he quickly showed considerable aptitude. He became a regular attender at the bridge club three nights a week. He developed a friendship with another man there and they became bridge partners – a relationship that continued for many years. After several months spent seriously developing their game, they began to enter and enjoy bridge competitions around the country.

After only two months of engaging in his new hobby, Phil was much brighter in his mood and had gained confidence. He learned of a local 'live role playing' group whose members enacted various fantasy dramas and staged battles several times a year. With his therapist's cautious encouragement Phil took the step to join this group too. They discussed the possibility that engaging in a fantasy world might cue unduly into Phil's old psychosis and precipitate another episode. On the other hand, Phil no longer took drugs and he had not had the slightest problem reading his science fantasy books. He accepted the need to monitor his mental state carefully. As it turned out, he enjoyed being with others who also had a strong interest in science fantasy. He developed his friendships with members of the group through corresponding by e-mail and going to their events.

### Points of discussion

- Phil's story highlights the importance of **the environment**, which can act in both positive and negative ways. After his illness, Phil was self-conscious about potentially negative community reactions. He feared being stigmatised. This perception (probably based on reality) created the conditions for him to withdraw, first socially and then geographically, from all his previous support systems. When he moved to the new town, the initial lack of social connections and support systems maintained his social withdrawal and exacerbated his depression. The impact of the environment was the key factor in Marco's therapeutic intervention: to encourage Phil to participate in activities involving different environments. The new environment of the bridge club allowed Phil to experience positive changes in his sense of self-efficacy and participation in meaningful roles and occupations.

- Phil's story also reminds us how occupational therapy interventions need to take into account a person's **long-term occupational participation and performance**. Simply treating Phil's acute illness and behaviour would have been insufficient. Arguably, Phil's enduring problems emerged as he was recovering from his illness. Had he not been adequately followed up and supported on his discharge, he could well have had a relapse of his psychosis or become clinically depressed. Belief in the importance of social inclusion combined with occupational participation and performance has reinforced the shift of mental health services into the community.

---

## CASE STUDY 9.9    ROSE

- **Problem issues** – Problems of independence and self-care; risk of falls in elderly people

### Summary of history

Rose, aged 85, has been referred to Social Services after being discharged home from hospital following a stroke. The referral has been made as there were some concerns about whether Rose could manage independently and safely at home. While she has largely recovered from the stroke, Rose has been left with some mobility, speech and visual perception problems. In addition, she has a history of falling. She clearly remains at risk.

Rose lives alone in a ground floor flat. She is fiercely independent and insists that she wants to remain in her own home despite finding it difficult to manage.

### Team approach

Rose's referral is discussed at the weekly team meeting. To help her remain independent at home, Rose seems likely to need equipment and a range of long-term care services. It is decided that the occupational therapist should co-ordinate Rose's care.

### Initial assessment

Within the first few minutes of meeting, Rose expressed some hostility and her suspicion that the occupational therapist was going to force her into residential care. Rose asserted that she was perfectly well – the hospital had been mistaken, she had not had a stroke. She attributed her collapse (and subsequent incontinence) to 'accidental food poisoning'.

To demonstrate to Rose that they would be working in partnership, the therapist decided to use the Canadian Occupational Performance Measure (COPM) as her main assessment tool. In this way she could show that she was primarily interested in hearing about Rose's own view of her situation, performance and level of satisfaction.

Using COPM Rose identified getting in and out of the bath, going shopping, dealing with correspondence and getting to the toilet as her biggest difficulties (see table below). Rose was insistent that she wanted to remain independent in her own home and that she could cope as long as she had a little help. The therapist accepted this, saying that it would be possible to create a 'care package' to suit Rose's needs but that they just needed to be absolutely clear about what was required.

## Initial COPM scores

| Problem | Performance | Satisfaction |
| --- | --- | --- |
| Getting in and out of the bath | 1 | 1 |
| Going out shopping | 1 | 1 |
| Getting to the toilet | 3 | 1 |
| Writing (dealing with correspondence, bills) | 3 | 3 |
| Dressing | 4 | 5 |
| Cooking | 5 | 6 |

Observing Rose make a cup of tea and put on her cardigan, the therapist was concerned about how unsteady Rose was on her feet. She had to negotiate a number of obstacles, such as rugs and trailing wires, on her way to the toilet and the kitchen, and the therapist could see that there was a high risk of her falling. Rose herself assured the therapist that this was 'not a problem'. Instead, Rose claimed that it was her 'slow movement and arthritis' that made it difficult to get to the toilet on time. Rose appeared mildly confused, in that explanations had to be repeated several times by the therapist. Her speech was also slightly slurred and she showed some visual perception problems. Constructional apraxia clearly impaired her dressing and writing.

## Treatment plan

The therapist made the following interventions:
1. **Provide equipment to increase Rose's mobility and independence in her daily tasks** – Supplying a walking frame, commode for night use, an electronic bath seat, and a stool and trolley for the kitchen.
2. **Give advice about preventing and managing falls** – Here, the therapist had to be more directive and advise Rose to give up her walking sticks. She instructed Rose on how to use the walking frame (which she happened to have with her). By emphasising the need to prevent falls in the future, thereby reducing the risk of hospitalisation or residential care, the therapist was able to persuade Rose to remove her extra rugs

and unnecessary furniture. She also organised the supply of an alarm system that Rose could activate in case of falls or emergencies.

3. **Organise a care package using a private agency and bringing in other volunteer services** – The therapist organised a care manager to come in to assess Rose's needs and a Social Services care worker to give Rose a fortnightly bath. meals-on-wheels would deliver a hot meal to Rose each day. The therapist also arranged, via Age Concern, for a 'shopper' to do Rose's weekly shopping.

4. **Assess cognitive function and identify any leisure/social needs towards ensuring a better quality of life** – Both Rose and her therapist agreed that it would be helpful for the therapist to visit Rose every week for the next month to see how she was managing and to talk through any problems as they arose. In these sessions the therapist planned to offer continuing support and to help Rose develop a realistic view of her abilities and the risk of falling.

## Progress

After assessing Rose, the care manager was able to offer Rose a care package involving five weekly morning sessions of only 20 minutes each. During these, the care workers would help Rose get up, wash and dress. The care manager said that, because of limited resources (i.e. staffing), they were unable to offer any more of a service. The occupational therapist remained concerned that this cover was too limited but the matter was out of her control.

The weekly (paid) 'shopper' provided by Age Concern was extremely helpful. Age Concern had also arranged for a (paid) cleaner to help Rose for a couple of hours a week. In addition, they provided an unpaid volunteer to visit Rose once a month to assist her with correspondence and help her put in a claim for extra benefits and Disability Allowance.

The therapist continue to work with Rose over the next month to help her improve her occupational functioning. As Rose's trust in the therapist developed she began to admit to her anxieties about falling. Together they talked about ways in which she could manage her daily occupations. The therapist encouraged Rose to speak more slowly and to practise walking with the frame. She also suggested there was a danger that Rose was unduly focused on her self-care and that her leisure and social contacts had been unnecessarily curtailed. The therapist persuaded Rose that attending the local day unit twice a week would offer both social and health benefits.

## Points of discussion

- In her capacity as a Social Services care co-ordinator, the therapist's main role was to organise a range of support systems. The **limited care resources** available made it necessary for the therapist to activate a range of other private and voluntary sector services. While Rose is likely to have benefited from more time with the care workers, it was not within the therapist's power to arrange this. Such realities often constrain our practice and we have to accept the need to offer a less than ideal service. Setting priorities for limited resources can be experienced as a challenging, if sometimes frustrating, part of our work.

- **The COPM** was a particularly suitable assessment but it was not without its challenges. Rose needed to be reassured that she would have some control over any intervention and the client-centred focus offered by the assessment provided this reassurance. The assessment was also suitable because it could be administered in the community and social care context. Here, Rose could be treated in her own home environment where she faced typical problems of daily living, as opposed to anticipating potential problems in an abstract future. However, applying such an assessment in these circumstances also poses dilemmas. While the therapist tried to be client-centred, believing Rose was at high risk of falling she found it necessary to be more directive at points. It was not possible to simply accept Rose's perceptions and assertions. The challenge lies in preserving the collaborative relationship while negotiating problems and helping the individual develop a realistic view of his or her occupational performance and needs.

## CASE STUDY 9.10    GERARD

- **Problem issues** – Learning disability; lack of independence; long-term concerns and implications

### Summary of history

Gerard is a 37-year-old man with a learning disability. He was a baby when his mother died and his grandmother came over from Mauritius to help his father look after him. His father died 10 years ago and since then Gerard's grandmother has been his main carer and legal guardian. Gerard's daily occupations are carried out with the grandmother's support except for the three mornings a week when he attends a local sheltered workshop by himself.

Recently, Gerard's grandmother was admitted to a Coronary Care Unit with angina. Gerard was temporarily placed in a care home – an event he found distressing and confusing. His grandmother has since come home from hospital and their normal lives have resumed. However, the grandmother has asked for help to provide for Gerard in the long term after she has died.

### Team approach

The occupational therapist became Gerard's care manager. On behalf of the community Learning Disabilities Team her aims were to evaluate his social, work, domestic and personal needs, to encourage greater independence training and to set up new social supports/contacts/activities for him.

### Initial assessment

The occupational therapist carried out two home visits to interview the grandmother and observe the interactions between her and Gerard. The therapist used the Life Experiences

Checklist to gain information on cognitive function, quality of life and environmental diffi-culties. She also visited the local sheltered workshop to liaise with the supervisor and observe Gerard's work skills and interactions.

Her observations suggested that Gerard was a shy but friendly, sociable man. Although he understood basic words in both English and French (his grandmother's mother tongue), he had limited language skills and was only able to engage in simple conversations. It was clear that Gerard and his grandmother had a strong emotional attachment. Gerard was reluctant to leave his grandmother's side and showed some anxiety about being taken away again.

In terms of self-care, Gerard was independent in eating, dressing and bathing on being given some support (e.g. the grandmother laid out his clothes). In terms of productivity, Gerard attended his local sheltered workshop three mornings a week. He showed himself to be a good, reliable worker able to perform basic repetitive tasks. Gerard also helped his grandmother with shopping, cooking and cleaning. She gave him basic instructions and tasks that he followed quite happily. He was unable to cook for himself but he could make a hot drink independently with prompting. In terms of leisure, Gerard watched a lot of television with his grandmother and he enjoyed playing some basic computer games.

### Treatment plan

The occupational therapist suggested that Gerard attend the local day centre (run by the Learning Disabilities Team) on the two days each week that he didn't go to his work placement. The planned day centre programme focused on: 1) teaching Gerard some additional basic independence and cooking skills; 2) encouraging new social interactions and activities; 3) developing new relationships. Alongside this programme, the grandmother agreed to work with Gerard's dressing skills and encouraging him to be more independent in his daily activities.

In the early stages of the programme, it was suggested that the grandmother attend the day centre with Gerard (to help his adjustment in a new environment) and then gradually withdrew. The staff and grandmother planned her level of participation/withdrawal each morning as Gerard set about his activities. They all agreed that Gerard would benefit from continuing to attend the day centre long-term. It was hoped that his new relationships and activities at the day centre would provide some support when he had to cope with his grandmother's death. While some members of the team thought that it would be preferable to settle Gerard into a new residential environment before his grandmother dies, the team respected the wishes of both Gerard and his grandmother to continue to live together.

Gerard's programme at the day centre included one-to-one cooking sessions with the occupational therapist, some group craft work and an end-of-day music/dance group. Occasionally, the service users went on outings, for instance to the park or local swimming baths.

### Progress

Initially, Gerard was reluctant to leave his grandmother's side. However, he soon began to enjoy the different activities and was content simply to have her in the room. After three months, Gerard was able to participate comfortably in the day centre activities without his grandmother.

Gerard enjoyed his one-to-one cooking sessions with the occupational therapist and he became quite attached to her. He learned how to cook cakes and biscuits using mixes. He also learned how to microwave prepared meals. He was encouraged to cook these meals at home for his grandmother.

Gerard's favourite group activity was the end-of-day music and dance session and he was an enthusiastic contributor. On recognising that music was a particular interest, the staff encouraged Gerard to listen to music on his newly acquired portable CD player. An outing to a music store to select a new CD became a regular, much anticipated, event. Gerard also enjoyed sharing treasured new CDs with his grandmother.

**Points of discussion**

- **Who is the service user** in this story? In some ways the grandmother was as much a service user as Gerard. Her co-operation and collaboration were crucial to the success of the intervention. She needed to be motivated to engage in the programme even more than Gerard. It was right that she was centrally involved in assessment, intervention and decisions about Gerard's future. As Gerard's legal guardian, her preferences and decisions about his welfare needed to be taken into account. While some team members suggested that Gerard might be better off being settled in a residential home before the grandmother died, the team accepted that both Gerard and his grandmother wanted to live together as long as it was possible. They respected this choice.
- It is often the **timing of interventions** that determines the success or failure of rehabilitation. This case illustration demonstrates the importance of a graded and gradual rehabilitation and change process. Gerard's history and his anxiety about being separated from his grandmother made it particularly important to have her attend the day centre with him initially – even although it was not common practice to accommodate relatives. Gerard needed time to settle in a new environment and her presence offered him a platform and feeling of security from which he could move on to new relationships.

## 9.2   CONCLUSION AND REFLECTIONS

In these 10 case studies I have tried to synthesise the different elements of occupational therapy practice discussed throughout the book. A summary of the problems, interventions and issues raised in each case study is offered in Table 9.1.

I am struck by the multiple problems, choices, issues and challenges confronting us in our work and how important it is to be flexible and responsive in our approach. I am also struck by the need to look more widely at the individual's environment and social relationships, drawing on this broader social context in our interventions. Sometimes our contributions are limited to a bit of

**Table 9.1** Summary of case studies

| Name | Age | Problems, issues, diagnosis | Assessment | Intervention | Points of discussion |
|------|-----|------------------------------|------------|--------------|----------------------|
| Catherine | 68 | Alcohol misuse; retirement; lack of productive occupations | OPHI-II; self-rating tools to explore roles, activities, values | Individual counselling; groupwork; activity programme | • Need for the individual to be motivated to engage in treatment<br>• Therapist's theoretical approach – opportunities and problems of combining models |
| Reg | 40 | Severe and enduring mental illness (chronic schizophrenia); rehabilitation | REHAB; Social Functioning Scale; general observation | Day hospital programme: art sessions, cookery, social skills training, social/domestic activities | • Role played by institutional racism<br>• Social construction of disability and the importance of having positive expectations that the individual can be occupationally satisfied and productive |
| Ifigenia | 50 | Mid-life crisis issues; loss of valued occupational roles; depression | Relationship-building interviews; observation; OCAIRS | Cooking; dressmaking and evening classes | • The limits of therapists' interventions and responsibilities<br>• Application of MOHO and therapeutic strategies of structuring activities, encouraging, advising, validating |
| Ed | 45 | Work rehabilitation; problematic behaviour; manic-depression | Observation; home visit; role-play | Containing structured activities; home tasks; work simulation | • Ethical dilemmas where service users' interests and society's interests may clash<br>• 'Falling in love with the therapist' – transference and disinhibition issues |
| Kevin | 8 | Anti-social behaviour; play therapy for limited play skills | Directive play using puppets, painting, dressing up | Individual play sessions structured to develop imagination; skateboarding with mother's support | • Choice of theoretical approach based on team decision-making and trial and error<br>• Importance of taking into account the wider environment and relationships |

**Table 9.1** Continued

| Name | Age | Problems, issues, diagnosis | Assessment | Intervention | Points of discussion |
|------|-----|------------------------------|------------|--------------|----------------------|
| Steve | 20 | Head injury; perceptual, motor and cognitive functional performance difficulties | COTNAB; AMPS; observation using computer and ADL activities | Dressing practice; social gym; computer games and college work | • Liaison psychiatry: the role of psychosocial OT in physical practice <br> • Value of outcome measures to motivate and monitor individual's progress |
| Sukhjeet | 18 | Anxiety; abuse and self-abuse; gender and race | Counselling interview | Individual counselling; group psychotherapy | • Being flexible enough to adapt or change approach <br> • Issues around culture, race and ethnicity and the importance of valuing individuals' background |
| Phil | 18 | Lack of life roles and interests; long-term implications of an acute psychotic episode | The Role Checklist; Modified Interest Checklist | Enabling new hobbies in the community: bridge and live role play | • Importance of environment which can have positive and negative effects <br> • The need to take into account a person's long term occupational participation |
| Rose | 85 | Problems of independence and self-care post-CVA; risk of falls in the elderly | COPM; observation making a cup of tea and dressing | Providing equipment; giving advice on preventing falls; organising a care package | • Realities of limited care resources which constrain our interventions <br> • Value and challenge of being client-centred and using COPM |
| Gerard | 37 | Learning disability; lack of independence: long term concerns and implications | Observation in different settings; interviewing a carer/family member; Life Experiences Checklist | Twice weekly attendance at a day centre encouraging new social contacts and activities | • Family members may need to be respected and worked with as service users themselves <br> • Timing of interventions – the importance of gradual/graded rehabilitation |

listening or practical common-sense to help people whose lives have been temporarily dislocated. Yet these small interventions can make a huge difference to a person's quality of life. This is what makes our work both satisfying and worthwhile.

# 10 EVALUATION

*The unexamined profession is not worth practising.*

Engelhardt

Our integrity, effectiveness and confidence as practitioners derive from our ability to evaluate what we do. Evaluation, then, must be a central component of our practice. Often considered to be the last stage of the occupational therapy process after assessment and treatment planning/implementation, evaluation in fact permeates every aspect of our work. In reality, it is much more than this. We evaluate continuously during our interventions in order to ensure what we are doing is sound. Our evaluations tell us when an intervention isn't working in the anticipated manner or when new emerging problems require attention. Evaluation also serves to safeguard good standards of practice in our service as a whole. The process applies throughout our professional development and constitutes our quality assurance.

Since the White Paper *A First Class Service* (Department of Health, 1998), we have been urged constantly to examine, monitor and improve the quality of our services. The advent of **clinical governance** (quality assurance) and the establishment of the National Institute for Clinical Excellence (NICE) have transformed care delivery. The search for 'quality' in our routine everyday practice has become a formal imperative rather than an ideal. **Evidence-based practice** and professional development are mandatory as we strive to improve the quality of our services and safeguard standards of our care through the use of regular clinical audit and other quality initiatives (Figure 10.1). We only have to look at the content of our professional journals to see how far the imperative of evidence-based practice has permeated our professional thinking.

These trends have put evaluation at the heart of our practice. Yet what precisely do we evaluate? And, how exactly do we evaluate? This chapter explores these questions by considering the different ways we can evaluate specific aspects of our work, including the progress made by individual clients, the interventions we make, ourselves as practitioners and the service as a whole. By exploring these different aspects in turn, I hope to show something of the multi-faceted, layered nature of our evaluation process.

## 10.1 EVALUATING INDIVIDUALS' PROGRESS

There are a number of ways to assess service users' progress during and after interventions. We might simply ask them if they feel any different or can recognise progress. Sometimes when dealing with mental health problems it is difficult to pinpoint exactly what has changed, but the person somehow 'feels'

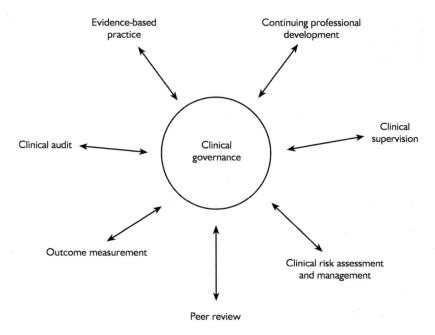

**Figure 10.1** Quality initiatives within clinical governance

better. We can also record tangible progress. For instance, the person may smile more and show greater spontaneity or enthusiasm to engage in activity.

Beyond these informal, and (it has to be said) largely unreliable, ways of monitoring progress we can use more concrete **outcome measures**. Outcome measures involve systematically measuring the results or outcomes of interventions by comparing measurements to pre-treatment objectives, earlier assessment results or established standards. This process may sound simple but it is not without challenges.

This section first explains the nature and challenges of employing outcome measures. Then it moves on to describe the different measures we might employ in practice.

### Challenges of 'measuring outcomes'

It is hard to pick up an occupational therapy journal today without reading something about outcome measures. Frequently we hear therapists pleading for more research to be done to find measures that appropriately reflect our values and practice concerns. This is because finding measures that are suitable for people with psychosocial problems is problematic. It is difficult enough to identify appropriate areas on which to focus but, even when that is done, there remains the challenge of identifying and devising the appropriate tools to measure progress.

Traditional management concepts of outcome measures derive from mechanical tasks, where 'laying 500 bricks per day' may be a suitable standard. Our goals and tasks are invariably more *complex* and defy reduction to such mechanistic measures. In our interventions we work with the physical, cognitive, emotional, social, spiritual and environmental dimensions of a person's health and well being. As Repper and Brooker (1998) point out, it is not sufficient to focus on changes in a person's clinical status or symptoms – we also need to examine the person's ability to care for themselves and how they function at work and in social situations. They cite the work of Hargreaves and Shumway (1989), which distinguishes between clinical, rehabilitative, humanistic and public safety goals. These goals are linked to different outcomes as the selected examples in Table 10.1 show.

***Table 10.1***   Treatment goals and outcomes

| Types of goal | Treatment aim | Example outcome |
|---|---|---|
| Clinical | To improve or cure illnesses or disorders and reduce its signs and symptoms | Reduction in anxiety |
| Rehabilitative | To improve social and vocational functioning | Increased occupational engagement |
| Humanistic | To maximise the well being of the person and their family | Positive change in self-reported quality of life |
| Public safety | To prevent injury to the individual and others | Stable engagement with appropriate services (e.g. maintaining appointments to receive medication) |

Having established our areas of focus, we then face the challenge of *measuring* progress or improvement. Can such things as 'well-being' or 'coping' be quantified and measured? If so, can the measures capture progress without overly focusing on small fragments of behaviour, thus ignoring gains of a more holistic nature? And who should be the judge? For instance, consider the situation where, after a therapy intervention, a person reports feeling more in control and having greater self-esteem, without having observably improved in their daily living skills or functioning. Outcome measures based on the individual's subjective perceptions would suggest that the intervention had been effective while more objective outcomes related to skill development might suggest otherwise.

Issues and questions such as these reveal the complexity underlying the use, purpose and value of outcome measures. However, despite the difficulties associated with using them, we need to strive to make them workable, not least because of what they can teach us about good practice.

So what appropriate measurement tools do we have at our disposal? Below, I distinguish between four different types:

- Objectives as outcome indicators
- Standardised measures

- Quality of life measures
- Subjective, person-centred measures.

While no single measure can capture all aspects of a person's progress, each has an important contribution to make and can be used (individually or in combination) in our occupational therapy evaluations.

### Objectives as outcome indicators

One way of measuring an individual's progress is to compare what has been achieved against behavioural objectives. The objective becomes a criterion for assessing the effectiveness of an intervention. Here the *criteria* for successful achievement are clearly stated, providing a marker against which we can measure actual outcomes. Vague aims of treatment, such as 'improve task performance', cannot act as outcome measures and are therefore less helpful for pinpointing progress. Table 10.2 identifies three aims and various associated objectives specifying outcomes that might be set in advance.

***Table 10.2***   Objectives as outcome indicators

| Aim | Objectives as outcome indicators |
| --- | --- |
| To increase social contacts with others | <ul><li>To attend a new evening class one night a week</li><li>To talk to at least one person in the group</li><li>To invite a friend to go out for the evening</li></ul> |
| To improve task performance | <ul><li>To concentrate on a task for up to half an hour until it is completed</li><li>To independently follow written instructions for a specified task</li><li>To complete a specified task successfully without prompting</li></ul> |
| To increase independence in feeding | <ul><li>To cut up food with a knife and fork with minimal assistance</li><li>To use a spoon appropriately and independently</li><li>To chew and swallow each mouthful before taking another mouthful</li></ul> |

In occupational therapy, the process of measuring a person's progress using objectives is not straightforward. Firstly, it is not always possible to set desired outcomes at the start of interventions. Commonly, in the early stages of treatment, a person's long term goals may remain vague or tentative as their prognosis could still be uncertain. Even when goals are fixed at the outset they may have to be modified over the course of treatment. Secondly, the success and usefulness of the process of measuring against objectives depends largely on how appropriate the objectives were in the first place. It is possible, for instance, to set relatively trivial and easily achieved objectives that, while demonstrating 'improvement', may not say anything useful about the individual's overall progress or the efficacy of the intervention. Care needs to be taken to ensure that the objectives set are meaningful and appropriate.

## Standardised measures

Standardised measures act as a mechanism to quantify improvements in a person's functioning. They offer the possibility of obtaining valid or reliable scores before treatment which can then be used as a basis for comparison during and after treatment. (See Donnelly and Carswell, 2002 for a good review of standardised and individualised outcome measures.)

If standardised outcome measures, such as the ones in Theory into practice 10.1, are used, then results from previous research studies and norm tables will be available. These allow us to compare the person's functioning with that of others in comparable situations (regarding, say, diagnosis, age, context). Such comparison offers an alternative opportunity to judge if a person has achieved *clinically significant* outcomes. Such comparisons can also be helpful for setting the standard for a local clinical audit. For instance, Cook and Spreadbury (2002) cite the example of individuals with anxiety who had attended a set number of group therapy sessions. Following therapy, they gained scores comparable to those reported in research on people who had had individual therapy. As the scores were similar it could be concluded that the group sessions were more efficient in terms of cost.

---

*Theory into practice 10.1* _____

**Two standardised assessments yielding functional measures**

Clifton Assessment Procedures for the Elderly (CAPE)

This test aims to assess cognitive and behavioural competence related to levels of dependency in elderly people. As an example, consider the use of the Behaviour Rating Scale which asks the 'carer' 18 questions about the elderly individual, such as whether:

He/she keeps him/herself occupied in a constructive or useful activity (works, reads, plays games, has hobbies, etc.):

Almost always occupied      0
Sometimes occupied      1
Almost never occupied      2

If the carer's responses total 20 (for the 18 items) before treatment and fall to 10 after treatment, then we have a clear-cut measure of improvement (e.g. using the norm tables we would interpret the score of 20 as indicating 'maximum dependency' while 10 indicates 'medium dependency').

Barthel ADL Scale

The Barthel is a popular standardised 'activities of daily living' scale which aims to measure independence in personal care. It covers 10 items including feeding, transfers, grooming/hygiene, etc. Items are scored on a scale of 1–10 (with 5 being given for assisted performance and 10 indicating maximum independence). Again, an improved numerical score (from, say, 55 to 80) offers an explicit measure of improvement in functional performance.

While such findings seem quite persuasive, we need to maintain a critical eye on the use of standardised measures. Firstly, measuring improvement using standardised assessment scores is not infallible in that no standardised assessment is completely valid and reliable. For one thing, the individual (or therapist) may perform in an uncharacteristic way during the test and bias the result; also, the scores have to be interpreted. The scoring of the Barthel Index, for instance, is problematic as the total score may disguise differences in independence due to the use of adaptive equipment. Professional judgement is required to contextualise the results and ensure that they are meaningful.

The use of standardised functional daily living assessments has been hotly debated (see, for instance, Hagedorn, 1995; Eakin, 1989). Often theses tests are limited in what they measure (e.g. perhaps over-emphasising personal care) and in their ability to predict how well a person will cope with life in general. Some therapists also find that the focus on practical functioning reduces their relevance in some mental health settings.

Spreadbury (1998) and others argue that clients have individual emotional, psychological and social needs that cannot always be categorised according to standardised formats. Individualised programmes of care result in variable outcomes and it may be not be appropriate to seek comparisons with norm tables. For this reason, some practitioners have sought measures that take greater account of an individual's quality of life.

## Quality of life measures

In an effort to do more to address broader emotional and social needs, some researchers have attempted to describe and quantify quality of life in general. Lawton (1991), for instance, offers a conceptual model of quality of life as the interaction of four domains: psychological well-being, perceived quality of life, behavioural competence (including occupational competence) and objective environment. Such models acknowledge the importance of the individual's own sense of performance and well-being, and as such they are valuable.

Attempting to measure quality of life becomes particularly important in fields such as mental health and learning disabilities where we often deal with individuals who have conditions that cannot be 'cured'. Our role, as part of the therapy team, is to enable improvement in quality of life. Yerxa makes a similar distinction between medicine and occupational therapy when she notes that 'medicine is concerned with preserving life; occupational therapy is concerned with the quality of life preserved' (Yerxa, 1990, p. 8).

Different theories of how to conceptualise quality of life have resulted in different tools to evaluate individual's progress – for instance, the Quality of Life

Interview (Lehman, 1988) and the Quality of Life Profile (Oliver, 1992). As these instruments tap a range of domains including participation in, or satisfaction with, work and leisure, they are valuable tools for measuring progress of individuals undergoing occupational therapy. Such tools are also useful in that they can be used in research to investigate the value of occupations.

Some occupational therapists would argue that we need to develop tools that are even more precise and sensitive than those above. For instance, Laliberte-Rudman *et al.* (2000) explored the perspectives of 35 individuals with schizophrenia on the meanings they associated with quality of life. The results suggests that quality of life assessments need to go further than simply examining what people do and their level of overall satisfaction with their activities. Individuals in the study highlighted the importance of exploring the extent to which people are able to *use activity* to manage time, connect with others, achieve a sense of belonging and gain a sense of control.

## Person-centred, subjective measures

One of the strengths of quality of life measures is that they, at least in part, attend to individuals' own perceptions. This is important as research suggests that professionals and service users may bring different concerns to bear. For instance, Sainfort *et al.* (1996) carried out a study involving 37 clients with schizophrenia together with their primary clinicians. They found that, although clients and clinicians gave similar ratings of satisfaction about the clients' symptoms and function, they diverged in terms of their views of social relations and occupational aspects of quality of life.

Writers on occupational therapy such as Whalley-Hammell (1998) have called for outcome measures that reflect our professional values and practice aims – i.e. ones that are both *person-centred* and *occupation-focused*. Spreadbury (1998) recommends that we recognise both subjective changes and individualised goals/outcomes related to particular clients. Here, she is contrasting subjective measures with objective behavioural ones, and also individualised measures with standardised outcomes (i.e. outcomes common to many individuals).

Person-centred, subjective measures aim to offer a way of measuring an individual's own perception of progress. Any self-rating assessments could be used, although, to maximise reliability and validity, well-researched published tools are recommended (see, for instance, the numerous tools associated with the Model of Human Occupation). The Canadian Occupational Performance Measure (COPM) is a currently popular tool that allows clients to identify their own priorities and levels of satisfaction related to occupational performance. For example, an individual might identify 'active recreation such as outings and travel' as their most important problem. The person would then rate this problem on a scale of 1–10 for both performance and satisfaction. This score offers a relatively clear-cut **baseline** from which to compare future scores (assuming that the client uses similar criteria the next time).

A growing pool of literature confirms the ability of COPM to provide useful measures of outcome (Research example 10.1). Chesworth *et al.* (2002), for instance, find it a useful tool for measuring clinical effectiveness in mental health. In their four-year study of 60 clients with mental health problems, they found that COPM detected significant changes in levels of performance and satisfaction. Other benefits resulted from using this measure routinely: other team members were better informed about the occupational therapy role, which resulted in more appropriate referrals; the focus of treatments shifted towards more individualised and community orientated interventions; and there was closer interagency collaboration.

---

*Research example 10.1*

**Outcome studies using the Canadian Occupational Performance Measure**

- Cresswell (1997) used COPM with 13 clients with a diagnosis of schizophrenia at the beginning of treatment and three months later. Quantitative analysis revealed that COPM identified statistically significant changes in performance and satisfaction over that time. Cresswell's study suggested that COPM offers useful outcome measures for community mental health occupational therapy.
- Bodium (1999) investigated the value of COPM with 17 clients having a variety of neurological disorders. Comparing scores before and after treatment showed a statistically significant increase in clients' ratings of performance and satisfaction. Improvements were higher for satisfaction than for performance in some clients (those with just physical, not cognitive, problems), suggesting that these individuals might have come to terms with their condition.

---

The use of subjective measures is not without critics, however. They argue that such measures lack reliability. The danger is that individuals might score themselves differently from day to day, depending on how they feel rather than on their objective performance. If they are feeling confused or lack insight and awareness, they may give inconsistent answers. Also, it is likely that the relationship between therapist and client will influence the scores and attitudes to the assessment. For this reason many practitioners prefer to stick to experimental evidence such as the randomised controlled trial.

## Randomised controlled trials

In complete contrast to subjective measures we have the randomised controlled experiment or trial (RCT). This experimental design, with double-blinding, is regarded as the 'gold standard' in health research. It is particularly used for testing the efficacy of drugs and other treatments. When used appropriately, it produces results that can be regarded with the most confidence in terms of validity, reliability and generalisability. The scientific basis of RCTs ensures their status as the preferred way to evaluate interventions. A glance at the content of the Cochrane Library databases used to search for evidence-based practice information or other internet based resources such as the Centre for Evidence Based Mental Health reveals the value placed on RCTs.

An RCT starts with a sample of people drawn from a particular population. How the sample is drawn and whether it is representative of a wider population are important considerations for the question of how far the results can be generalised. Once a pool of participants have been assembled they are divided *at random* into groups. They are then assessed, using highly standardised measures and protocols, before and after treatment.

Accumulated findings from several studies provide objective evidence that can be both powerful and persuasive (Research example 10.2). On the other hand, if we are to be truly person-centred, it could be argued that subjective measures have the most relevance for our work as occupational therapists. Ideally, to be truly evidence-based practitioners, we need to use both objective and subjective evidence in combination.

---

### Research example 10.2

**Randomised controlled trials on treatments for people diagnosed with borderline personality disorder**

- Linehan *et al.* (1993) carried out a follow-up study of a cognitive behavioural treatment for chronically parasuicidal borderline patients. A RCT was conducted to evaluate whether the superior performance of dialectical behaviour therapy (DBT), a psychosocial treatment for borderline personality disorder, compared with treatment-as-usual in the community, was maintained over a one-year post-treatment follow-up. A total of 39 women meeting the criteria for borderline personality disorder were randomly assigned to either one year of DBT (combining individual psychotherapy with group behavioural skills training) or treatment-as-usual. Efficacy was measured using a range of standardised assessments (Parasuicide History Interview, Global Assessment Scale, Treatment History Interview, Social Adjustment Scale, State–Trait Anger Scale, Social Adjustment Scale – Interview and Self-Report). Results revealed that DBT subjects had significantly higher Global Assessment Scale scores, less parasuicidal behaviour, less anger, fewer psychiatric inpatient days and better social adjustment.
- Linehan *et al.* (1999) conducted a RCT comparing drug-dependent women who had received DBT and treatment-as-usual in the community. Subjects assigned to DBT had significantly greater reductions in drug abuse measured both by structured interviews and urinalyses throughout

---

the treatment year and at follow-up. Subjects assigned to DBT had significantly greater gains in global and social adjustment at follow-up.

- Telch *et al.* (in press) evaluated the use of DBT adapted for binge-eating disorder. A total of 44 women with binge-eating disorder were randomly assigned to group DBT or a wait-list control condition. They were administered the Eating Disorder Examination in addition to measures of weight, mood, and affect regulation at baseline and post-treatment. Treated women evidenced significant improvement on binge-eating and eating pathology measures and 89% of the women had stopped binge-eating by the end of treatment. The findings on the measures of weight, mood, and affect regulation were not significant.

## 10.2 EVALUATING INTERVENTIONS

In addition to using outcome measures, we engage in evaluation routinely and continuously as part of the therapy process. This can be seen in the way we formally record an evaluation of how a treatment session went. Here, we can draw on our own observations, impressions and judgement, as well as those of service users, to evaluate the impact and efficacy of interventions.

### Therapist's evaluations

Therapists record and evaluate treatments/interventions in different ways. Case examples 10.1 and 10.2 present two different forms of evaluation carried out on the same group treatment. The first example uses a *subjective* narrative approach while the second attempts *quantify* something about the group dynamics. Accounts like these will often be made in addition to recording specific information about individuals' performance and progress. Both examples show the therapist as actively observing, reasoning, analysing and evaluating the dynamics of a group session. Both accounts offer a useful record of what occurred and contain information which can be used to evaluate a group's progress over time.

---

**Case example 10.1   A narrative approach to evaluating a group session**

The cooking group was initially tense as Karen vetoed everyone's suggestions. Eventually she agreed to spaghetti bolognese and apple crumble. Mario was elected as 'chief chef' as he had a special family recipe. He asked Bill to chop the vegetables and Sam and Kim to make the dessert. Karen stormed out saying there wasn't any point in her being there. Mario followed her to encourage her back to do the actual cooking.

Karen returned to cook the sauce and the group mood lifted. Karen flirted with Mario while he reminisced about his childhood in Italy. Bill was quiet but seemed to enjoy listening. Sam and Kim worked independently and well at the other cooker, although they isolated themselves from the group conversation.

---

**Group evaluation**

The meal worked well in the end and the group was productive. I facilitated some discussion about the group process, suggesting that a sense of group/group spirit was still lacking. We discussed their individual roles, for instance that Mario was a positive leader and Bill a positive contributor while Karen remained self-absorbed. Karen acknowledged that she became attention-seeking if she didn't get her own way. Sam and Kim understood that their close, supportive relationship was potentially destructive to the rest of the group as they could be seen as an exclusive clique.

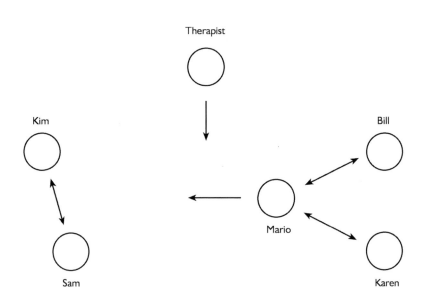

**Figure 10.2**   Sociogram of interactions

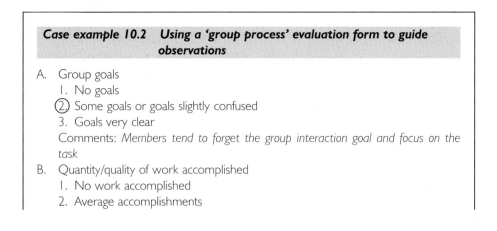

**Case example 10.2   Using a 'group process' evaluation form to guide observations**

A.  Group goals
   1. No goals
   ② Some goals or goals slightly confused
   3. Goals very clear
   Comments: *Members tend to forget the group interaction goal and focus on the task*
B.  Quantity/quality of work accomplished
   1. No work accomplished
   2. Average accomplishments

③ Great deal of quality work accomplished
Comments: *Good lunch produced*
C.  Group atmosphere
①  Hostile, uncomfortable, negative
2.  Average, reasonable
3.  Highly supportive, co-operative, warm
Comments: *Initially uncomfortable when Karen blocked suggestions, then ran out upset*
D.  Group cohesion/trust
①  Group fragmented or lacking in trust
2.  Average
3.  Strong sense of belonging and trust
Comments: *Group split into sub-groups*
E.  Participation
①  Limited and uneven
2.  Average
3.  Great deal of group member involvement
Comments: *Mario needed to encourage and support Karen to keep her in the group; Bill largely silent but encouraging*
F.  Sensitivity
1.  Group members self absorbed, insensitive
②  Average
3.  Outstanding empathy and listening
Comments: *Karen self-absorbed; Sam and Kim isolated; Mario shows good empathy and facilitating skill*
G.  Group decisions
1.  No decisions or decisions made by a few
②  Majority decisions accepted
3.  Full participation and consensus achieved
Comments: *Eventually consensus achieved*

## User evaluations

Any evaluation of a treatment or intervention needs to take into account the service user's (or their carer's) own views. They are, after all, the 'experts'. They are the ones at the receiving end and we need to be responsive to their experience. In practice, we will commonly involve users in monitoring their own performance and experience of particular interventions. We might even turn this **feedback** into something more structured. For example, at the end of a group session we might ask each member to share 'one thing they have found difficult' and 'one thing gained from the session'. At a more formal level, we might ask users to fill out specific **evaluation forms**. Research example 10.3 offers a couple of examples of what could be included on such a form. This example also shows how such data can eventually be turned into a more comprehensive research project designed to evaluate a programme – the topic of the next section.

### Research example 10.3

**Rating the usefulness of a group treatment**

Heather (2003, p. 28) describes a series of structured supportive group psychotherapy sessions for 6 clients with severe and enduring mental health problems. Clients were asked to rate their experience of each group session, using a six-point Likert scale, in terms of enjoyment, interest and helpfulness. For example:

| *Session: 'Road map of my life'* | Enjoyment | Interest | Helpfulness |
|---|---|---|---|
| Male, 37 years | 4 | 3 | 4 |
| Male, 59 years | 6 | 6 | 5 |
| Female, 36 years | 6 | 6 | 6 |
| Female, 43 years | 3 | 4 | 3 |
| Male, 47 years | 6 | 6 | 5 |
| Male, 59 years | 5 | 5 | 4 |

Clients were then asked to rate the group attributes according to certain statements. Heather (2003, p. 29) tabulated these scores to gain an overall view of group members' experience ($n = 6$):

| Attribute | Not true | Partly true | Very true |
|---|---|---|---|
| The group has helped me to gain confidence | | 3 | 3 |
| The group has enable me to talk to others more easily | | 3 | 3 |
| The group has helped me to relax | | 3 | 3 |
| The group has relieved my anxiety | 1 | 2 | 3 |
| The group has lifted my mood | | 3 | 3 |
| I have been able to share my needs | | 3 | 3 |
| I have learnt about myself | | 2 | 4 |
| I have learnt about other people | | 1 | 5 |

## 10.3 EVALUATING OURSELVES

Sometimes we are so busy evaluating and caring for service users that we forget to evaluate and care for ourselves. Critically reflecting on our own performance, attitudes and actions is an anxiety-provoking business but it is crucial to our ability to work effectively in the long term. 'The most important prerequisite to being an effective helper is self-knowledge' (Hopkins and Tiffany, 1983, p. 94). In essence, we need to monitor ourselves to evaluate our past actions, gain support (if needed) for present activity and learn for the future.

The advent of clinical governance has ensured that **continuing professional development (CPD)** is centrally on the agenda. It has become policy to reflect on our practice, identify our learning needs, access opportunities to keep up to date and provide evidence of learning and development.

This section discusses some different ways in which we can evaluate ourselves and enhance our professional development. In particular, it explores:

- Reflection
- Reflexivity
- Supervision and CPD.

### Reflection

Reflection can be defined as 'thinking about' or, as Hagedorn more poetically puts it, as 'emotion and action recollected in tranquillity' (Hagedorn, 1995, p. 191). Since Schön's (1983) seminal work on how professionals think, the concepts of reflection and **reflective practice** have been put firmly on the thera-pist's agenda. The example in Case example 10.3 shows Dan being a reflective practitioner. We see him thinking carefully about, and trying to learn from, a difficult situation. The idea of such reflection is to think about a piece of practice from different angles, and over a period of time, in order to gain new insight and improve future practice.

---

**Case example 10.3    Reflecting on a critical incident**

During an art session, Stephanie suddenly screams, tears up her painting, smashes the paint pots and threatens Dan, her therapist, with a pair of scissors. After the incident, in a team meeting, Dan reflects on what happened. He acknowledges his frustration and irritation in the face of what he sees as Stephanie's 'game playing' and 'provocative taunts'. Dan recognises that his feelings stopped him listening to Stephanie and caused him to be somewhat brusque with her. In retrospect he can see how his behaviour may have seemed rejecting and how that would have contributed to escalating Stephanie's aggression. He takes an opportunity in his supervision session to explore some more gentle ways in which he could have responded. When he next approaches Stephanie he asks her if, together, they can look at the violent incident and consider how they might prevent such a thing happening again.

---

Schön (1983) distinguished between *reflection-on-action* (after-the-event thinking) and *reflection-in-action* (thinking while doing) – the latter being seen as the core of professional artistry. As we become more expert in our practice, we develop the skill of being able to monitor and adapt our practice simultaneously, perhaps even intuitively. Novice practitioners, focused as they are on following rules and procedures more mechanically, need to step back and take time to think situations through more. However, regardless of whether we are novices or experts, we all need to have time to reflect on our practice – both in general and with regard to specific situations. In the midst of busy therapy sessions, too many things are happening. There is often no time to think. It is only after the event that we might identify subtle dynamics or nuances in the situation, as the above case of Dan shows.

Numerous models of reflection (arising particularly from the education and nursing fields) have been created over the last decade to help us reflect more effectively, particularly about problem situations. In their review of the extensive literature on reflection, Atkins and Murphy (1993) present reflection in terms of a series of stages:

- **Self-awareness** – which involves an honest examination of how we are feeling and the extent to which we understand our role in a given situation
- **Description** – where we give a comprehensive account of the situation
- **Critical analysis** – which aims to examine the components of the situation where we both challenge our assumptions and explore alternatives
- **Synthesis** – which comes when we integrate new understandings and old knowledge about thinking ahead and finding ways to solve problems creatively
- **Evaluation** – which involves making judgements about our actions and using known standards to judge our practice.

Johns (1996) offers a more prescriptive, detailed structure consisting of guided questions to help practitioners learn from the process of reflecting on experiences (Figure 10.3).

## Reflexivity

In contrast to reflection (which can be understood as 'thinking about something'), reflexivity involves a more immediate, dynamic and continuing *self*-awareness (a process more akin to Schön's reflection-in-action). It involves critically examining the way our emotions, assumptions, values, social background and behaviour impact on the therapy process and relationships (Finlay and Gough, 2003).

All too often we ignore our **subjective** responses. Yet, they may well play a significant role in the therapy process and our attending to them can be highly informative. Sometimes our emotions can act as a useful barometer. For example, when we use a psychodynamic approach a key source of information involves analysing clients' transferences and our own counter-transferences.

Consider, for instance, the following quotation from a therapist reflexively explaining how some of her patients can feel so 'demanding and dependent' that

**Core question: What information do I need access to in order to learn through this experience?**

**Cue questions**

1.0 *Description of experience*
     1.1 *Phenomenon* – describe the 'here and now' experience
     1.2 *Causal* – what essential factors contributed to this experience?
     1.3 *Context* – what are the significant background factors to this experience?
     1.4 *Clarifying* – what are the key processes (for reflection) in this experience?
2.0 *Reflection*
     2.1 What was I trying to achieve?
     2.2 Why did I intervene as I did?
     2.3 What were the consequences of my actions for
         – myself?
         – the patient/family?
         – the people I work with?
     2.4 How did I feel about this experience when it was happening?
     2.5 How did the patient feel about it?
     2.6 How do I know how the patient felt about it?
3.0 *Influencing factors*
     3.1 What internal factors influenced my decision-making?
     3.2 What external factors influenced my decision-making?
     3.3 What sources of knowledge did/should have influenced my decision-making?
4.0 *Could I have dealt better with the situation?*
     4.1 What other choices did I have?
     4.2 What would be the consequences of those choices?
5.0 *Learning*
     5.1 How do I **now** feel about this experience?
     5.2 How have I made sense of this experience in the light of past experiences and future practice?
     5.3 How has this experience changed my ways of knowing:
         – empirics?
         – aesthetics?
         – ethics?
         – personal?

***Figure 10.3*** Johns's model of structured reflection

she likens them to children. She struggles not to respond like an authoritarian parent and she has to remind herself to be empathetic.

**Jenny**: She is still very, very dependent on people . . . .
**Interviewer**: . . . What does it feel like to have somebody like that be so dependent on you?
**Jenny**: It's very weird at times . . . . If I'm stood talking to my colleague, she doesn't like it, especially if it's one of the younger, more attractive nursing staff. She doesn't like it and woe betide me . . . . I get messages like . . . 'You were talking to so and so and you didn't acknowledge me.' . . . What she reminds me of, very much in the way she handles things and the way she behaves, is a child. And having a 4-year-old daughter, the comparisons are quite similar, in that, if things don't go her way, you can almost see the

tantrum arriving. And sometimes its very difficult for me not to treat her in the same manner as I do a 4-year-old in the supermarket .... And she is extremely trying and she's extremely wearing because its like one step forward, 10 steps back . . . .

**Interviewer:** ... She's clearly a difficult person, but it also sounds like you've got a fondness for her(?)

**Jenny:** Oh, most definitely.

Finlay, 2004a, p. 103.

It may be equally valuable to examine our subjective reactions when working alongside co-therapists. Consider Case example 10.4, where a female group therapist reflects on her relationship with a male co-leader who is a doctor.

---

**Case example 10.4   A therapist critically self-reflects on group dynamics and the relationship with her co-leader**

I went into the group with some feelings of competition as my co-leader was a doctor. I was also ambivalent – grateful he wanted to work with me yet annoyed that he viewed being a group leader as a research exercise rather than an opportunity to care for the members. In the first group session, I had been going gently, trying to build up trust with this group of vulnerable women. Near the end of the session, Michael (the co-leader) suddenly came out with what I perceived as a critical, insensitive remark. A female group member had just talked of her frustration that men responded to her only in sexual terms. Michael confronted her, saying she had a responsibility for this as she had even been giving him those messages. At this point the women in the group (including myself) felt furious! That feeling continued into the next group where the women were quite aggressive towards Michael and I colluded by letting this happen. To a degree, I was pleased they were saying things I wanted to say but had not felt able to do so. After the group, however, I thought things over and realised I had been unfair to Michael. We sat down and properly shared our respective feelings. By doing so, our relationship as co-leaders was strengthened – an important step for the group as a whole.

---

Reflexivity also involves being aware of the ways in which we 'represent' and position ourselves and others in our discourses and choice of words. Of particular concern is the way we exert professional power over service users, which can be benign and facilitative but can also be negative and destructive (Finlay, 2004b). Understanding the complex dynamics involved can enable us to build a greater element of egalitarianism into situations which inevitably involve an unequal distribution of power. 'Working reflexively', Opie advises 'includes acknowledging the inevitability of differential power relations between clients and health professionals and the development, and on-going critique, of modes of interaction that seek explicitly to minimise that difference' (Opie, 1997, p. 273). (See Research example 6.3 in Chapter 6.)

## Supervision and continuing professional development

It is only by acknowledging and attending to our need for support and learning that we are able to sustain the emotional and physical demands inherent in our work. Supervision can meet these needs. It can also offer us an opportunity to reflect upon, and evaluate, our own performance. While engaging in such tasks requires considerable trust between colleagues, putting effort in will often pay off in terms of strengthening teamwork.

Ideally a formal supervision session (preferably with a senior colleague) should occur on a regular basis – say, once a month (or more often if working psychotherapeutically). The supervisor would usually be a senior colleague who is either an occupational therapist or multidisciplinary team member. Therapists may need additional supervision to help them reflect on, and be supported through, particularly difficult encounters. Hunter and Blair (1999) suggest that, to be effective, supervision should be supportive, challenging and supervisee-led. They emphasise the value of the supervisor being non-judgemental, allowing opportunities for the supervisee to share, reflect on and critically evaluate their work.

Research pinpoints inadequate supervision as a key factor in stress and burn-out among therapists. Allan and Ledwith (1998) investigated self-reported levels of stress in 211 senior occupational therapists practising in Britain. They linked levels of stress with perceived needs for supervision and future job intentions. Roughly one-third of the staff reported high or very high levels of stress and 19% reported that they intended to leave occupational therapy within five years. Only 25% reported feeling satisfied with the level of supervision they received. Those wanting to leave the profession were seen to lack opportunities to off-load feelings and gain support.

As part of the wider supervision structure, therapists can benefit from a range of **peer review** meetings. Regular team meetings (be they case reviews, journal clubs or staff sensitivity groups, etc.) offer opportunities for both support and learning. Through discussion, team members can examine their practice and gain valuable feedback. Such a process forms the foundation of CPD geared to enhancing our knowledge and skills.

Continuing professional development is an essential part of career development and the idea of 'life-long learning' advanced by successive government papers and quality initiatives. It is also laid down as an essential dimension of professional codes of practice where we are seen as being personally responsible for actively maintaining and developing our competence (see, for instance, the document *Professional Standards for Occupational Therapy* produced by COT).

In practice, there are multiple routes for CPD by which we can take up opportunities for work-based learning and formal learning. Work-based learning includes a range of activities including:

- Maintaining a developing a **portfolio** to provide evidence of accomplishments and learning outcomes

- Taking part in **journal clubs** to explore and evaluate current research
- **Supervising students** and perhaps even becoming an accredited fieldwork educator.

Formal learning opportunities include participating in conferences, going on training courses and undertaking modules at higher-degree level.

One direction of CPD currently being stressed is the need to develop the skills of an evidence-based practitioner (Taylor, 2000). Aims here include being able to:

- Explain the clinical reasoning behind our interventions
- Develop appropriate information technology skills to allow us to access current research to support our interventions
- Critically evaluate research evidence.

This ability to actively **use research** and evidence develops over time (Cusick and McCluskey, 2000). The process starts by being prepared to critically read research and learn how to search databases for information. The next step is to take up opportunities for learning how to do research, for instance, doing a master's level course. The next section focuses further on the process of doing research.

## 10.4   EVALUATING A SERVICE

There are two routes to formally evaluating a service as a whole: clinical (or service) audit and research. Each is discussed briefly below, illustrated by examples from actual practice.

### Clinical (or service) audit

Clinical audit is a systematic process undertaken to assess the quality of treatment interventions or, more generally, of the service provided. It has become a necessary part of managing a service as purchasers and health care policy makers demand evidence that services provided are effective and efficient. Increasingly, we are being asked to specify the value of what we do and to demonstrate that the best outcome has been achieved for the least cost.

Audit examines the clinical practices and standards of organisations. Specifically, it asks critical questions (Theory into practice 10.2) relating to:

- **Structure** – e.g. staff training and support, physical resources, lines of communication, numbers of service users treated
- **Process** – e.g. referral system, assessment procedures, therapeutic interventions and techniques, relationships
- **Outcome** – e.g. whether or not therapy objectives are appropriate and have been met (Cook and Spreadbury, 2002).

---

*Theory into practice 10.2*_____

**The focus of clinical audit**

The kinds of question we might want to answer in a clinical audit relate to four issues:

- **Quality** – e.g. Are the clinical services offered appropriate for meeting the needs of local people? How long do users have to wait between referral and treatment? Does the unit have the time or resources to deliver the quality of service it aspires to? What mix of service delivers a balanced and beneficial product?
- **Effectiveness** – e.g. Which therapy procedure produces a consistent increase in functional performance? How many therapy sessions are required to gain a satisfactory outcome? Are staff used in their most valuable and rewarding roles? Are staff being given sufficient resources, support and training to implement the service to the required standard?
- **Efficiency** – e.g. Which assessment best defines key problem areas quickly? Can some information be given to users in a written form to increase time for therapy interventions? Can communications between staff, units and agencies be improved? Is the time/resource balance of the unit priorities appropriately split between therapy services, team liaison, support, research, record keeping and audit?
- **Value** – e.g. Do the treatment gains result in reduced costs (e.g. reduced hospital stay), greater quality of life or higher user satisfaction? What are the predicted future costs of failing to deliver an improved service? Can costs be saved by streamlining systems?

---

Once the problem or focus of the audit has been agreed, measures need to be identified to act as a baseline for investigation. For example, outcome measures using results of standardised assessments giving pre- and post-treatment scores might be used. Alternatively the process of service delivery might be evaluated against set service *standards* or *protocols* (e.g. a home visit is to be made within four weeks of referral). Then, various methods of collecting information can be used (such as a review of case notes or a user satisfaction survey) to identify strengths and shortfalls in the service. This information is analysed either quantitatively or qualitatively. Findings are used to improve the service and the cycle begins again (Figure 10.4 and the examples of audits in Case example 10.5).

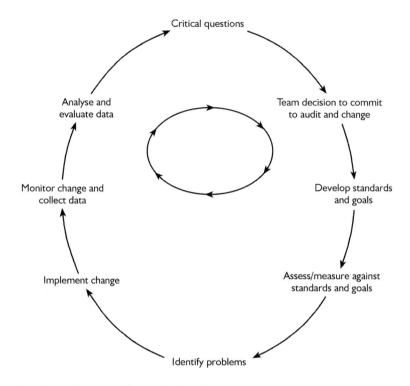

**Figure 10.4** Cyclical process of clinical audit

---

**Case example 10.5   Examples of audits**

**Audit example A**

*Aim*
To check that home visit report documentation meets required standard

*Method*
Peer review of case notes from the last four months, checking that a report has been submitted and when. Usefulness and quality of the report to be checked against a list of criteria that reflect departmental standards.

*Analysis*
Each home visit report is scored against a checklist of criteria (e.g. that the report was written within 2 weeks of the visit and that future recommendations for action are clearly indicated).

*Action*

Criteria not being met are identified and staff training on how to write reports to be implemented.

**Audit example B**

*Aim*

To check users' satisfaction with the service.

*Method*

1    User satisfaction survey given to all users attending outpatients on four specified days
2    In-depth interview of eight clients.

*Analysis*

1    Survey results analysed statistically
2    Interview results analysed qualitatively.

*Action*

Suggestions to improve the service made by users are tabulated in preparation to being discussed by staff. Staff team to audit review findings and any implement changes deemed appropriate.

**Audit example C**

*Aim*

To evaluate the effectiveness of a 10-week group therapy anxiety management programme (run on three separate occasions) for users living in the community.

*Method*

1    Use of standardised assessments of anxiety – namely, the Beck Anxiety Inventory (BAI) and State–trait Anxiety Inventory (STA) – administered to users before and after the programme
2    Standards set using published outcomes for other similar anxiety management programmes and results checked against these.

*Analysis*

1    Statistical test to determine if there are significant differences between the before and after values
2    Statistical comparison with other evidence to ensure comparable norms achieved.

*Action*

After evaluating outcomes decide if the group should continue or not.

It takes time, skill, experience and other resources to carry out clinical/service audits in a meaningful, useful way. First, appropriate standards need to be in place (set nationally, locally by providers/purchasers or by the individual therapists), against which the service can be audited. Then, numerous decisions need to be taken to do with the focus and method of the audit. Research knowledge and skills are then needed to carry out the audit effectively. Finally, management systems need to be put into place to implement and review changes. Each of these stages needs to be given due attention and handled carefully.

It is important that evaluation and audit processes are seen as inherently valuable rather than resented as a chore. Ideally, staff should embrace a participative and mutually supportive process of personal and unit evaluation as part of an non-intrusive, ongoing programme to improve service delivery. This can only be achieved if the tedious aspects of data collection and analysis are achieved relatively painlessly and if the good work done is regularly recognised and rewarded.

For staff relatively new to the audit process, it can be useful to work with others who are more experienced (e.g. using the local clinical governance department or carrying out the audit in conjunction with other professional groups). Increasingly, useful 'Audit Packs' are being published – e.g. the College of Occupational Therapists' *Guidelines for the Collaborative Rehabilitative Management of Elderly People Who Have Fallen* (CSP/COT, 2001). Information on clinical governance and audit is also available on the Internet. For instance, information on cost effectiveness and good practice (concerning medicines, clinical guidelines for patients with particular disorders, and therapeutic interventions) is available on the site for the National Institute of Clinical Excellence (NICE): www.nice.org.uk/.

## Researching the effectiveness of a service

In this era of **evidence-based practice** (Taylor, 2000), we are increasingly required to ground our practice in research findings and established theoretical knowledge. Figure 10.5 shows how practice, research and theory are linked. This means we need to *do* research to demonstrate the efficacy of our interventions. It also means we need to *draw on* research findings systematically and rigorously. If we are planning a new treatment, for instance, it can be informative to carry out a literature search to see if any previous research has been carried out in this, or another relevant, area. Research example 10.4 shows how research can be undertaken to investigate practice which has been informed by evidence.

---

*Research example 10.4*

**Researching the benefits of an early intervention programme**

Fisher and Savin-Baden (2001) provide a good example of evidence-based practice. Using a pluralistic model of evaluation (Salmon, 2003), they investigated the perspectives of consumers and providers of a specially designed early intervention programme for young people who had recently experienced psychosis. The programme, known as 'TIME', integrated a range of psychosocial therapies the efficacy of which had been previously researched

---

and documented, including occupational therapy, cognitive–behavioural therapy and family intervention. The precise therapy offered was negotiated collaboratively with each individual.

In-depth qualitative interviews were used to explore the experiences of the young people and service providers. Results showed positive evaluations of the programme. Users, for instance, perceived TIME to be a place where they had a 'voice' and could be supported. The importance of being engaged in meaningful occupations was highlighted and the young people's stories reflected the value of having a supportive environment where they could share their experiences of psychosis.

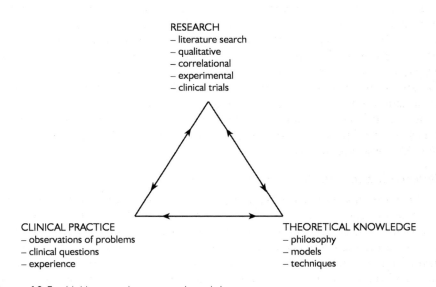

**Figure 10.5** Linking practice, research and theory

In order to show something of the complexity and range of activities that can be involved when researching the effectiveness of a service, I offer one example taken from Cook's (2001) PhD research. I chose this research because I think this is an excellent, comprehensive example of what can (and arguably should) be done. If you are particularly interested in these findings, I recommend that you consult the actual thesis for details.

**Evaluating a primary-care-based occupational therapy and care management service for people with severe and enduring mental health problems**
In this study, Cook (2001) researched a primary care scheme based in a GP's surgery. This aimed to improve the quality of life of a group of people with severe and enduring mental health problems. The newly developed service

consisted of care management and occupational therapy and included assertive outreach work, the education of carers, cognitive–behavioural interventions and different community initiatives primarily delivered by one senior occupational therapist (Cook herself) and a part-time support worker. After careful baseline functional assessment, a range of interventions was offered, from the use of thera-peutic activities (e.g. gardening and social skills training) to developing partner-ships in the local community (e.g. developing a befriending scheme and providing information about mental health).

An important step in Cook's research was to carry out an extensive **literature review**. Here she investigated what services were available for people with severe and enduring mental health problems. She compared the results of several studies and reviews of Assertive Community Treatment with traditional care and care management programmes. Research example 10.5 gives a flavour of some of the findings.

---

*Research example 10.5*

**Two studies comparing the effectiveness of Assertive Community Teams versus traditional care**

- **Monach *et al*. (2000)** demonstrated how the use of Assertive Community Teams in Sheffield (UK) improved the health and social functioning of people with severe and enduring mental health problems. They studied clients with psychosis and social disability who were at risk, poorly engaged and high users of services over time. Both clients and carers were found to value the service. Significantly, there was a reduction in hospital bed use from 5045 days to 929 days.
- **Marshall and Lockwood (2000)** reviewed 17 studies comparing the impact of Assertive Community Treatment and traditional care for people with severe mental disorder. They found that those treated by Assertive Community Teams were more likely to remain in contact with services and less likely to be admitted to hospital. While there were significant improvements on some social outcomes (e.g. employment), no significant differences were found in terms of mental state. Reduced costs of hospital care were counterbalanced with community care costs.

---

Adopting a case study design, Cook employed six different methods in her research to evaluate the effectiveness of the service:

- Quantitative comparison of groups (those that had and those that had not lost contact with psychiatric services prior to the intervention) on a range of variables
- Measurement of individuals' engagement with the new service

- Single group quasi-experimental study of clinical and social outcomes for those receiving one year's intervention
- Measurement of patient satisfaction using a standardised questionnaire delivered by interviewers who were users
- Cost-consequence analysis of mental health-care costs
- Qualitative investigation of the views of key staff involved.

Cook's research demonstrated that the new primary care scheme was effective in engaging people at risk, reducing their symptoms and problems, increasing their social functioning and offering opportunities for social inclusion. The new service was viewed as highly satisfactory by the recipients and key staff were enthusiastic about the benefits. Estimates of costs suggested that direct costs were comparatively low and were reasonable considering the improved outcomes. While Cook concedes the limitations of the research in terms of generalisability and attribution, she recommends that her model of a service should be further developed and tested.

## 10.5 CONCLUSION AND REFLECTIONS

In this era of clinical governance and evidence-based practice, we are required to continuously monitor and improve the quality of our service, using a range of initiatives from outcome measures and clinical audit to peer review and professional development. The challenge we face is how to turn the rhetoric into a valued and purposeful reality.

This chapter has shown something of the multilayered and complex process of evaluation. I have described some of the different ways in which we can evaluate users' progress, the impact of interventions, ourselves and the service as a whole.

I have argued for using standardised (objective) and person-centred (subjective) measures in combination. The key point is that, irrespective of the evaluation tool used, it should be deployed critically, pragmatically and selectively. Such tools must be consistent with our professional values and aims. Our evaluations also need to be informative and worth the time and effort they involve.

Some say that it is essential for occupational therapists to *prove their worth* in order to survive as a profession. My own view is that the survival of the profession needs to take second place to critically evaluating both clients' progress and how well our services meet users' needs. By doing so, we affirm – to ourselves and others – that we are making a difference.

In this and the preceding chapters, I have tried to unravel some of the complexities of our occupational therapy process. I have also tried to explore some of the debates, dilemmas and issues that arise in our practice as we deal with people who are damaged and situations that are invariably difficult.

Through the examples offered from practice I hope that something of the interest, excitement and satisfaction of our work has been revealed. Psychosocial occupational therapy can indeed be difficult, ambiguous, contradictory, frustrating and stressful. We have few definite answers to give individuals facing huge emotional trauma and social struggle. Where we do have answers, the impact of our interventions is often hard to see. There are also practical limits to what we can do, given the system we work in and the pressures on our time and resources. For all that, the experience of sharing in someone's growth and development makes our work deeply worthwhile. The gains experienced by service users as a result of our interventions may not appear glamorous but, for individuals now better able to cope with day-to-day life, such gains are often profound.

# REFERENCES

Ager, A. (1990) *Life Experiences Checklist*. NFER-Nelson, Windsor, Berkshire.

Allan, F. and Ledwith, F (1998) Levels of stress and perceived need for supervision in senior occupational therapy staff. *British Journal of Occupational Therapy*, **61**(8), 346–350.

Allen, C. K. (1985) *Occupational therapy for psychiatric diseases: measurement and management of cognitive disabilities*. Little, Brown & Co., Boston, MA.

Atkins, T. W. and Murphy, K. (1993) Reflection: a review of the literature. *Journal of Advanced Nursing*, **18**, 1188–1192.

Atkinson, K. and Wells, C. (2000) *Creative therapies: a psychodynamic approach within occupational therapy*. Stanley Thornes, Cheltenham.

Axline, V. (1989) *Play Therapy*. Churchill Livingstone, Edinburgh.

Ballinger, C. (2003) Navigating multiple research identities: reflexivity in discourse analytic research, in *Reflexivity: a practical guide for researchers in health and social sciences* (eds L. Finlay and B. Gough). Blackwell Science, Oxford.

Ballinger, C. and Payne, S. (2000) Falling from grace or into expert hands? Alternative perspectives about falls in older people. *British Journal of Occupational Therapy*, **63**, 573–579.

Bandura, A. (1977) *Social learning theory*. Prentice Hall, Englewood Cliffs, NJ.

Baron, K. B.(1994) Clinical interpretation of 'the Assessment of Motor and Process Skills of persons with psychiatric disorders'. *American Journal of Occupational Therapy*, **48**, 781–782.

Barris, R. and Kielhofner, G. (1986) Beliefs, perceptions and activities of psychosocial occupational therapy educators. *American Journal of Occupational Therapy*, **40**(8), 535–541.

Bauer, B. and Hall, S. S. (1986) *Essentials of health care planning and intervention*. W. B. Saunders, Philadelphia, PA.

Beck, A. T. (1976) *Cognitive therapy and emotional disorders*. International Universities Press, New York.

Bion, W. R. (1961) *Experiences in groups and other papers*. Tavistock, London.

Birchwood, M., Smith, J., Cochrane, R. *et al.* (1990) The Social Functioning Scale: the development and validation of a new scale of social adjustment for use in the Family Intervention Programme with schizophrenic patients. *British Journal of Psychiatry*, **157**, 853–859.

Blom-Cooper, L. (1989) *Occupational Therapy: an emerging profession in health care*. Duckworth, London.

Bodium, C. (1999) The use of the Canadian Occupational Performance Measure for the assessment of outcome on a neurorehabilitation unit. *British Journal of Occupational Therapy*, **62**(3), 123–126.

Borg, B. and Bruce, M. A. (1997) *Occupational therapy stories: psychosocial interaction in practice*. Slack, Thorofare, NJ.

Bowlby, J. (1988) *A secure base: clinical applications of attachment theory*. Routledge, London.

Brayman, S. J., Kirby, T. F., Misenheimer, A. M. and Short, M. J. (1976) Comprehensive occupational Therapy Evaluation scale. *American Journal of Occupational Therapy*, 30, 94–100.

Brechin, A. (2000) The challenge of caring relationships, in *Critical practice in health and social care* (eds A. Brechin, H. Brown and M. A. Eby). Sage, London.

Briggs, A. K., Duncombe, L. W., Howe, M. C. and Schwartzberg, S. L. (1979) *Case simulations in psychosocial occupational therapy*. F. A. Davis, Philadelphia.

Bruner, J. (1990) *Acts of meaning*. Harvard University Press, Cambridge, MA.

Burke, J. P. and Cassidy, J. C. (1991) Disparity between reimbursement-driven practice and humanistic values of occupational therapy. *American Journal of Occupational Therapy*, 45, 173–176.

Canadian Association of Occupational Therapists (1991) *Occupational therapy guidelines for client-centred practice*. Canadian Association of Occupational Therapists Publications, ACE, Toronto, Ontario.

Canadian Association of Occupational Therapists (1997) *Enabling occupation: an occupational therapy perspective*. CAOT Publications, ACE, Ottawa.

Cara, E. and MacRae, A. (1998) *Psychosocial occupational therapy: a clinical practice*. Delmar Publishers, Albany, NY.

Charmaz, K. (2000) Experiencing chronic illness, in *The handbook of social studies in health and medicine* (eds G. L. Albrecht, R. Fitzpatrick and S. C. Scrimshaw). Sage, London.

Chern, J., Kielhofner, G., Heras, C. and Magalhaesi, L. (1996) The Volitional Questionnaire: psychometric development and practical use. *American Journal of Occupational Therapy*, 50(7), 515–525.

Chesworth, C., Duffy, R., Hodnett, J. and Knight, A. (2002) Measuring clinical effectiveness in mental health: is the Canadian Occupational Performance an appropriate measure? *British Journal of Occupational Therapy*, 65(1), 30–34.

Christiansen, C. (1996) Three perspectives on balance in occupation, in *Occupational science: the evolving discipline* (eds R. Zemke and F. Clark). F. A. Davis, Philadelphia, PA.

Christiansen, C. and Baum, C. (1997) Understanding occupation: definition and concepts, in *Enabling function and well-being*, 2nd edition (eds C. Christiansen and C. Baum). Slack, Thorofare, NJ.

Chugg, A. and Craik, C. (2002) Some factors influencing occupational engagement for people with schizophrenia living in the community. *British Journal of Occupational Therapy*, 65, 67–74.

Clark, D. M. (1986) A cognitive approach to panic. *Behaviour Research and Therapy*, 24, 461–470.

Clark, F. (1993) Occupation embedded in a real life: Interweaving occupational science and occupational therapy. *American Journal of Occupational Therapy*, 47(12), 1067–1078.

Clark, D. M., Salkovskis, P. M., Hackmann, A. *et al.* (1994) A comparison of cognitive therapy, applied relaxation and imipramine in the treatment of panic disorder. *British Journal of Psychiatry*, 164, 759–769.

College of Occupational Therapists (2001) *Guidelines for the collaborative rehabilitative management of elderly people who have fallen*. CSP/COT, London.

Cook, S. (2001) The effectiveness of primary care based occupational therapy and care management for people with severe and enduring mental health problems: a case study. Unpublished PhD thesis, University of Sheffield.

Cook, S. (2003) Generic and specialist interventions for people with severe mental health problems: can interventions be categorised? *British Journal of Occupational Therapy*, 66(1), 17–24.

Cook. S. and Spreadbury, P. (2002) Clinical governance and clinical audit, in *Occupational therapy and mental health*, 3rd edn (ed. J. Creek). Churchill Livingstone, Edinburgh.

Corring, D. and Cook, J. (1999) Client-centred care means that I am a valued human being. *Canadian Journal of Occupational Therapy*, 66(2), 71–82.

Coupland, K., Macdougall, V. and Davis, E. (2002) Group work for psychosis. *Mental Health Nursing*, 22(6), 6–9.

Crabtree, J. L.(1998) The end of occupational therapy. *American Journal of Occupational Therapy*, **52**, 205–214.

Crabtree, M. and Lyons, M. (1997) Focal points and relationships: a study of clinical reasoning. *British Journal of Occupational Therapy*, **60**, 57–64.

Craik, C. and McKay, E. A. (2003) Consultant therapists: recognising and developing expertise. *British Journal of Occupational Therapy*, **66**(6), 281–283.

Craik, C., Austin, C., Chacksfield, J. D. and Schell, D. (1998a) College of Occupational Therapists: position paper on the way ahead for research, education and practice in mental health. *British Journal of Occupational Therapy*, **61**(9), 390–392.

Craik, C., Chacksfield, J. D. and Richards, G. (1998b) A survey of occupational therapy practitioners in mental health. *British Journal of Occupational Therapy*, **61**(5): 227–234.

Craik, C., Austin, C. and Schell, D. (1999) A national survey of occupational therapy managers in mental health. *British Journal of Occupational Therapy,* **62**(5), 220–228.

Creek, J. (ed.) (1997) *Occupational therapy and mental health*, 2nd edn. Churchill Livingstone, Edinburgh.

Creek, J. (1998) Purposeful activity, in *Occupational therapy: new perspectives* (ed. J. Creek). Whurr Publishers, London.

Creek, J. and Feaver, S. (1993) Models for practice in occupational therapy, part 1: defining terms. *British Journal of Occupational Therapy*, **56**(1), 4–6.

Creek, J. and Ormston, C. (1996) The essential elements of professional motivation. *British Journal of Occupational Therapy*, **59**, 7–10.

Crepeau, E. B. (1991) Achieving intersubjective understanding: examples from an occupational therapy treatment session. *American Journal of Occupational Therapy*, **45**, 1016–1025.

Cresswell, M. K. M. (1997) A study to investigate the utility of the Canadian Occupational Performance Measure as an outcome measure in community mental health occupational therapy. Unpublished MSc thesis, University of Exeter.

Csikszentmihalyi, M. (1992) Flow: the psychology of happiness. Rider Press, London.

Csikszentmihalyi, M. (1993) Activity and happiness: towards a science of occupation. *Occupational Science Australia*, **1**, 38–42.

Csikszentmihalyi, M. (1999) If we are so rich, why aren't we happy? *American Psychologist*, **October**, 821–827.

Cusick, A. and McCluskey, A. (2000) Becoming an evidence-based practitioner through professional development. *Australian Occupational Therapy Journal*, **47**, 159–170.

Dalgleish, T. (2002) Posttraumatic stress disorder (PTSD), in *Applying psychology* (eds N. Brace and H. Westcott). Open University Press, Buckingham.

De Clive-Lowe, S. (1996) Outcome measurement, cost-effectiveness and clinical audit: the importance of standardised assessment to occupational therapists in meeting these new demands. *British Journal of Occupational Therapy*, **59**(8), 357–362.

Deegan, P. E. (2001) Recovery as a self-directed process of healing and transformation. *Occupational Therapy in Mental Health*, **17**(3–4).

De las Heras, C. G., Geist, R., Kielhofner, G. and Li, Y. (2002) *The Volitional Questionnaire* (VQ) (Version 4.0). University of Illinois at Chicago, Chicago, IL.

Devereaux, E. B. (1984) Occupational therapy's challenge: the caring relationship. *American Journal of Occupational Therapy*, **38**, 791–798.

Department of Health (1998) *A First Class Service*. Department of Health, London.

Department of Health (1999) *National Service Framework for Mental Health: modern standards and service models*. Department of Health, London.

Department of Health (2000) *Manual of cancer service standards*. Stationery Office, London.

Department of Health (2003) *Mental health: fast-forwarding primary care mental health*. Stationery Office, London.

Doble, S. E., Fisk, J. D., Lewis, N. and Rockwood, K. (1999) Test-retest reliability of the

Assessment of Motor and Process skills in elderly adults. *Occupational Therapy Journal of Research*, **19**, 203–215.

Donnelly, C. and Carswell, A. (2002) Individualized outcome measures: a review of the literature. *Canadian Journal of Occupational Therapy*, **69**(2), 84–94.

Donnelly, S. M., Hextell, D. and Matthey, S. (1998) The Rivermead Perceptual Assessment Battery: its relationship to selected functional activities. *British Journal of Occupational Therapy*, **61**(1): 27–32.

Donohue, M. V. (1999) Theoretical bases of Mosey's group interaction skills. *Occupational Therapy Interntional*, **6**(1), 35–51.

Doyal, L. and Cameron, A. (2001) Professions allied to medicine: continuity and change in a complex workforce, in *Health and disease: a reader*, 3rd edn (eds B. Davey, A. Gray and C. Seale). Open University Press, Buckingham.

Duncan, E. A. S. (1999) Occupational therapy in mental health: it is time to recognise that it has come of age. *British Journal of Occupational Therapy*, **62**(11), 521–522.

Durham, T. (1997) Work-related activity for people with long-term schizophrenia: a review of the literature. *British Journal of Occupational Therapy*, **60**(6), 248–252.

Eakin, P. (1989) Problems with assessments of activities of daily living. *British Journal of Occupational Therapy*, **52**(2), 50–54.

Eaton, P. (2002) Psychoeducation in acute mental health settings: is there a role for occupational therapy. *British Journal of Occupational Therapy*, **65**(7), 321–326.

Egan, G. (1982) *The skilled helper: model, skills, and methods for effective helping*, 2nd ed. Brooks Cole, Monterey, CA.

Egan, G. (1986) *The skilled helper*, 3rd edn. Brooks Cole, Monterey, CA.

Elliot, M. and Barris, R. (1987) Occupational role performance and life satisfaction in elderly persons. *Occupational Therapy Journal of Research*, **7**, 215–224.

Ellis, A. (2000) *Rational Emotive Behaviour Therapy: a therapist's guide*. Impact Publishers, San Luis Obispo, CA.

Ellis, R. and Whittington, D. (1981) *A guide to social skills training*. Croom Helm, London.

Emerson, H. A., Cook, J., Polatajko and Segal, R. (1998) Enjoyment experiences as described by persons with schizophrenia: a qualitative study. *Canadian Journal of Occupational Therapy*, **65**(4), 183–192.

Erikson, E. (1977) *Childhood and society*. Triad Paladin, St. Albans.

Everett, T., Donaghy, M. and Feaver, S. (2003) *Interventions for mental health: an evidence-based approach for physiotherapists and occupational therapists*. Butterworth-Heinemann, Edinburgh.

Falardeau, M. and Durand, M. J. (2002) Negotiation-centred versus client-centred: which approach should be used? *Canadian Journal of Occupational Therapy*, **69**(3), 135–142.

Fanchiang, S. P. C. (1996) The other side of the coin: Growing up with a learning disability. *American Journal of Occupational Therapy*, **50**(4), 277–285.

??Fidler, G. (1985) In *A model of human occupation – theory and application* (ed. G. Kielhofner). Williams & Wilkins, Baltimore.

Fidler, G. S. and Fidler, J. W. (1963) *Occupational therapy: a communication process in psychiatry*. Macmillan, New York.

Fidler, G. and Fidler, J (1983) Doing and becoming: the occupational therapy experience, in *Health through occupation: theory and practice in occupational therapy* (ed. G. Kielhofner). F. A. Davis, Philadelphia, PA.

Fieldhouse, J. (2003) The impact of an allotment group on mental health clients' health, wellbeing and social networking. *British Journal of Occupational Therapy*, **66**(7),286–296.

Finlay, L. (1997a) Good patients and bad patients: how occupational therapists view their patients/clients. *British Journal of Occupational Therapy*, **60**, 440–446.

Finlay, L. (1998) The lifeworld of the occupational therapist: meaning and motive in an uncertain world. Unpublished PhD thesis, The Open University, Milton Keynes.

Finlay, L. (2000) The challenge of working in teams, in *Critical practice in health and social care* (eds A. Brechin, H. Brown and M. A. Eby). Sage, London.

Finlay, L. (2001) Holism in occupational therapy: elusive fiction and ambivalent struggle. *American Journal of Occupational Therapy*, 55(3), 268–276.

Finlay, L. (2002) Groupwork, in *Occupational therapy and mental health*, 3rd edn (ed. J. Creek). Churchill Livingstone, Edinburgh.

Finlay, L. (2004a) Feeling powerless: therapists' battle for control, in *Communication, relationships and care: a reader* (eds M. Robb, S. Barrett, C. Komaromy and A. Rogers). London, Routledge.

Finlay, L (2004b) *Challenging 'power-full' relationships, K205 Communication and relationships in health and social care*. Open University Press, Buckingham.

Finlay, L. and Gough, B. (2003) (eds) *Reflexivity: a practical guide for qualitative researchers in health and social sciences*. Blackwell Sciences, Oxford.

Fisher, A. G. (1999) *Assessment of motor and process skills, 3rd edn – unpublished test manual.* Three Star Press, Fort Collins, CO.

Fisher, A. and Savin-Baden, M. (2001) The benefits to young people experiencing psychosis, and their families, of an early intervention programme: evaluating a service from the consumers' and providers' perspectives. *British Journal of Occupational Therapy*, 64(2), 58–65.

Forsyth, K., Salamy, M., Simon, S. and Kielhofner, G. (1998) *The Assessment of Communication and Interaction Skills (Version 4.0)*. Department of Occupational Therapy, University of Illinois at Chicago, Chicago, IL.

Forsyth, K., Lai, J. and Kielhofner, G. (1999) The Assessment of Communication and Interaction Skills (ACIS): measurement properties. *British Journal of Occupational Therapy*, 62(2), 69–74.

Fortune, T. (1999) Students' fieldwork stories: Reflecting on supervision, in *Thinking and reasoning in therapy: narratives from practice* (eds S. E. Ryan and E. A. McKay). Stanley Thornes, Cheltenham.

Fortune, T. (2000) Occupational therapists: is our therapy truly occupational or are we merely filling gaps? *British Journal of Occupational Therapy*, 63(5), 225–230.

Fossey, E. (1996) Using the Occupational Performance History Interview (OPHI): therapists' reflections. *British Journal of Occupational Therapy*, 59(5) 223–228.

Fox, K. R. (2000) The effects of exercise on self-perceptions and self-esteem, in *Physical activity and psychological well-being* (eds S. J. H. Biddle, K. R. Fox and S. H. Boutcher). Routledge, London.

Frank, G. (1996) Life histories in occupational therapy clinical practice. *American Journal of Occupational Therapy*, 50(4), 251–264.

Frank, A. W. (1998) Just listening: narrative and deep illness. *Families, Systems and Health*, 16(3), 197–212.

Frank, G. (2000) *Venus on wheels: two decades of dialogue, on disability, biography, and being female in America*. University of California Press Berkeley, CA.

Freud, S. (1936) *The ego and the mechanisms of defence*. Hogarth Press, London.

Gage, M. (1999) Physical disabilities: meeting the challenges of client-centred practice, in *Client-centred practice in occupational therapy: a guide to implementation* (ed. T. Sumsion). Churchill Livingstone, Edinburgh.

Godschalx, S. M. (1989) Experiencing life with a psychiatric disability, in *Chronic mental illness: coping strategies* (ed. J. T. Maurin). Slack, Thorofare, NJ

Goffman, E. (1959) *The presentation of self in everyday life*. Penguin, New York.

Golledge, J. (1998a) Distinguishing between occupation, purposeful activity and activity, part 2: Why is the distinction important? *British Journal of Occupational Therapy,* **61**(4), 157–60.

Golledge, J. (1998b) Is there unnecessary duplication of skills between occupational therapists and physiotherapists? *British Journal of Occupational Therapy,* **61**(4), 161–162.

Golledge, J. (1998c) Distinguishing between occupation, purposeful activity and activity, part 1: Review and explanation. *British Journal of Occupational Therapy,* **61**(3), 100–105.

Good, B. (1992). A body in pain: the making of a world of chronic pain, in *Pain as human experience: an anthropological perspective* (eds M. Delvecchio-Good, P. Brodwin, B. Good and A. Kleinman). University of California Press, Berkeley, CA.

Green, S. (2003) Occupation as a quality of life domain for vulnerable elderly people. Unpublished PhD Thesis, University of Liverpool.

Hagedorn, R. (1995) *Occupational therapy: perspectives and processes.* Churchill Livingstone, Edinburgh.

Hagedorn, R. (1997) *Foundations for practice in occupational therapy.* 2nd edn. Churchill Livingstone, Edinburgh.

Haig, J. (1997) Assessment tools used by occupational therapists with head injured patients in a rehabilitation setting. *British Journal of Occupational Therapy,* **60**(12): 541–545.

Hargie, O. D. W. (1997) Training in communication skills: research, theory and practice, in *The handbook of communication skills,* 2nd edn (ed. O. D. W. Hargie). Routledge, London.

Harries, P. A. (2002) CMHTs: specialist versus generalist roles (letter). *British Journal of Occupational Therapy,* **65**(1), 40–41.

Harries, P. and Caan, A. W. (1994) What do psychiatric inpatients and ward staff think about occupational therapy? *British Journal of Occupational Therapy,* **57**, 219–233.

Harries, P. A. and Gilhooly, K. (2003) Generic and specialist occupational therapy casework in community mental health teams. *British Journal of Occupational Therapy,* **66**(3), 101–109.

Harrison, D. (2003) The case for generic working in mental health occupational therapy. *British Journal of Occupational Therapy,* **66**(3), 110–112.

Hart, L. (1994) *Phone at nine just to say you're alive.* Douglas Elliot Press, London.

Hasselkus, B. R. (2002) T*he meaning of everyday occupation.* Slack, Thorofare, NJ.

Health Professions Council (2003) *Standards in conduct, performance and ethics.* Health Professions Council, London.

Heather, F. (2003) Pro-motion: a positive way forward for clients with severe and enduring mental health problems living in the community, part 2. *British Journal of Occupational Therapy,* **66**(1), 25–30.

Helfrich, C. and Kielhofner, G. (1993) Volitional narratives and the meaning of therapy. *American Journal of Occupational Therapy,* **48**(4), 319–326.

Hobson, S. J. G. (1999) Using a client-centred approach with elderly people, in *Client-centred practice in occupational therapy: a guide to implementation* (ed. T. Sumsion). Churchill Livingstone, Edinburgh.

Hopkins, H. (1983) An historical perspective on occupational therapy, in *Willard and Spackmans occupational therapy,* 6th edn (eds H. L. Hopkins and H. D. Smith). J. B. Lippincott, Philadelphia, PA.

Hopkins, H. L. and Tiffany, E. G. (1983) Occupational therapy: a problem-solving process, in *Willard and Spackmans occupational therapy,* 6th edn (eds H. L. Hopkins and H. D. Smith). J. B. Lippincott, Philadelphia, PA.

Hughes, J. L. (2002) Illness narrative and chronic fatigue syndrome/myalgic encephalomyelitis: a review. *British Journal of Occupational Therapy,* **65**(1), 9–14.

Hugman, R. (1991) *Power in caring professions.* Macmillan Press, Basingstoke.

Hunter, E. P. and Blair, S. E. E. (1999) Staff supervision for occupational therapists. *British Journal of Occupational Therapy,* **62**(8), 344–350.

Hyde, P. J. (2002) Organisational dynamics of mental health teams. Unpublished PhD, University of Manchester.

Jenkins, M., Mallett, J., O'Neill, C. *et al.* (1995) Insights into 'practice' communication: an interactional approach. *British Journal of Occupational Therapy*, **57**(8), 297–302.

Jensen, C. M. and Blair, S. E. E. (1997) Rhyme and reason: the relationship between creative writing and mental wellbeing. *British Journal of Occupational Therapy*, **60**(12), 525–530.

Johns, C. (1996) Visualising and realizing caring in practice through guided reflection. *Journal of Advanced Nursing*, **24**, 1135–1143.

Kanas, N.(1996) *Group therapy for schizophrenic patients*. American Psychiatric Association, Washington, DC.

Kaplan, K. and Kielhofner, G. (1989) *Occupational Case Analysis Interview and Rating Scale*. Slack, Thorofare, NJ.

Karp, D. A. (1996) *Speaking of sadness: depression, disconnection, and the meaning of illness*. Oxford University Press, New York.

Kashner, T. M., Rosenheck, R., Campinell, A. B. *et al.* (2002) Impact of work therapy on health status among homeless substance-dependent veterans: a randomised controlled trial. *Archives of General Psychiatry*, **59**, 938–944.

Kaur, D., Seager, M., Orrell, M. (1996) Occupation or therapy? The attitudes of mental health professionals. *British Journal of Occupational Therapy*, **59**(7), 319–322.

Keable, D.(1996) Managing stress, in *Occupational therapy in short-term psychiatry* (ed. M. Willson). Churchill Livingstone, Edinburgh.

Kelly, G. A. (1955) *The psychology of personal constructs*, vol. 1. Norton, New York.

Kielhofner, G. (1992) *Conceptual foundations of occupational therapy*. F. A. Davis, Philadelphia, PA.

Kielhofner, G. (ed.) (1995) *A model of human occupation: theory and application*, 2nd edn. Williams & Wilkins, Baltimore, MD.

Kielhofner, G. (ed.) (2002a) *Model of human occupation: theory and application*, 3rd edn. Lippincott Williams & Wilkins, Baltimore, MD.

Kielhofner, G. (2002b) The environment and occupation, in *Model of human occupation: theory and application*, 3rd edn (ed. G. Kielhofner). Lippincott Williams & Wilkins, Baltimore, MD.

Kielhofner, G. (2002c) Dimensions of doing, in *Model of Human Occupation: theory and application*, 3rd edn (ed. G. Kielhofner). Lippincott Williams & Wilkins, Baltimore, MD.

Kielhofner, G. and Burke, K. (1977) Occupational therapy after 60 years: an account of changing identity and knowledge. *American Journal of Occupational Therapy*, 31, 657–689.

Kielhofner, G. and Forsyth, K. (2002) Therapeutic strategies for enabling change, in *Model of Human Occupation: theory and application*, 3rd edn (ed. G. Kielhofner). Lippincott Williams & Wilkins, Baltimore, MD.

Kielhofner, G. and Neville, A. (1983) The Modified Interest Checklist – unpublished manuscript. University of Illinois at Chicago, Chicago.

Kielhofner, G., Henry, A., Walens, D. (1989) *A user's guide to the Occupational History Interview*. American Occupational Therapy Association, Rockville, MD.

Kielhofner, G., Mallison, T., Crawford, C. *et al.* (1998) *A user's guide to the Occuptional Performance History Interview – II (OPHI-II) (version 2.0)*. University of Illinois at Chicago, Chicago, IL.

Kielhofner, G., Mallison, T., Forsyth, K. and Lai, J. (2001) Psychometric properties of the second version of the Occupational Performance History Interview (OPHI-II). *American Journal of Occupational Therapy*, 55, 260–267.

Kielhofner, G., Borell, L., Freidheim, L. *et al.* (2002) Crafting occupational life, in *Model of Human Occupation: theory and application*, 3rd edn (ed. G. Kielhofner). Lippincott Williams & Wilkins, Baltimore, MD.

Kinebanian, A. and Stomph, M. (1992) Cross-cultural occupational therapy: a critical reflection. *American Journal of Occupational Therapy*, **46**(8), 751–757.

Kitwood, T. (1997) *Dementia reconsidered: the person comes first*. Open University Press, Buckingham.

Klein, M. (1975) *Love, guilt and reparation*. Hogarth Press, London.

Kleinman, A. (1988) *The illness narratives: suffering, healing and the human condition*. Basic Books, New York.

Klyczek, J., Mann, W. (1986) Therapeutic modality comparisons in day treatment. *American Journal of Occupational Therapy*, **40**, 606–611.

Kortman, B. (1994) The eye of the beholder: models in occupational therapy. *Australian Occupational Therapy Journal*, **41**, 115–122.

Kremer, E. R. H., Nelson, D. and Duncombe, L. (1984) Effects of selected activities on affective meaning in psychiatric patients. *American Journal of Occupational Therapy*, **38**(8), 552–528.

Kuznir, A. and Scott, E. (1999) The challenges of client-centred practice in mental health settings, in *Client-centred practice in occupational therapy: a guide to implementation* (ed. T. Sumsion). Churchill Livingstone, Edinburgh.

Laliberte-Rudman, D. L., Cook, J. V. & Polatajko, H. (1997) Understanding the potential of occupation: a qualitative exploration of seniors' perspectives on activity. *American Journal of Occupational Therapy*, **51**, 640–650.

Laliberte-Rudman, D., Betty Y., Scott, E. and Pajouhandeh, P. (2000) Explorations of the perspectives of persons with schizophrenia regarding quality of life. *American Journal of Occupational Therapy*, **54**(2), 137–147.

Laver, A. J. and Hutchinson, S. (1994) The performance and experience of normal elderly people on the COTNAB. *British Journal of Occupational Therapy*, **57**, 137–42.

Law, M., Baptiste, S., Carswell-Opzoomer, A. *et al.* (1991) *Canadian Occupational Performance Measure*. Canadian Association of Occupational Therapists Publication, Toronto, Ontario.

Law, M., Baptiste, S., Carswell-Opzoomer, A. *et al.* (1994) *Canadian Occupational Performance Measure*, 2nd edn. Canadian Association of Occupational Therapists Publication, Toronto, Ontario.

Law, M., Baptiste, S., Mills, J. (1995) Client-centred practice: what does it mean and does it make a difference? *Canadian Journal of Occupational Therapy*, **62**(5), 250–257.

Law, M., Baum, C. and Dunn, W. (2001) *Measuring occupational performance: supporting best practice in occupational therapy*. Slack, Thorofare, NJ.

Lawlor, D. A. and Hopker, S. W. (2001) The effectiveness of exercise as an intervention in the management of depression,: systematic review and meta-regression analysis of randomised controlled trials. *British Medical Journal*, **322**, 1–8.

Lawton, M. P. (1991) A multidimensional view of quality of life in frail elders, in *The concept and measurement of quality of life in frail elders* (ed. J. Birren). Academic Press, San Diego, CA.

Lehman, A. F. (1988) A quality of life interview for the chronically mentally ill. *Evaluation and program planning*, **11**, 51–62.

Linehan, M. M., Heard, H. L. and Armstrong, H. E. (1993) Naturalistic follow-up of a behavioral treatment for chronically parasuicidal borderline patients. *Archives of General Psychiatry*, **50**, 971–974.

Linehan, M. M., Schmidt, H., Craft, J. C. *et al.* (1999) Dialectical behavior therapy for patients with borderline personality disorder and drug-dependence. *American Journal on Addiction*, **8**, 279–292.

Lloyd, C., King, R. and Bassett, H. (2002) Mental health: how well are occupational therapists equipped for a changed practice environment? *Australian Occupational Therapy Journal*, **49**, 163–166.

Lyons, M. (1997) Understanding professional behaviour: experiences of occupational therapy students in mental health settings. *American Journal of Occupational Therapy*, **51**, 686–692.

Lyons, M., Orozovic, N., Davis, J. and Newman, J. (2003) Doing–being–becoming: occupational experiences of persons with life-threatening illnesses. *American Journal of Occupational Therapy*, **56**(3), 285–295.

McDermott, A. (1988) The effect of three group formats on group interaction patterns, in *Group process and structure in psycho-social occupational therapy* (ed. D. Gibson). Haworth Press, New York.

McKay, E. A. (2002) 'Rip that whole book up – I've changed': life and work narratives of mental illness. Unpublished PhD thesis, University of Strathclyde

McKay, E. and Ryan, S. (1995) Clinical reasoning through story telling: examining a student's case story on a fieldwork placement. *British Journal of Occupational Therapy*, **58**(6), 234–238.

McNulty, M. C. and Fisher, A. G. (2001) Validity of using the Assessment of Motor and Process Skills to estimate overall home safety in persons with psychiatric conditions. *American Journal of Occupational Therapy*, **55**(6), 649–655.

Mallinson, T., Kielhofner, G. and Mattingly, C. (1996) Metaphor and meaning in a clinical interview. *American Journal of Occupational Therapy*, **50**(5), 338–346.

Managh, M. F. and Cook, J. V. (1993) The use of standardized assessment in occupational therapy: the BaFPE-R as an example. *American Journal of Occupational Therapy*, **47**(10), 877–884.

Marshall, M. and Lockwood, A. (2000) Assertive community treatment for people with severe mental disorders (Cochrane Review), in *The Cochrane Library, Issue 3 (2000)*. Update Software, Oxford.

Maslow, A. H. (1954) *Motivation and personality*. Harper & Row, New York.

Maslow, A. H. (1973) *The farther reaches of human nature*. Penguin, Harmondsworth.

Matsutsuyu, J. (1969) The interest checklist. *American Journal of Occupational Therapy*, **23**, 323–328.

Mattingly, C. (1998) *Healing dramas and clinical plots: the narrative structure of experience*. Cambridge University Press, Cambridge.

Mattingly, C. and Fleming, M. H. (1994) *Clinical reasoning: forms of enquiry in a therapeutic practice*. F. A. Davis, Philadelphia, PA.

May, R. (1983) The discovery of being: writings in existential psychology. Norton, New York.

Mayers, C. (1990) A philosophy unique to occupational therapy. *British Journal of Occupational Therapy*, **53**(9), 379–380.

Mayers, C. (2000) Quality of life: priorities for people with enduring mental health problems. *British Journal of Occupational Therapy*, **63**(12), 591–597.

Mayers, C. A. (2003) The development and evaluation of the Mayers' Lifestyle Questionnaire. *British Journal of Occupational Therapy*, **66**(9), 388–395.

Meeson, B. (1998) Occupational therapy in community mental health teams: generic or specialist? *British Journal of Occupational Therapy*, **61**(1), 7–12.

Melton, J. (1998) How do clients with learning disabilities evaluate their experience of cooking with the occupational therapist? *British Journal of Occupational Therapy*, **61**(3), 106–110.

Mitchell, L. (1977) *Simple relaxation*. John Murray, London.

Mocellin, G. (1995) Occupational therapy: a critical overview, part 1. *British Journal of Occupational Therapy*, **58**(12), 502–506.

Mocellin, G. (1996) Occupational therapy: a critical overview, part 2. *British Journal of Occupational Therapy*, **59**(1), 11–16.

Molineux, M. (2002) The age of occupation: an opportunity to be seized. *Mental Health OT*, **7**(1), 12–14.

Molineux, M. and Rickard, W. (2003). Storied approaches to understanding occupation. *Journal of Occupational Science*, **10**(1), 52–60.

Moll, S. and Cook, J. V. (1997) 'Doing' in mental health practice: therapists' beliefs about why it works. *American Journal of Occupational Therapy*, **51**(8), 662–670.

Monach, J., Repper, J., Roberts, J. *et al.* (2000) Sheffield Outreach Team (SORT) Evaluation Report, ScHARR. University of Sheffield, Sheffield.

Moore, C. and Bracegirdle, H. (1994) The effects of a short-term low-intensity exercise programme on the psychological wellbeing of community-dwelling elderly women. *British Journal of Occupational Therapy*, **57**(6), 213–216

Morgan, A. (2000) *What is narrative therapy? An easy to read introduction*. Dulwich Centre Publications, Adelaide, South Australia.

Mosey, A. C. (1970) *Three frames of reference for mental health*. Charles B. Slack, Thorofare, NJ.

Mosey, A. (1974) An alternative: the biopsychosocial model. *American Journal of Occupational Therapy*, **28**, 137–140.

Mosey, A. (1981) *Occupational therapy: configuration of a profession*. Raven Press, New York.

Mosey, A. C. (1986) *Psychosocial components of occupational therapy*. Raven Press, New York.

Mostert, E., Zacharkiewicz, A. and Fossey, E. (1996). Claiming the illness experience: Using narrative to enhance theoretical understanding. *Australian Occupational Therapy Journal*, **43**, 125–132.

Mozley, C. G. (2001) Exploring connections between occupation and mental health in care homes for older people. *Journal of Occupational Science*, **8**(3), 14–19.

Mutrie, N. and Faulkner, G. (2003) Physical activity and mental health, in *Interventions for mental health: an evidence-based approach for physiotherapists and occupational therapists* (eds. T. Everett, M. Donaghy and S. Feaver). Butterworth-Heinemann, Edinburgh.

Nagle, S., Cook, J. V. and Polatajko, H. J. (2002) I'm doing as much as I can: occupational choices of persons with severe and persistent mental illness. *Journal of Occupational Science*, **9**(2), 72–81.

Oakley, F. (1981) *The Role Checklist*. National Institutes of Health, Bethesda, MD.

Oakley, F., Kielhofner, G., Barris, R. and Reichler, R. K. (1986) The Role Checklist: development and empirical assessment of reliability. *Occupational Therapy Journal of Research*, **6**, 157–170.

Oliver, J. (1992) The social care directive: development of quality of life profile for use in community services for the mentally ill. *Social Work and Social Services Review*, **3**, 5–45.

O'Loughlin, A. (1999) On living with chronic pain, in *Nursing and the experience of illness: phenomenology in practice* (eds I. Madjar and J. A. Walton). Routledge, London.

O'Neill, S. A. (1999) Living with obsessive-compulsive disorder: a case study of a woman's construction of self. *Counselling Psychology Quarterly* **12**(1), 73–86.

Opie, A. (1997) Thinking teams thinking clients: issues of discourse and representation in the work of health care teams. *Sociology of Health and Illness*, **19**(3), 259–280.

Oxley, C. (1995) Work and work programmes for clients with mental health problems. *British Journal of Occupational Therapy*, **58**(11), 465–468.

Parker, D. M. (1999) Implementing client-centred practice. In *Client-centred practice in occupational therapy: a guide to implementation* (ed. T. Sumsion). Churchill Livingstone, Edinburgh.

Payne, S. (2002) Standardised tests: an appropriate way to measure the outcome of paediatric occupational therapy? *British Journal of Occupational Therapy*, **65**(3), 117–122.

Peloquin, S. M. (1990) The patient-therapist relationship in occupational therapy: understanding visions and images. *American Journal of Occupational Therapy*, **44**, 13–21.

Peloquin, S. M. (1993) The depersonalizatyion of patients: a profile gleaned from narratives. *American Journal of Occupational Therapy*, **47**, 830–837.

Peloquin, S. M. (1995) The fullness of empathy: reflections and illustrations. *American Journal of Occupational Therapy*, **49**(19), 24–31.

Perls, F. (1973) *The gestalt approach and eyewitness to therapy*. Bantam Books, New York.

Pieris, Y. (2002) A study to investigate what leisure means to clients with enduring mental health problems. Unpublished MSc thesis, Brunel University.

Polkinghorne, D. E. (1996) Transformative narratives: From victimic to agentic life plots. *American Journal of Occupational Therapy*, **50**(4), 299–305.

Pollock, N., McColl, M. A. and Carswell, A. (1999) The Canadian Occupational Performance Measure, in *Client-centred practice in occupational therapy: a guide to implementation* (ed. T. Sumsion). Churchill Livingstone, Edinburgh.

Potter, J. and Wetherell, M. (1995) Discourse analysis, in *Rethinking methods in psychology* (eds J. A. Smith, R. Harré and L. van Langenhove). Sage, London.

Predretti, L. W. (1996) Occupational performance: a model for practice in physical dysfunction, in *Occupational therapy: practice skills for physical dysfunction*, 4th edn (ed. L. W. Predretti). C. V. Mosby, St Louis, MO.

Ravetz, C. (1984) Leisure, in *Occupational therapy in short-term psychiatry* (ed. M. Willson). Churchill Livingstone, Edinburgh.

Rebeiro, K. L. and Allen, J. (1998) Voluntarism as occupation. *Canadian Journal of Occupational Therapy*, **66**, 279–285.

Rebeiro, K. L. and Cook, J. V. (1999) Opportunity, not prescription: an exploratory study of the experience of occupational engagement. *Canadian Journal of Occupational Therapy*, **66**, 176–187.

Reed, K. (1984) *Models of practice in occupational therapy*. Williams & Wilkins, Baltimore, MD.

Reed, K. L. and Sanderson, S. R. (1999) *Concepts of occupational therapy*, 4th edn. Lippincott Williams & Wilkins, Philadelphia, PA.

Reilly, M. (1962) Occupational therapy can be one of the greatest ideas of 20th century medicine. *American Journal of Occupational Therapy*, **16**, 1–9.

Repper, J. and Brooker, C. (1998) Difficulties in the measurement of outcome in people who have serious mental health problems. *Journal of Advanced Nursing*, **23**, 75–82.

Repper, J., Perkins, R. and Owen, S. (1998) 'I wanted to be a nurse ... but I didn't get that far': women with serious ongoing mental health problems speak about their lives. *Journal of Psychiatric and Mental Health Nursing*, **5**, 505–513.

Reynolds, F. (1997) Coping with chronic illness and disability through creative needlecraft. *British Journal of Occupational Therapy*, **60**(8), 352–356.

Robinson, S. E. and Fisher, A. G. (1996) A study to examine the relationship of the Assessment of Motor and Process Skills (AMPS) to other tests of cognition and function. *British Journal of Occupational Therapy*, **59**, 260–263.

Rogers, C. (1961) *On becoming a person*. Houghton Mifflin, Boston, MA.

Rogers, C. (1970) *Client-centered therapy*. Constable, London

Rogers, J. C. (1983) Eleanor Clarke Slagle Lecture – Clinical reasoning: the ethics, science, and art. *American Journal of Occupational Therapy*, **37**, 601–6.

Rosa, S. A. and Hasselkus, B. R. (1996) Connecting with patients: the personal experience of professional helping. *Occupational Therapy Journal of Research*, **16**(4), 245–260.

Rosier, C., Williams, H. and Ryrie, I. (1998) Anxiety management groups in a community mental health team. *British Journal of Occupational Therapy*, **61**(5), 203–206.

Ross, J. C. (1997) The relationship between occupational roles and life satisfaction in young adults with serious mental disorders. Unpublished MSc Thesis, University of Exeter.

Ryan, S. (1995) The study and application of clinical reasoning research. *British Journal of Therapy and Rehabilitation*, **2**(5), 265–271.

Ryan, S. and McKay, E. A. (eds) (1999). *Thinking and reasoning in therapy: Narratives from practice*. Stanley Thornes, Cheltenham.

Sainfort, R., Becker, M. and Diamond, R. (1996) Judgements of quality of life of individuals with severe mental disorders: patient self-report versus provider perspectives. *American Journal of Psychiatry*, **153**, 497–503.

Salmon, N. (2003) Service evaluation and the service user: a pluralistic solution. *British Journal of Occupational Therapy*, **66**(7), 311–316.

Salo-Chydenius, S. (1996) Changing helplessness to coping: an exploratory study of social skills training with individuals with long-term illness. *Occupational Therapy International*, **3**(3), 174–189.

Scaffa, M. (1991) Alcoholism: an occupational behaviour perspective. *Occupational Therapy in Mental Health*, **11**, 99–111.

Schell, B. A. (1998) Clinical reasoning: the basis of practice, in *Willard and Spackman's occupational therapy*, 9th edn (eds M. E. Neistadt and E. B. Crepeau). J. B. Lippincott, Philadelphia, PA.

Schell, B. A. and Cervero, R. M. (1993) Clinical reasoning in occupational therapy: an review. *American Journal of Occupational Therapy*, **47**, 605–610.

Schkade, J. K. and Schultz, S. (1992) Occupational adaptation: toward a holistic approach for contemporary practice, part 1. *American Journal of Occupational Therapy*, **46**, 829–837.

Schon, D. (1983) *The reflective practitioner: how professionals think in action*. Basic Books, New York.

Schultz, S. and Schkade, J. K. (1992) Occupational adaptation: toward a holistic approach for contemporary practice, part II. *American Journal of Occupational Therapy*, **46**, 917–916.

Schwartzberg, S. (2002) *Interactive reasoning in the practice of occupational therapy*. Prentice Hall, New York.

Shimitras, L., Fossey, E. and Harvey, C. (2003) Time use of people living with schizophrenia in a North London catchment area. *British Journal of Occupational Therapy*, **66**(2), 46–54.

Slater, R. (2000) A photography group as a mental health intervention: a pilot study. Unpublished MSc Thesis, Middlesex University.

Smith, N., Kielhofner, G., Watts, J. (1986) The relationship between volition, activity pattern and life satisfaction in the elderly. *American Journal of Occupational Therapy*, **40**, 278–283.

Solomon, A. (2001) The noonday demon: an atlas of depression. Scribner, New York.

Spreadbury, P. (1998) 'You will measure outcomes', in *Occupational therapy: new perspectives* (ed. J. Creek). Whurr Publishers, London.

Stevens, R. (2002) Person psychology: psychoanalytic and humanistic perspectives, in *Mapping psychology* (2) (eds D. Miell, A. Phoenix and K. Thomas). Open University Press, Buckingham.

Steward, B. (1997) Employment in the next millennium: the impact of changes in work on health and rehabilitation. *British Journal of Occupational Therapy*, **60**(6), 268–272.

Strong, J., Gilbert, J., Cassidy, S. and Bennett, S. (1995) Expert clinicians' and students' views on clinical reasoning in occupational therapy. *British Journal of Occupational Therapy*, **58**(3), 119–123.

Sumsion, T. (ed.) (1999a) *Client-centred practice in occupational therapy: a guide to implementation*. Churchill Livingstone, Edinburgh.

Sumsion, T. (1999b) The client-centred approach, in *Client-centred practice in occupational therapy: a guide to implementation* (ed. T. Sumsion). Churchill Livingstone, Edinburgh.

Sumsion, T. (1999c) Overview of client-centred practice, in *Client-centred practice in occupational therapy: a guide to implementation* (ed. T. Sumsion). Churchill Livingstone, Edinburgh.

Taylor, M. C. (2000) *Evidence-based practice for occupational therapists*. Blackwell Science, Oxford.

Taylor, A. and Rubin, R. (1999) How do occupational therapists define their role in a community mental health setting. *British Journal of Occupational Therapy*, **62**(2), 59–63.

Telch, C. F., Agras, W. S., and Linehan, M. M. (2001) Dialectical behavior therapy for binge eating disorder: a promising new treatment. *Journal of Consulting and Clinical Psychology*, 69(6), 1061–1065.

Toomey, M., Nicholson, D., Carswell, A. (1995) The clinical utility of the Canadian Occupational Performance Measure. *Canadian Journal of Occupational Therapy*, 62(5), 242–249.

Velde, B. and Fidler, G. (2002) *Lifestyle performance: a model for engaging the power of occupation*. Slack, Thorofare, NJ.

Velozo, C., Kielhofner, G and Fisher, G. (1998) A user's guide to the Worker Role Interview (WRI) (version 9.0). Department of Occupational Therapy, University of Illinois at Chicago, Chicago, IL.

Waller, D. (1993) *Group interactive art therapy: its use in training and treatment*. Routledge, London.

Walton, J. A. (1999) On living with schizophrenia, in *Nursing and the experience of illness: phenomenology in practice* (eds I. Madjar and J. A. Walton). Routledge, London.

Waters, D. (1995) Recovering from a depressive episode using the Canadian Occupational Performance Measure. *Canadian Journal of Occupational Therapy*, 62(4), 278–282.

Wetherell, M., Taylor, S. and Yates, S. (eds) (2001) *Discourse theory and practice*. Sage/Open University, London.

Whalley-Hammell, K. (1998) Client-centred occupational therapy: collaborative planning, accountable intervention, in *Client-centred occupational therapy* (ed. M. Law). Slack, Thorofare, NJ.

Whiteford, G. (2000) Occupational deprivation: global challenge in the new millennium. *British Journal of Occupational Therapy*, 63(5), 200–204.

Whiting, S., Lincoln, N. B., Bhavnani, G. and Cockburn, J. (1985) *The Rivermead perceptual assessment battery*. NFER-Nelson, Windsor.

Wilcock, A. (1998) *An occupational perspective of health*. Slack, Thorofare, NJ.

Wilcock, A, (1999) The Doris Sym Memorial Lecture: developing a philosophy of occupation for health, *British Journal of Occupational Therapy*, 62(5), 192–198.

Wilkins, S., Pollock, N., Rochon, S. and Law, M. (2001) Implementing client-centred practice: why is it so difficult to do? *Canadian Journal of Occupational Therapy*, 68(2), 70–79.

Williams, C. C. and Collins, A. A. (2002) The social construction of disability in schizophrenia. *Qualitative Health Research*, 12(3), 297–309.

Yakobina, S., Yakobina, S. and Tallant, B. (1997) I came, I thought, I conquered: cognitive behaviour approach applied in occupational therapy for the treatment of depressed (dysthymic) females. *Occupational Therapy in Mental Health*, 13(4), 59–73.

Yalom, I. D. (1975) *The theory and practice of group psychotherapy*, 2nd ed. Basic Books, New York.

Yerxa, E. J. (1967) Eleanor Clarke Slagle Lecture: authentic occupational therapy. *American Journal of Occupational Therapy*, 21, 1–9.

Yerxa, E. J. (1980) Occupational therapy's role in creating future climate of caring. *American Journal of Occupational Therapy*, 34, 529–534.

Yerxa, E. J. (1983a) Audacious values: the energy source for occupational therapy practice, in *Health through occupation – theory and practice in occupational therapy* (ed. G. Kielhofner). F. A. Davis, Philadelphia, PA.

Yerxa, E. J. (1983b) The occupational therapist as a researcher, in *Willard and Spackman's occupational therapy*, 6th edn (eds H. L. Hopkins and H. D. Smith). J. B. Lippincott, Philadelphia, PA.

Yerxa, E. J. (1987) Quotations taken from talks given by Professor E. Yerxa at a conference in Exeter on, Occupational therapy: a foundation for practice, 2–4 April.

Yerxa, E. J. (1993) Occupational science: a new source of power for participants in occupational therapy. *Occupational Science*, **1**(1).

Young, M. and Quinn, E. (1992) *Theories and principles of occupational therapy*. Churchill Livingstone, Edinburgh.

# INDEX